Clinical Nutrition for Oncology Patients

Mary Marian, MS, RD, CSO

Clinical Nutritionist, Curriculum Specialist, and Clinical Lecturer
University of Arizona
College of Medicine and Department of Nutritional Sciences
Arizona Cancer Center and Center for Excellence in Integrative Medicine
Tucson, AZ

Susan Roberts, MS, RD, LD, CNSD

Assistant Director of Clinical Nutrition and Nutrition Support Team Coordinator
Baylor University Medical Center
Dallas, TX

JONES AND BARTLETT PUBLISHERS
Sudbury, Massachusetts
BOSTON   TORONTO   LONDON   SINGAPORE

World Headquarters
Jones and Bartlett Publishers
40 Tall Pine Drive
Sudbury, MA 01776
978-443-5000
info@jbpub.com
www.jbpub.com

Jones and Bartlett Publishers
Canada
6339 Ormindale Way
Mississauga, Ontario L5V 1J2
Canada

Jones and Bartlett Publishers
International
Barb House, Barb Mews
London W6 7PA
United Kingdom

Jones and Bartlett's books and products are available through most bookstores and online booksellers. To contact Jones and Bartlett Publishers directly, call 800-832-0034, fax 978-443-8000, or visit our website www.jbpub.com.

Substantial discounts on bulk quantities of Jones and Bartlett's publications are available to corporations, professional associations, and other qualified organizations. For details and specific discount information, contact the special sales department at Jones and Bartlett via the above contact information or send an email to specialsales@jbpub.com.

The authors, editor, and publisher have made every effort to provide accurate information. However, they are not responsible for errors, omissions, or for any outcomes related to the use of the contents of this book and take no responsibility for the use of the products and procedures described. Treatments and side effects described in this book may not be applicable to all people; likewise, some people may require a dose or experience a side effect that is not described herein. Drugs and medical devices are discussed that may have limited availability controlled by the Food and Drug Administration (FDA) for use only in a research study or clinical trial. Research, clinical practice, and government regulations often change the accepted standard in this field. When consideration is being given to use of any drug in the clinical setting, the health care provider or reader is responsible for determining FDA status of the drug, reading the package insert, and reviewing prescribing information for the most up-to-date recommendations on dose, precautions, and contraindications, and determining the appropriate usage for the product. This is especially important in the case of drugs that are new or seldom used.

Production Credits
Publisher: Michael Brown
Production Director: Amy Rose
Acquisitions Editor: Katey Birtcher
Editorial Assistant: Catie Heverling
Senior Production Editor: Tracey Chapman
Associate Production Editor: Kate Stein
Marketing Manager: Jessica Faucher

Manufacturing and Inventory Control
Supervisor: Amy Bacus
Composition: Cape Cod Compositors, Inc.
Art: Accurate Art, Inc.
Cover Design: Scott Moden
Cover Image: © Kyle Smith/ShutterStock, Inc.
Printing and Binding: Malloy, Inc.
Cover Printing: Malloy, Inc.

Library of Congress Cataloging-in-Publication Data
Clinical nutrition for oncology patients / [edited by] Mary Marian and Susan Roberts.
    p. ; cm.
  Includes bibliographical references.
  ISBN-13: 978-0-7637-5512-6 (hardcover)
  ISBN-10: 0-7637-5512-5 (hardcover)
  1. Cancer—Diet therapy. 2. Cancer—Nutritional aspects. I. Marian, Mary, 1956– II. Roberts, Susan, 1951–
  [DNLM: 1. Neoplasms—diet therapy. 2. Nutrition Therapy. QZ 266 C64178 2010]
  RC271.D52C65 2010
  616.99'40654—dc22

2008046220

6048

Printed in the United States of America
13 12 11 10 09   10 9 8 7 6 5 4 3 2 1

*This book is dedicated to our families
for their support and love,*

*to our authors and colleagues
for their valuable time and contributions to this project,*

and

*to all cancer survivors and their caregivers
that we may continue to support you on your journey.*

Contents

Chapter 1   Introduction to the Nutritional
            Management of Oncology Patients   1

Mary Marian, MS, RD, CSO
Susan Roberts, MS, RD, LD, CNSD

Chapter 2   Nutrition Screening and Assessment
            in Oncology 21

Pamela Charney, PhD, RD
Andreea Cranganu, RD, LD, CNSD

Chapter 3   Nutrition Support for Oncology Patients . . . 45

M. Patricia Fuhrman, MS, RD, LD, FADA, CNSD

Chapter 4   Medical and Radiation Oncology 65

Carole Havrila, RD, CSO
Paul W. Read, MD, PhD
David Mack, MD

Chapter 5   Surgical Oncology 101

Maureen B. Huhmann, DCN, RD, CSO
David August, MD

Chapter 6   Nutrition and Cancer Prevention 137

Nicole Stendell-Hollis, MS, RD

Cancer is the second leading cause of death in the United States for adults. While everyone diagnosed with cancer reacts differently, the diagnosis is often associated with fear, anger, hopelessness, and a range of other emotions. The American Cancer Society states that as many as one third of cancer deaths in the United States could be prevented if Americans consumed a diet rich in plants and maintained a healthy body weight.[1] Scientific evidence has shown consumption of a diet that consists mostly of plant-based foods such as vegetables, fruits, whole grains, and legumes together with restricting intake of saturated and trans fats and added sugars, and maintaining a body mass index (BMI) < 25, is associated with a reduced risk for chronic diseases such as cancer.[1] Evidence strongly suggests that obesity is associated with an increased risk for breast, colorectal, endometrial, esophageal, and kidney cancer; obesity is also linked with cancers of the cervix, gallbladder, ovary, pancreas, and thyroid; multiple myeloma, Hodgkin's lymphoma, and aggressive prostate cancer are also associated with excess body fat.[1] Alcohol consumption is associated with cancers of the mouth, larynx, pharynx, esophagus, and liver. Smoking is the leading cause of lung cancer, laryngeal and oral cavity and pharyngeal cancers; cancers of the mouth, esophagus, kidney, bladder, cervix, pancreas, and acute myelogenous leukemia are also linked with tobacco use.[2] Inadequate physical activity is strongly associated with the risk for developing many types of cancer. Sun exposure is another lifestyle habit influencing the risk for cancer. The World Health Organization (WHO) expects worldwide cancer rates to continue increasing because of lifestyle choices, including poor dietary intake and the increasing incidence of overweightness, obesity, physical inactivity, and tobacco use.[3]

The number of cancer survivors in the United States is over 11 million people[4]; therefore, healthcare clinicians are likely to care for someone with cancer or who has had cancer. Many cancer survivors become interested in changing their diets and lifestyle habits after being diagnosed with cancer. During treatment for cancer, many face a number of challenges, including trying to consume adequate food or liquid in order to maintain nutrition and hydration status. After treatment, some survivors continue to struggle with intake while others strive to improve their diets to promote recovery and prevent cancer recurrence.

Because of the significant relationship between lifestyle and cancer, it is imperative for healthcare providers to serve as knowledgeable resources. This book is written by a variety of clinicians who not only care for cancer survivors and their caregivers but are also experts in the field of nutritional oncology. The goal of this text is to provide all clinicians interacting with cancer survivors with information to help their patients make informed choices and improve long-term outcomes. The chapters provide nutritional management recommendations for care prior to, during, and after treatment. Given the prevalence of widely available misinformation regarding nutrition and cancer, this text also serves as a reliable and accurate resource. Our hope is that the information provided by this text will assist all clinicians caring for cancer survivors to promote not only survivorship but also optimal quality of life.

Mary Marian and Susan Roberts

REFERENCES

1. The American Cancer Society. Nutrition and Cancer. http://www.cancer.org. Accessed September 21, 2008.
2. Centers for Disease Control and Prevention 2008. New Report Estimates More than 2 million Cases of Tobacco-related Cancers Diagnosed in the United States During 1999-2004. http://www.cdc.gov/media/pressrel/2008/r080904a.htm. Accessed September 21, 2008.
3. World Health Organization. Global cancer rates could increase by 50% to 15 million by 2020. http://www.who.int/mediacentre/news/releases/2003/. Accessed September 20, 2008.
4. The National Cancer Institute. Science Serving People: Why Cancer Research is Important. http://www.cancer.gov/aboutnci/servingpeople/WhyItIsImportant/. Accessed September 20, 2008.

Recent advantages in the recognition and treatment of many malignancies have allowed the development of effective and curative treatments for numerous patients with cancer. More than ever, patients who were diagnosed with cancer can say they have been cured. The mainstay of treatment involves chemotherapy, radiation, and surgery. Typically, these treatment modalities impair a patient's capacity to maintain adequate nutrition.

Chemotherapy utilized to eliminate cancer cells takes advantage of the growth preferential of malignant cells over normal cells. This implies, however, that normal healthy cells are also going to be affected by these therapies. Abnormalities of the mucosal lining or gastrointestinal tract are a major problem in the delivery of effective chemotherapy and radiotherapy. This results in significant mucositis, esophagitis, gastritis, and enteritis, with the end result of nausea, vomiting, abdominal pain, diarrhea, and often malabsorption.

Maintaining adequate nutrition during treatment for cancer is often a major ordeal. Treating physicians may have difficulty completing or keeping a patient on schedule due to the known side effects of the treatment. Also, it is not uncommon for cancer therapies to severely impair a patient's nutritional status.

In this book, leading experts in the field of cancer and nutrition provide insight into the challenges associated with the evaluation and maintenance of cancer patients' nutritional status. It is certainly a welcome asset to all health professionals who treat patients with cancer.

Luis Piñeiro, MD, FACP
Hematopoietic Stem Cell Transplant Program
Director of Marrow and Apheresis Laboratory
Baylor University Medical Center
Sammons Cancer Center
Dallas, TX

Mary Marian has been practicing as a clinical dietitian in Tucson, Arizona, for over 20 years. She is currently employed at the University of Arizona as a clinical lecturer and nutritionist at the College of Medicine and Sunstone Cancer Resource Centers. Mary is also a faculty member at the University of Arizona's Center for Excellence in Integrative Medicine. Her current practice focuses on preventive medicine, cancer, and specialized nutrition support. Mary is also a faculty member at the University of Phoenix in Tucson. She is widely published and has given numerous lectures locally, nationally, and internationally. Additionally, she is involved in several professional organizations, including the American Dietetic Association and the American Society of Parenteral and Enteral Nutrition (A.S.P.E.N.). She is married to her husband, Jim, and has two adult children, Scott and Brittney.

Susan Roberts has been a registered dietitian for 20 years and has 14 years of experience with oncology and hematopoietic stem cell transplant patients. Susan's current roles at Baylor University Medical Center are Assistant Director of Clinical Nutrition, Nutrition Support Coordinator, and Dietetic Internship Director. She has numerous publications and presentations and is also involved as a professional volunteer with the American Dietetic Association, Dietitians in Nutrition Support, the American Society for Parenteral and Enteral Nutrition (A.S.P.E.N.), and the North Texas Society for Parenteral and Enteral Nutrition. Susan is married to her husband, Chris, and has two young boys, Ross and Griffin.

Contributors

David August, MD
Professor, Department of Surgery and Oncology
Robert Wood Johnson Medical School—University of Medicine and
    Dentistry, New Jersey
Chief, Surgical Oncology
The Cancer Institute of New Jersey
New Brunswick, NJ

Jayne M. Camporeale, MS, RN, OCN, APN-C
Adult Nurse Practitioner
The Cancer Institute of New Jersey
New Brunswick, NJ

Pamela Charney, PhD, RD
Clinical Coordinator
Graduate Coordinated Program in Dietetics
Lecturer, Department of Epidemiology
Nutrition Sciences Program
School of Public Health and Community Medicine
Affiliate Associate Professor
School of Pharmacy
University of Washington
Seattle, WA

Andreea Cranganu, RD, LD, CNSD
Clinical Dietitian
Baylor University Medical Center
Dallas, TX

M. Patricia Fuhrman, MS, RD, LD, FADA, CNSD
National Director of Nutrition Services
DCRX Infusion
Ballwin, MO

Dawn E. Goetz, PharmD, BCOP
Clinical Pharmacist
H. Lee Moffitt Cancer Center and Research Institute
Tampa, FL

Carole Havrila, RD, CSO
Registered Dietitian
University of Virginia Cancer Center
Charlottesville, VA

Heather Hendrikson, RD, CSP, LD
Clinical Dietitian
Baylor University Medical Center
Dallas, TX

Maureen B. Huhmann, DCN, RD, CSO
Assistant Professor, Department of Nutrition Sciences, School of Health
    Related Professions
University of Medicine and Dentistry, New Jersey
Clinical Dietitian
The Cancer Institute of New Jersey
New Brunswick, NJ

Elisabeth Isenring, PhD, AdvAPD
NHMRC Postdoctoral Fellow, Institute of Health and Biomedical
    Innovation, School of Public Health
Queensland University of Technology
Australia

Natalie Ledesma, MS, RD, CSO
Oncology Dietitian
UCSF Helen Diller Family Comprehensive Cancer Center
University of California
Cancer Resource Center
San Francisco, CA

David Mack, MD
Assistant Professor of Medicine
Duke Oncology Network
Durham, NC

Todd W. Mattox, PharmD, BCNSP
Coordinator, Nutrition Support Team
H. Lee Moffitt Cancer Center and Research Institute
Tampa, FL

Paul W. Read, MD, PhD
Associate Professor
University of Virginia Department of Radiation Oncology
UVA Medical Center
Department of Radiation Oncology
Charlottesville, VA

Kim Robien, PhD, RD, CSO, FADA
Assistant Professor
Division of Epidemiology and Community Health, School of Public Health
    and Population Sciences Program, Masonic Cancer Center
University of Minnesota
Minneapolis, MN

Cathy Scanlon, MS, RD, LD
Clinical Dietitian
University of Iowa Hospitals and Clinics
Iowa City, IA

Nicole Stendell-Hollis, MS, RD
Nutritional Sciences Department
University of Arizona
Tucson, AZ

Deborah Straub, MS, RD
Integrative Medicine Nutritionist
Canyon Ranch Health
Tucson, AZ

Kelay Trentham, MS, RD, CD
Oncology Dietitian
MultiCare Regional Cancer Center
Tacoma, WA

Reviewers

Susan Brantley, MS, RD, LDN, CNSD
Metabolic Support Nutritionist
University of Tennessee
Knoxville, TN

Paula Charuhas Macris, MS, RD, FADA, CNSD
Nutrition Education Coordinator/Pediatric Nutrition Specialist
Clinical Nutrition Program
Seattle Cancer Care Alliance
Seattle, WA

Deana Cox, RD, LD, CNSC
Clinical Dietitian
Baylor University Medical Center
Dallas, TX

Andreea Cranganu, RD, LD, CNSD
Clinical Dietitian
Baylor University Medical Center
Dallas, TX

Lindsey R. Curtis, PharmD
Clinical Pharmacist
Allogeneic Bone Marrow/Stem Cell Transplant Clinic
   Seattle Cancer Care Alliance
University of Washington Medical Center
Seattle, WA

Jennifer Duffy, MS, RD, LD, CNSD
Clinical Dietitian
Baylor University Medical Center
Dallas, TX

Laura Elliott, MPH, RD, CSO, LD
Clinical Dietitian
Mary Greeley Medical Center
Ames, IA

Stacey Dunn-Emke, MS, RD
Owner, NutritionJobs.com
San Francisco, CA
Nutrition Consultant
Preventative Medicine Research Institute
Sausalito, CA

Ami Gaarde, RN, BSN, OCN
Assistant Nurse Manager
Chemotherapy Infusion Suite
Holden Comprehensive Cancer Center
University of Iowa Hospitals and Clinics
Iowa City, IA

Edwina Hall, PharmD
Clinical Pharmacist
Northwest Medical Center
Tucson, AZ

Kathryn Hamilton, MA, RD, CSO
Clinical Oncology Dietitian
Atlantic Health Carol G. Simon Cancer Center
Morristown Memorial Hospital
Morristown, NJ

Dianne Kiyomoto, RD
Oncology Dietitian
California Cancer Center
Fresno, CA

Jessica Monczka, RD, LD/N, CNSC
Clinical Dietitian
Arnold Palmer Hospital for Children
Orlando, FL

Eric Nadler, MD, MPP
Medical Oncologist
Baylor Sammons Cancer Center
Dallas, TX

Mary K. Russell, MS, RD, LDN, CNSD
Director of Nutrition Services
University of Chicago Hospitals
Chicago, IL

Cynthia A. Thomson, RD, PhD, FADA, CSO
Associate Professor
Nutritional Sciences, Medicine, and Public Health
Member Arizona Cancer Center
University of Arizona
Tucson, AZ

Ching Ueng, PharmD
Clinical Pharmacist
Baylor University Medical Center
Dallas, TX

Chapter 1

Introduction to the Nutritional Management of Oncology Patients

Mary Marian, MS, RD, CSO
Susan Roberts, MS, RD, LD, CNSD

INTRODUCTION

Although the precise number of new cases of cancer that occur each year is unknown, the incidence in the United States was greater than 1.4 million cases in 2007.[1] This number does not include diagnoses of carcinoma in situ (with the exception of urinary cancer), nor does it include basal and squamous cell cancers of the skin.[2] Cancer is the cause of death in approximately 23% of deaths each year in the United States[2] and is currently estimated to be the leading cause of mortality for American adults younger than the age of 85. The current lifetime risk for Americans is estimated as one in three among women and one in two among men.[2] Table 1.1 shows the estimated number of deaths by cancer site and by gender in the United States in 2008.

The lifetime probability of developing cancer is greater for men (46%) than for women (38%), although many young women are diagnosed with breast cancer, thereby placing women at a higher risk of developing cancer before the age of 60.[1] While cancer rates differ greatly throughout the world, rates are projected to more than double by the year 2030.[3] Projected increases are due to several factors:

- Growth of the worldwide population
- Aging of the population
- Improved screening, detection, and treatments, resulting in higher survival rates
- Projected increases in tobacco use
- Increases in the number of individuals with HIV/AIDS in some countries[3]

Table 1.1   *Estimated Cancer Deaths in the United States, 2008*

Men		Women	
Lung and bronchus	31%	Lung and bronchus	26%
Prostate	10%	Breast	15%
Colon and rectum	8%	Colon and rectum	9%
Pancreas	6%	Pancreas	6%
Liver, intrahepatic, and bile ducts	4%	Ovary	6%
Leukemia	4%	Non-Hodgkin's lymphoma	3%
Esophagus	4%	Leukemia	3%
Urinary bladder	3%	Uterine corpus	3%
Non-Hodgkin's lymphoma	3%	Liver, intrahepatic, and bile ducts	2%
Kidney and renal	3%	Brain/other nervous system	2%
All other sites	24%	All other sites	25%

Source: Data from American Cancer Society, www.cancer.org.

Worldwide, the most commonly diagnosed cancers (excluding skin cancers) are lung, breast, and colorectal cancers, with lung cancer being the primary cancer cause of death.[3] In developed countries, hormonal-related cancers are the most prevalent types of cancer; in underdeveloped areas, the most common cancers are those arising from infectious agents. In men, prostate cancer is the most common type of cancer in high-income countries, followed by lung, stomach, and colorectal cancers. In men in underdeveloped countries, lung cancer prevalence exceeds esophageal, stomach, and liver cancer prevalence. In women residing in developed countries, breast cancer is the most commonly diagnosed cancer, followed by lung, colorectal, and endometrial cancers. In underdeveloped countries, breast cancer is also the most prevalent cancer diagnosed in women, followed by lung, stomach, and cervical cancers.[3]

This chapter provides an overview of how cancer and oncological therapies affect individuals' nutritional status. A brief introduction to nutrition intervention is also given.

Cancer Development

Cancer is actually a cluster of more than 100 diseases that arise due to uncontrolled cellular growth. Normal cellular growth and differentiation are controlled by a myriad of complex systems, which involve a number of physiologic functions such as cell signaling and gene expression that influence cellular development and communication, as well as cell death. The development of cancer is a multistep process that occurs in three stages: initiation, promotion, and progression.

Initiation is the first step in the development of precancerous cells. In this stage, the cell has been exposed to stress, such as oxidative stress, or to endogenous or exogenous carcinogens; precancerous cells form when the cell undergoes such exposure and either fails to repair itself or fails to die. Subsequently, the cell forms DNA adducts (intermediates formed during phase I metabolism in the liver that may be carcinogenic and bind to DNA), which in turn distort the DNA, disrupting its replication and possibly its translation.[3] Carcinogenic activation can occur through the interaction between dietary and/or environmental components and the enzymes involved in the detoxification phase of metabolism, where phase II enzymes are responsible for producing by-products that can be excreted in the bile or urine. Any of the enzymes that participate in phase I and II metabolism represent potential targets for carcinogenesis, which can be either promoted or prevented during the initiation phase. Initiation alone is not enough for a cell to become cancerous; the cell must then go through the promotion stage. However, the more precancerous cells that are initiated, the greater the risk for developing cancer.

During stage 2, the initiated cancer cell is further stimulated through cell signaling, which allows for cellular replication and growth leading to excess DNA damage that is beyond the capacity of the cell to repair the damage. This process, called cellular proliferation or promotion, is critical in the carcinogenesis process. As the expression of cellular receptors for growth factors increases, intracellular exposure of such growth factors also increases, such that division and growth of the abnormal cell are perpetuated. Further damage to the cell results in alterations in gene expression and cellular proliferation. Clusters of abnormal cells develop, subsequently resulting in tumor formation. Consequently tumor types can be characterized by specific genetic lesions that develop during each step of the carcinogenesis pathway. Nevertheless, there may be significant individual variability in the sequence of genetic lesions or in the quantity of clusters "required" to develop a tumor.

During the promotion stage, precancerous lesions (versus precancerous cells associated with initiation) can usually be detected, although the degree to which a given precancerous lesion evolves into a cancer is not always known. In the final stage, known as progression, the cluster of abnormal cells (i.e., the tumor) may grow into a larger lesion and/or translocate into other areas of the body, resulting in metastasis of cancer cells to other parts of the body.

An understanding of cancer biology is important to understand the impact of diet and other lifestyle components on cancer. An in-depth discussion of this topic is beyond the scope of this chapter, however.

Causes of Cancer

A number of exogenous factors are known to cause cancer, including the following:[3]

- Tobacco use
- Infectious agents (e.g., bacteria, parasites, viruses)
- Medications
- Radiation
- Chemical exposure (e.g., polychlorinated biphenyls, organic compounds used in plastics, paints, adhesives)
- Carcinogenic components found in foods and beverages (e.g., aflatoxins, heterocyclic amines, polycyclic aromatics hydrocarbons, N-nitroso compounds)

Endogenous causes of cancer include inherited germ-line mutations, oxidative stress, inflammation, and hormones. Most cancer experts believe that the majority of cancers are not inherited, but rather arise from alterations in gene expression that promote changes in DNA; over many years, these mutations develop into cancerous tumors. Many nutrients have been shown to influence cell-cycle progression and proliferation.[3] For example, vitamin A can result in cell-cycle arrest. Likewise, retinoids can inhibit cellular proliferation of initiated cells by inducing apoptosis or inducing differentiation of abnormal cells back to normal.[4] Conversely, heme iron has been found to promote cellular proliferation of colonocytes.[5]

Because both exogenous and endogenous factors promote the initiation and progression of cancer, it is often difficult to determine the precise etiology of specific cancers. Many of these factors interact with one another, as modifiers or precursors, potentially resulting in either an increase or a decrease in cancer risk.

In addition to single nutrients' effects on cellular functions, energy intake and physical activity have been noted to alter pathophysiology. In animal studies, energy restriction has been found to prevent cancer to a significant extent.[6, 7] Suppression of tumor development in mice and an increase in lifespan in rodents have been observed with energy restriction.[6] Energy restriction results in reduced circulating levels of insulin-like growth factor 1 (IGF-1) and insulin, both of which serve as growth factors for many cancer cells. Other inflammatory markers also decline with energy restriction. To date, these observations have not been confirmed in human studies, and further research is needed to explore the specific mechanistic effects in humans. Physical activity (PA) has been found to improve insulin sensitivity and reduce insulin levels.[8] Additionally, PA decreases serum estrogen and androgen levels in both premenopausal and postmenopausal women, thereby potentially providing a protective effect against hormone-related cancers.

Lifestyle Factors

Historically, as populations have evolved from a primarily agricultural society to an urbanized culture, the quality of foods and beverages consumed has changed rapidly—as have their impact on the risk for disease. Since the second half of the twentieth century, more and more evidence has accrued showing that diet plays a significant role in the development of many of the primary causes of death in the United States, including heart disease, some types of cancers, diabetes, stroke, and kidney disease. Although cessation of tobacco use is the most critical modifiable risk factor in preventing cancer, body weight, diet, and PA are thought to play prominent roles in both the primary and tertiary prevention of breast, colorectal, ovarian, endometrial, and prostate cancers.[3]

Paralleling the change in dietary habits that tends to accompany economic development and urbanization, profound changes in PA patterns have also occurred with industrialization: Populations have become extremely sedentary as urbanization and technologic advancements have been integrated into societies. PA is thought to play a key role in the development of chronic disease and some types of cancers. Strong evidence suggests that increased levels of PA reduce the risk for colorectal and breast cancers.[9] Evidence is also accruing that regular PA is beneficial for reducing risk for cancer in cancer survivors.[10–13]

These subsequent lifestyle changes have resulted in another problem that is becoming a global epidemic—namely, obesity. Since the 1980s, the number of people worldwide who have become overweight or obese has skyrocketed. In the United States, more than 66% of the population is considered overweight or obese. In the United Kingdom, 65% of men and 56% of women are overweight, and 22% of men and 23% of women are obese. In China, more than 20% of the population is considered overweight in some cities, while the number of people considered obese has increased to 7% of the population. Although the latter rate is considered low in comparison to the obesity rates observed in other countries, it represents a tripling in obesity from 1992 to 2006.[3] Obesity is projected to continue increasing within the worldwide population.

Body Composition

In addition to diet and PA, the supporting evidence that the presence of excess body fat increases the risk for developing certain types of cancers is convincing.[3] As previously described, the number of overweight and obese individuals worldwide is increasing at an alarming rate. Excess body weight—and particularly excess body fat—increases the risk not only for certain cancers, but also for heart disease, stroke, type II diabetes, hypertension, and many other medical conditions. Given the prevalence of overweight and obesity, both conditions are likely to have a significant impact on the incidence of obesity-related cancers in years to come as the number of individuals with excess body weight and fat continues to increase.

In their recent systemic review of the literature, Renehan and colleagues[14] found that a higher body mass index (BMI) is associated with an increased risk for the following cancers: thyroid, renal, colon, adenocarcinoma of the esophagus, multiple myeloma, leukemia, and non-Hodgkin's lymphoma. Rectal and malignant melanoma cancers are increased in men with a higher BMI, while incidence of cancers of the gallbladder, pancreas, endometrium, and breast (postmenopausal women) is greater in women with a higher BMI. Obesity is also associated with a poorer prognosis in cases of breast, colon, prostate, endometrial, and ovarian cancers.[14]

Although the precise mechanisms of how excess body weight increases the risk for cancer are poorly understood, potential mechanisms that have been cited include changes in circulating endogenous hormones such as insulin, insulin-like growth factors, and sex steroids, as well as changes in the metabolism of adipokines, localized inflammation, oxidative stress, altered immune response, hypertension, and lipid peroxidation.[14] Much speculation surrounds the insulin–cancer hypothesis in particular: Chronic hyperinsulinemia is known to reduce circulating levels of insulin-like growth hormone (IGF) binding protein 1 and IGF-binding protein 2, thereby increasing the availability of IGF, which in turn promotes an environment that favors tumor formation. Adiponectin, which is primarily secreted by adipocytes, is the most abundant circulating adipokine. Its secretion is inversely correlated with BMI; women typically have greater concentrations of adiponectin than men. The benefits of greater adiponectin concentrations lie in its anti-inflammatory, antioxidant, antiangiogenic, and insulin-sensitizing properties. Although some studies have noted inverse correlations between cancer risk and adiponectin levels,[15, 16] further research is needed to delineate this relationship given the early stages of these observations.

Cancer and Nutritional Status

The continuum of cancer survival includes treatment and recovery as well as living with advanced cancer. Each stage is associated with different needs and challenges for the patient, caregivers, and clinicians. Both cancer and the oncological therapies utilized for its treatment can have profound effects on an individual's nutritional status, thereby making nutrition an important component of medical care. Malnutrition is characterized by a variety of clinical symptoms, including weight loss, poor wound healing, electrolyte and fluid imbalances, depressed immune function, and increased morbidity and mortality.

Although all patients with cancer are at nutritional risk, not all patients with cancer become malnourished. Therefore, nutrition screening and the nutrition care process—including nutrition assessment, ongoing monitoring, and follow-up—are crucial for preventing or minimizing the development of malnutrition at all stages of treatment. This plan of care allows for the implementation of the appropriate intervention to target problem areas as warranted. Long-term follow-up upon completion of therapy is also recommended, as nutrition-impact symptoms may be experienced even as long as 12 months following commencement of therapy and have been associated with reductions in quality of life.[17]

Cancer and Malnutrition

One of the most significant nutritional issues that can arise during cancer treatment is malnutrition. Malnutrition may result from the disease process, from the use of antineoplastic therapy, or from both. Side effects related to common oncological therapies, including chemotherapy, radiation, immunotherapy, and surgery, are key contributors in promoting a deterioration in nutritional status. Additionally, deteriorations in nutritional status have been found to predict outcome prior to the initiation of therapy. Dewys and colleagues found that as little as a 6% weight loss predicted response to therapy.[18] These researchers also noted that overall survival rates, performance status, productivity, and quality of life declined concurrently with weight loss in cancer patients. Of note, approximately 80% of the study patients presented with weight loss before being diagnosed with cancer.

Malnutrition also has a detrimental effect on quality of life. Patients with cancer cachexia reported that alterations in body image negatively affected their self-esteem, relationships, spirituality, physical activity, and social functioning.[19]

Cancer Cachexia

Cancer cachexia is a multifactorial syndrome that encompasses a spectrum ranging from early weight loss to significant deteriorations in body fat and lean muscle tissue resulting in death. The term "cachexia" is derived from the Greek words *kakos*, meaning "bad," and *hexis*, meaning "condition."[19] Although no precise definition has been established for cancer cachexia, also known as cancer anorexia–cachexia syndrome (CACS), cachexia is manifested by weight loss and loss of lean body mass. The wasting exhibited by people with cancer and some other conditions (such as cardiac cachexia and chronic obstructive pulmonary disease) is significantly different from that seen in patients with simple starvation: The former individuals experience profound weight loss and loss of lean tissue mass, whereas in persons with starvation lean body mass is generally preserved until the late stages of starvation. Reportedly, 50% of patients with cancer lose some body weight, with one third losing more than 5% of their original body weight and as many as 20% of cancer deaths resulting from cachexia.[20, 21]

Reductions in oral intake alone do not explain why malnutrition often occurs in people with cancer; indeed, cachexia may occur in patients who consume apparently sufficient calories.[20] Moreover, nutrition support does not successfully restore the loss of lean body mass with CACS.

Mediators of Malnutrition

Although the mechanisms leading to cachexia arise from complex tumor–host interactions, a number of metabolic abnormalities that result in catabolism rather than anabolism have been identified. Known factors contributing to the development of CACS include anorexia, early satiety, taste changes, nausea, diarrhea/constipation, fatigue, and anemia. Cachexia also results from an imbalance between pro-inflammatory and anti-inflammatory cytokines. Pro-inflammatory cytokines, including tumor necrosis factor (TNF), interleukins 1 and 6 (IL-1 and IL-6), and interferon gamma (IFN-γ), are thought to be the primary mediators associated with the development of CACS.[22] Cytokines are glycoproteins and cell signaling proteins secreted by a wide variety of hematopoietic and non-hematopoietic cell types (e.g., macrophages, monocytes, lymphocytes, and endothelial and epithelial cells) in response to malignancy, injury, or infection. These cytokines are thought to work in concert, rather than individually, in promoting catabolism and malnutrition.

Figure 1.1 illustrates the array of factors contributing to the development of malnutrition and cachexia. The infusion of pro-inflammatory cytokines in animal studies was found to produce anorexia, weight loss, proteolysis and

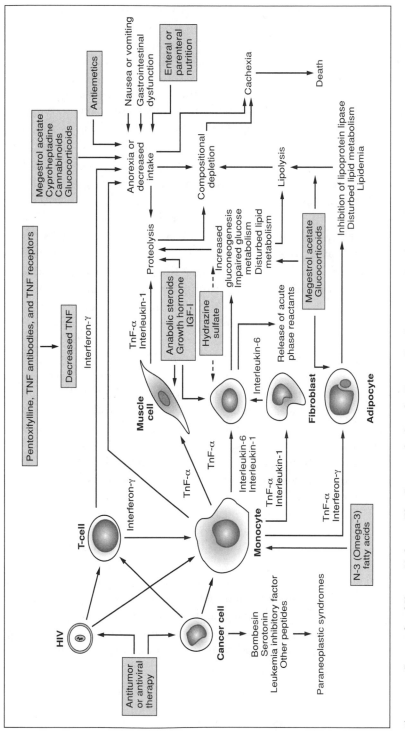

Figure 1.1 *Proposed and Known Mediators That Promote the Complex Tumor-Host Interactions Resulting in Cancer Cachexia*

Adapted from Tchekmedyian NS. Clinical approaches to nutritional support in cancer. *Curr Opin Oncol.* 1993;5(4):633-638.

lipolysis, and elevations in cortisol and glucagon levels in addition to increasing energy expenditure.[23]

Leptin and ghrelin are two hormones that influence appetite and oral intake. Ghrelin increases appetite, whereas leptin reduces appetite. In cancer patients, increases in ghrelin levels and reductions in leptin levels have not resulted in increases in oral intake.[24] Downregulation of leptin production and expression of leptin receptors in the hypothalamus by tumor necrosis factor have been reported, however.[24] Reductions in gastric production of ghrelin synthesis by various cytokines have also been noted. While the relationship between the cytokines, leptin, and ghrelin in regard to CACS requires further investigation, alterations in neurohormonal balance are hypothesized to contribute to CACS.[24]

Another mediator thought to play a role in the development of cancer cachexia is proteolysis-inducing factor (PIF), a glycoprotein that has been isolated from the urine of weight-losing cancer patients. Interestingly, PIF has not been found in persons losing weight from other causes.[25] Additionally, several neurotransmitter systems within the hypothalamus are thought to contribute to the development of CACS. For example, increases in serotonin result in the activation of melanocortin neurons, which are thought to cause anorexia, although their precise role requires further study.[24]

Changes in energy, carbohydrate, protein, and lipid metabolism have also been cited as causes of weight loss in patients with cancer. Alterations in carbohydrate metabolism have been noted in patients with CACS, including both glucose intolerance and insulin resistance, although this effect varies with the type of cancer.[26] Glucose intolerance has been noted to increase with increases in tumor burden, leading to increasing insulin resistance and weight loss.[26] Increases in glucose utilization combined with the energy demands of the tumor may subsequently increase the patient's energy needs, leading to depletion of protein and fat stores in the face of anorexia and other factors that suppress oral intake.

Increased glucose utilization by both the host and the tumor results in increased lactate production. In the Cori cycle, glucose released by peripheral tissues is metabolized to lactate; in the liver, lactate is synthesized back to glucose. In patients with advanced cancer, an increased rate of the Cori cycle has been observed.[27] Gluconeogenesis from lactate is a very energy-inefficient process that requires an increased number of adenosine triphosphate (ATP) molecules to complete the cycle. Ultimately, this futile cycle increases energy needs further, thereby contributing to weight loss. Enhanced glucose consumption and elevated lactate levels are strongly negatively correlated with patient outcome.[28–30] Mitochondrial defects have also been reported to increase glycolysis.[31] Lastly, increases in glucose utilization are thought to be necessary for cancer progression.[31]

Similar to alterations in glucose metabolism, abnormalities in lipid metabolism are thought to contribute to weight loss in patients with cancer. Body fat is lost when lipolysis and fatty acid oxidation increase and lipogenesis decreases. In noncancer states, infusions of glucose generally suppress lipolysis; in some cancer patients, this process is diminished.[32] Furthermore, the reduction in lipogenesis is thought to reflect the influence of the cytokines. Lipid-mobilizing factor, which is produced by both the tumor and adipose tissue, induces lipolysis by promoting an increased in cyclic adenosine monophosphate production.[33] Of interest, lipid-mobilizing factor has been found in the serum of patients with CACS but not in healthy individuals. Levels of this factor have also been noted to parallel the degree of weight loss experienced.[33, 34] Other alterations in cellular metabolism related to lipid metabolism have also been reported, such as overexpression of the enzymes fatty acid synthase and choline kinase.

Tumor type and stage of disease also affect the nutritional status of cancer patients, with more advanced stages being associated with greater incidence of malnutrition. The heterogeneity of the population with CACS demonstrates that tumor phenotype and host response likely play key roles in the development of cachexia, as patients with similar cancer type and disease stage may vary significantly in terms of developing malnutrition. For example, patients with gastric, esophageal, head/neck, and pancreatic cancers develop malnutrition to a greater degree than do individuals with breast cancer and hematologic malignancies.[18] Patients with colon, prostate, lung and unfavorable non-Hodgkin's lymphoma often experience moderate weight loss (48–61%). Not surprisingly, people with advanced cancer experience the greatest degree of malnutrition.[35] Interestingly, weight gain following diagnosis and treatment has been associated with reduced survival in patients with breast cancer.[36]

Classification of cachexia as primary or secondary is important, as the treatment can differ depending on the type. The etiology of primary cachexia is not well understood and the condition is difficult to treat due the complex nature of CACS. By comparison, the causes of secondary cachexia (a functional inability to achieve an adequate intake) may be more amenable to treatment. Secondary cachexia often develops as a result of mechanical factors (e.g., obstruction) or related to the side effects of the various treatment modalities.

Although ameliorating the factors influencing the inability to consume adequate nutrition is critical for the prevention and treatment of malnutrition, curing the underlying cancer is the only intervention known to be successful in reversing true CACS. Pharmacologic management of cancer-associated symptoms may also be successfully employed to maintain or improve nutritional status (e.g., Megace, steroids). The bottom line is that the preservation of nutritional status can prevent or at least delay the onset of CACS for many patients.

Oncological Treatment Modalities and Malnutrition

Oncological treatment modalities (e.g., chemotherapy, radiation, surgery) can have a profound impact on oral intake, leading to poor nutritional status and malnutrition (see Table 1.2).

Alterations in gastrointestinal absorptive area due to surgical procedures can induce malnutrition secondary to reductions in nutrient absorption or increased metabolic demands for postoperative healing concurrent with inadequate nutrition intake or nutrition support. Chemotherapy can produce a multitude of problems, including mucositis, taste changes, early satiety, diarrhea, constipation, anorexia, nausea, and emesis—all of which can have a profound impact on nutritional intake. Radiation therapy resulting in esophageal stricture, reflux, gastritis, radiation enteritis, xerostomia, dysphagia, odynophagia, diarrhea, and enteritis can also promote deteriorations in nutritional status. The presence of such treatment impact symptoms should be aggressively treated. Table 1.3

Table 1.2 *Antineoplastic Therapies That May Impact Nutritional Status*

Treatment	*Potential Nutritional Impact*
Surgery	Increased nutrient needs for recovery and wound healing, malabsorption, early satiety, dehydration, abdominal cramping, diarrhea, bloating/gas, fluid/electrolyte imbalance, lactose intolerance, hyperglycemia
Chemotherapy	
Cytotoxic	Nausea, vomiting, anorexia, diarrhea, immunosuppression, fatigue, mucositis, peripheral neuropathy, dysgeusia, heightened sensitivity to tastes, metallic taste
Hormonal (glucocorticoids, anti-androgens/estrogens, gonadotropin-releasing hormone analog)	Hyperglycemia, edema, osteoporosis, nausea, vomiting, bone pain, hot flashes, hypercalcemia
Immunotherapy (interleukins, interferon alfa, monoclonal antibodies)	Anorexia, nausea, vomiting, diarrhea, fatigue, immunosuppression
Radiation	Thorax area: anorexia, dysphagia, esophagitis, heartburn, early satiety, fatigue
	Abdomen/pelvic area: nausea, vomiting, diarrhea, abdominal cramping/bloating/gas, lactose intolerance, malabsorption, chronic colitis and enteritis

Table 1.3   *Nutritional Strategies for Management of Treatment-Related Symptoms*

Symptom	Etiology	Recommendations
Alterations in taste/smell, anorexia	Radiation, chemotherapy, cytokines, oncological therapy, pain, depression	Small, frequent, nutrient-dense meals; drinking fluids with meals; avoid low-calorie filler foods; increase physical activity; appetite stimulants
Constipation, diarrhea	Antineoplastic therapies	Low-fat, lactose-free diet; increase soluble fiber intake; avoid spicy foods; avoid caffeine; drink plenty of liquids; probiotics
Dysphagia	Tumor burden, antineoplastic therapies	Thickened, moist, soft or ground/pureed foods
Early satiety	Antineoplastic therapies	Small, frequent, nutrient-dense meals; avoid drinking fluids with meals
Fatigue	Tumor burden, antineoplastic therapies, anemia, dehydration, chronic pain, medications, stress, depression, poor nutrition	Small, frequent, nutrient-dense meals; physical activity; meal planning/assistance with shopping/meal preparation; manage stress and depression
Nausea/vomiting	Antineoplastic therapies	Small, frequent, low-fat, low-fiber meals; avoid spicy foods and caffeine; try not to eat 1–2 hours before treatment; antiemetics; hypnosis, acupuncture, music therapy also effective
Stomatitis, mucositis	Antineoplastic therapies	Soft, nonirritating foods; nutrient-dense liquids/nutritional supplements; Miracle Mouth/viscous lidocaine swishes; lemon/glycerine swabs
Weight loss	Tumor burden, cytokines, antineoplastic therapies	Small, frequent, nutrient-dense meals; try liquid/powder nutritional supplements; consume high-calorie, high-protein foods
Weight gain	Antineoplastic therapies, edema	Low-fat diet with lean meats; low-fat dairy products; whole grains, fruits, and vegetables
Xerostomia	Tumor burden, antineoplastic therapies	Drink/swallow small amounts of food at one time; sip water/fluid after each bite; try sweet or tart foods, soft/pureed foods; suck on hard candies; artificial saliva

outlines strategies that can be employed for managing treatment-related side effects that impact on nutritional intake.

Nutrition Intervention

Maintenance or improvement in nutrition status is the key goal of medical nutrition therapy for individuals undergoing treatment for cancer. Although many patients tolerate therapy well and experience few or no side effects, malnutrition is still a common entity that affects quality of life and survival for many persons with cancer. As previously described, many contributing factors have been implicated in promoting the deterioration in nutrition status. To maintain or improve nutritional status, all barriers associated with oral intake should be aggressively addressed unless aggressive intervention is not warranted.

Modifications in diet and eating habits may be necessary during treatment to reduce or eliminate the side effects of therapy. Weight maintenance is strongly recommended during therapy, with weight gain or loss being recommended based on the individual's nutritional status. Calorie and protein requirements may increase during treatment. Although there is no consensus regarding the optimal calorie and protein requirements for cancer patients, current guidelines recommend a caloric range of 25–35 kcal/kg/day and 1.0–1.5 g/kg/day protein for preserving or improving nutritional status.[37]

Given that many patients with cancer suffer severe alterations in nutritional intake, specialized nutrition support should be considered not only for improving and/or maintaining nutritional status, but also for improving quality of life. For patients undergoing blood or marrow transplantation, nutrition support—both enteral and parenteral—is life saving. For patients with cancer undergoing major surgical procedures, perioperative nutrition support appears beneficial for both adequately nourished and malnourished patients. Braga and colleagues[38] found that patients with cancer who had experienced a weight loss of more than 10% in the past 6 months and who consumed 1 liter/day of a diet enriched with arginine, omega-3 fatty acids (Ω-3), and nucleotides both preoperatively (for 5 days prior to surgery) and postoperatively (administered via jejunostomy) experienced fewer postoperative complications compared to the other study groups for whom perioperative nutrition was not provided.

In a separate study, Gianotti et al.[39] enrolled 305 well-nourished and malnourished patients scheduled to undergo resection of the stomach, pancreas, or colon. Patients were randomized to 1 of 3 groups: (1) consume 1 liter/day for 5 days preoperatively of the same immune-enriched diet as used in the Braga study; (2) receive the study diet preoperatively and postoperatively;

or (3) receive no nutrition support (this group received only IV fluids post-operatively until advancement to an oral diet). In comparison to the group receiving no nutrition support, the preoperative-diet-only group experienced a reduction in septic complications (30% versus 14%; $p = 0.009$) and length of stay (14.0 ± 7.7 days versus 11.6 ± 4.7 days). Complications and length of stay were also significantly reduced in the perioperative-diet group.

The authors from both studies note that the preoperative period may be an important time in which to modify the host response by using an immune-enhancing diet to maximally stimulate the immune system. In the Gianotti study,[39] BMI was also associated with outcomes, as patients with a BMI ranging from 18 to 25 experienced less morbidity; the risk for postoperative complications was found to increase as body weight increased.

Enteral or parenteral nutrition is often indicated for patients with cancer who are unable to consume adequate oral nutrition or in whom oral intake is contraindicated. Patients with head and neck cancers commonly require enteral nutrition via the percutaneous placement of a gastrostomy tube to prevent significant deteriorations in nutritional status during therapy and thereafter. Parenteral nutrition is also often indicated in patients with intestinal failure, which frequently results from severe malabsorption or malignant bowel obstructions. For patients with advanced cancers, however, the initiation of parenteral nutrition can be controversial. Home parenteral nutrition (HPN) support has been associated with long-term survival in select patients with advanced cancers with acceptable complication rates.[40, 41] Additionally, patients with a Karnofsky score greater than 50 reportedly experience an increase in survival when receiving HPN compared with patients scoring lower than 50.[42]

Hoda and colleagues recommend that HPN should be utilized only after an in-depth clinical assessment is completed on a patient-by-patient basis.[40] In general, nutrition support is not indicated for patients who are not expected to survive for more than three months. In many cases, patients must also meet the requirements established by insurance companies to obtain reimbursement for HPN expenses.

Dietary Supplements

Dietary supplements and complementary and alternative therapies are heavily advertised for cancer prevention and immune support. Many cancer survivors also take dietary supplements, more so than individuals without cancer.[43] Many oncological nutrition experts, however, recommend avoiding dietary supplements, and particularly ingestion of pharmacologic levels of antioxidants, during treatment.

Similar to other disease states, whether benefits can be derived from post-treatment efforts to prevent cancer recurrence is unclear, although some studies have found an increase in morbidity and mortality with the use of some supplements.[44, 45] Additionally, the use of some herbal supplements has been associated with a reduction in the levels of chemotherapeutic agents in the body, which is of great concern given that patients hope to gain the maximal benefits related to treatment.[46, 47] Oral nutritional supplements, by contrast, can serve an important role in meeting nutritional needs in the face of adverse effects such as anorexia, early satiety, and fatigue associated with cancer. Deterioration of nutritional status not only plays a major role in the development of the cancer cachexia syndrome, but also leads to alterations in quality of life.[19, 48]

Concerns surrounding the influence of nutrition on tumor growth have long been voiced. For example, women with estrogen receptor-positive breast cancers often worry about consumption of soy protein, which is a rich source of isoflavones. The chemical structure of isoflavones is similar to that of estrogen, with isoflavones having the ability to bind to estrogen receptors. Under experimental conditions, isoflavones have been found to exert estrogen-like effects.[49] For this reason, they are commonly classified as selective estrogen-receptor modulators. Although the consumption of soy products has been linked with possibly reducing the risk for breast cancer, in some animal and in vitro studies, the soy isoflavone genistein has been observed to stimulate the growth of estrogen-sensitive tumors.[50–54] Thus, from a public health viewpoint, there is a critical need to discern whether the ingestion of soy products is safe for women with these types of tumors. To date, the results of neither animal nor clinical studies have allowed definitive conclusions to be made.

In a study investigating the influence of parenteral nutrition on tumor growth, Pacelli and colleagues recently reported that this type of nutrition did not stimulate tumor proliferation in malnourished patients with gastric cancer.[55] Conversely, when single nutrients have been studied, some have shown the ability to play a dual role in both cancer prevention and promotion. Folic acid is an example of one such nutrient: It may protect against cancer initiation, yet also promote the growth of preneoplastic cells. Some studies have shown that concentrations of serum folate levels are associated with a reduced risk for breast and colorectal cancer,[56, 57] particularly in individuals who consume alcohol.

Other studies have found an increased risk for prostate, breast, and ovarian cancers related to folic acid intake.[58–60] Notably, the rates of colorectal cancer incidence had been declining in the United States and Canada prior to the establishment of those countries' mandatory food folic acid fortification programs.[61] Mason and colleagues[61] reviewed the data sets from the Surveillance, Epidemiology and End Result registry and Canadian Cancer Statistics and found that incidence rates began to reverse in parallel with the implementation of the food fortification programs in both countries. In their recent review of the literature, Smith et al.[62] concluded that the evidence is mounting suggesting that increasing folate levels in some people increases the risk for cancer. Clearly, further research is needed to determine the precise relationship between folic acid intake and the prevention and promotion of cancer.

SUMMARY

This chapter provided a brief discussion of many of the key elements that contribute to maintaining or improving the nutritional status of individuals with cancer. Cancer is not just a major cause of death—it is also becoming a chronic illness as more individuals are living with cancer longer, as they experience intermittent periods of active cancer with remission. The number of individuals who are cured of cancer is also increasing. Subsequent chapters of this book provide a more in-depth discussion of the nutrition care process and medical nutrition therapy for individuals with many of the different types of cancers as well as nutrition recommendations for cancer survivors.

REFERENCES

1. Pickle LW, Hao Y, Jemal A, et al. A new method of estimating United States and state-level cancer incidence counts for the current calendar year. *CA Cancer J Clin.* 2007;57(1):30–42.
2. American Cancer Society. Cancer facts and figures 2008. http://www.cancer.org/downloads/STT/2008CAFFfinalsecured.pdf. Accessed December 18, 2008.
3. American Institute for Cancer Research. Food, nutrition, physical activity, and the prevention of cancer: A global perspective. http://www.aicr.org. Accessed April 15, 2008.
4. Butterworth C Jr, Hatch K, Gore H, et al. Improvement in cervical dysplasia associated with folic acid therapy in users of oral contraceptives. *Am J Clin Nutr.* 1982;35:73–82.
5. Sesink AL, Termont DS, Kleibeuker JH, et al. Red meat and colon cancer: The cytotoxic and hyperproliferative effects of dietary heme. *Cancer Res.* 1999;59:5704–5709.
6. Tannenbaum A. The dependence of tumour formation on the degree of caloric restriction. *Cancer Res.* 1945;5:609–615.
7. Tucker MJ. The effect of long term food restriction on tumours in animals. *Int J Cancer.* 1979;23:803–807.
8. Irwin ML, Mayer-Davis EJ, Addy CL, et al. Moderate-intensity physical activity and fasting insulin levels in women: The Cross-Cultural Activity Participation Study. *Diabetes Care.* 2000;23(4):449–454.

9. Kushi LH, Byers T, Doyle C, et al., for the American Cancer Society 2006 Nutrition and Physical Activity Guidelines Advisory Committee. American Cancer Society guidelines on nutrition and physical activity for cancer prevention: Reducing the risk of cancer with healthy food choices and physical activity [published correction appears in *CA Cancer J Clin.* 2007;57(1):66]. *CA Cancer J Clin.* 2006;56 (5):254–281.

10. Holmes MD, Chen WY, Feskanich D, Kroenke CH, Colditz GA. Physical activity and survival after breast cancer diagnosis. *JAMA.* 2005; 293(20):2479–2486.

11. Meyerhardt JA, Giovannucci EL, Holmes MD, et al. Physical activity and survival after colorectal cancer diagnosis. *J Clin Oncol.* 2006;24(22):3527–3534.

12. Meyerhardt JA, Heseltine D, Niedzwiecki D, et al. Impact of physical activity on cancer recurrence and survival in patients with stage III colon cancer: Findings from CALGB 89803. *J Clin Oncol.* 2006;24(22):3535–3541.

13. Demark-Wahnefried W. Cancer survival: Time to get moving? Data accumulate suggesting a link between physical activity and cancer survival. *J Clin Oncol.* 2006;24(22):3517–3518.

14. Renehan AC, Tyson M, Egger M, Heller RF, Zwahlen M. Body-mass index and incidence of cancer: A systematic review and meta-analysis of prospective observational studies. *Lancet.* 2008;371:569–578.

15. Rose DP, Komninou D, Stephenson GD. Obesity, adipocytokines, and insulin resistance in breast cancer. *Obes Rev.* 2004;5:153–165.

16. Tian YF, Chu CH, Wu MH, et al. Anthropometric measures, plasma adiponectin, and breast cancer risk. *Endocr Relat Cancer.* 2007;14(3):669–677.

17. Tong H, Isenring E, Yates P. The prevalence of nutrition impact symptoms and their relationship to quality of life and clinical outcomes in medical oncology patients [published online ahead of print June 13, 2008]. *Support Care Cancer.*

18. Dewys WD, Begg C, Lavin PT, et al. Prognostic effect of weight loss prior to chemotherapy in cancer patients: Eastern Cooperative Oncology Group. *Am J Med.* 1980;69:491–497.

19. Fearon KC. Cancer cachexia: Developing multimodal therapy for a multidimensional problem. *Eur J Cancer.* 2008. In press.

20. Skipworth RJ, Steart GD, Dejong CH, et al. Pathophysiology of cancer cachexia: Much more than host–tumour interaction? *Clin Nutr.* 2007;26:667–676.

21. Stewart GD, Skipworth RJ, Fearon KC. Cancer cachexia and fatigue. *Clin Med.* 2006;6:140–143.

22. Fearon KC, Moses AG. Cancer cachexia. *Int J Cardiol.* 2002;85(1):73–81.

23. Martignoni ME, Kunze P, Friess H. Cancer cachexia. *Mol Cancer.* 2003:2:36.

24. Bennani N, Davis MP. Cytokines and cancer anorexia cachexia syndrome. *Am J Hosp Palliat Care.* 2008. In press.

25. Todorov P, Cariuk P, McDevitt T, et al. Characterization of a cancer cachectic factor. *Nature.* 1996;379:739–742.

26. Young CD, Anderson SM. Sugar and fat—that's where it's at: Metabolic changes in tumors. *Breast Cancer Res.* 2008;10(1):202.

27. Holyrode CP, Reichard GA. Carbohydrate metabolism in cancer cachexia. *Cancer Treat Rep.* 1987;65(suppl 5):55–59.

28. Gambhir SS, Czernin J, Schwimmer J, Silverman DH, Coleman RE, Phelps ME. A tabulated summary of the FDG PET literature. *J Nucl Med.* 2001;42(suppl 5): 1S–93S.

29. Brizel DM, Schroeder T, Scher RL, et al. Elevated tumor lactate concentrations predict for an increased risk of metastases in head-and-neck cancer. *Int J Radiat Oncol Biol Phys.* 2001;51:349–353.
30. Walenta S, Wetterling M, Lehrke M, et al. High lactate levels predict likelihood of metastases, tumor recurrence, and restricted patient survival in human cervical cancers. *Cancer Res.* 2000;60:916–921.
31. Gillies RJ, Robey I, Gatenby RA. Causes and consequences of increased glucose metabolism of cancers. *J Nucl Med.* 2008;49(suppl 2):24S-42S.
32. Shaw JH, Wolfe RR. Glucose and urea kinetics in patients with early and advanced gastrointestinal cancer: The response to glucose infusion, parenteral feeding, and surgical resection. *Surgery.* 1987;101:181–191.
33. Guirao X. Impact of the inflammatory reaction on intermediary metabolism and nutrition status. *Nutrition.* 2002;18:949–952.
34. Beck SA, Mulligan HD, Tisdale MJ. Lipolytic factors associated with murine and human cancer cachexia. *J Natl Cancer Inst.* 1990;82:1922–1926.
35. Teunissen SC, Wesker W, Kruitwagen C, et al. Symptom prevalence in patients with incurable cancer: A systematic review. *J Pain Symptom Manage.* 2007;34: 94–104.
36. Cleveland RJ, Eng SM, Abrahamson PE, et al. Weight gain prior to diagnosis and survival from breast cancer. *Cancer Epidemiol Biomarkers Prev.* 2007;16:1803–1811.
37. Nitenberg G, Raynard B. Nutritional support of the cancer patient: Issues and dilemmas. *Crit Rev Oncl Hematol.* 2000;34:137–168.
38. Braga M, Gianotti L, Nespoli L, Radaelli G, Di Carlo V. Nutritional approach in malnourished surgical patients: A prospective randomized study. *Arch Surg.* 2002;137(2):174–180.
39. Gianotti L, Braga M, Nespoli L, Radaelli G, Beneduce A, Di Carlo V. A randomized controlled trial of preoperative oral supplementation with a specialized diet in patients with gastrointestinal cancer. *Gastroenterology.* 2002;122:1763–1770.
40. Hoda D, Jatoi A, Burnes J, Loprinzi C, Kelly D. Should patients with advanced, incurable cancers ever be sent home with total parenteral nutrition? A single institution's 20-year experience. *Cancer.* 2005;103(4):863–868.
41. Fan BG. Parenteral nutrition prolongs the survival of patients with malignant gastrointestinal obstruction. *JPEN.* 2007;31(6):508–510.
42. Soo I, Gramich L. Use of parenteral nutrition in patients with advanced cancer. *Appl Physiol Nutr Metab.* 2008;33(1):102–106.
43. Velicer CM, Ulrich CRM. Vitamin and mineral supplement use among US adults after cancer diagnosis: A systematic review. *J Clin Oncol.* 2008;26:665–673.
44. Watkins ML, Erickson JD, Thun MJ, et al. Multivitamin use and mortality in a large prospective study. *Am J Epidemiol.* 2000;152:149–162.
45. Stevens VL, McCullough ML, Diver WR, et al. Use of multivitamins and prostate cancer mortality in a large cohort of US men. *Cancer Causes Control.* 2005;16: 643–650.
46. Mathijssen RH, Verweij J, de Bruijn P, et al. Effects of St. John's wort on irinotecan metabolism. *J Natl Cancer Inst.* 2002;94:1247–1249.
47. Meijerman I, Beijnen JH, Schellens JHM. Herb–drug interactions in oncology: Focus on mechanisms of induction. *Oncologist.* 2006;11(7):742–752.
48. Nourissat A, Vasson MP, Merrouche Y, et al. Relationship between nutritional status and quality of life in patients with cancer. *Eur J Cancer.* 2008;44(9):1238–1242.

49. Rice S, Whitehead SA. Phytoestrogens and breast cancer: Promoters or protectors? *Endocr Relat Cancer*. 2006;13(4)995–1015.
50. Shao ZM, Wu J, Shen ZZ, Barsky SH. Genistein exerts multiple suppressive effects on human breast carcinoma cells. *Cancer Res*. 1998;58:4851–4857.
51. Zava DT, Duwe G. Estrogenic and antiproliferative properties of genistein and other flavonoids in human breast cancer cells in vitro. *Nutr Cancer*. 1997;27:31–40.
52. Petrakis NL, Barnes S, King EB, et al. Stimulatory influence of soy protein isolate on breast secretion in pre- and postmenopausal women. *Cancer Epidemiol Biomarkers Prev*. 1996;5:785–794.
53. Wang C, Kurzer MS. Effects of phytoestrogens on DNA synthesis in MCF-7 cells in the presence of estradiol or growth factors. *Nutr Cancer*. 1998;31:90–100.
54. Allred CD, Ju YH, Allred KF, Chang J, Helferich WG. Dietary genistein stimulates growth of estrogen-dependent breast cancer tumors similar to that observed with genistein. *Carcinogenesis*. 2001;22:1667–1673.
55. Pacelli F, Bossola M, Teodori L, et al. Parenteral nutrition does not stimulate tumor proliferation in malnourished gastric cancer patients. *JPEN*. 2007;31(6):451–455.
56. Kato I, Dnistrian AM, Schwartz M, et al. Serum folate, homocysteine and colorectal cancer risk in women: A nested case-control study. *Br J Cancer*. 1999;79:1917–1922.
57. Sellers TA, Kushi LH, Cerhan JR, et al. Dietary folate intake, alcohol, and risk of breast cancer in a prospective study of postmenopausal women. *Epidemiology*. 2001;12(4):420–428.
58. Hultdin J, Van Guelpen B, Bergh A, Hallmans G, Stattin P. Plasma folate, vitamin B12, and homocysteine and prostate cancer risk: A prospective study. *Int J Cancer*. 2005;113:819–824.
59. Stolzenberg-Solomon RZ, Chang SC, Leitzmann MF, et al. Folate intake, alcohol use, and postmenopausal breast cancer risk in the Prostate, Lung, Colorectal, and Ovarian Cancer Screening Trial. *Am J Clin Nutr*. 2006;83:895–904.
60. Tworoger SS, Hecht JL, Giovannucci E, Hankinson SE. Intake of folate and related nutrients in relation to risk of epithelial ovarian cancer. *Am J Epidemiol*. 2006;163:1101–1111.
61. Mason JB, Dickstein A, Jacques PF, et al. A temporal association between folic acid fortification and an increase in colorectal cancer rates may be illuminating important biological principles: A hypothesis. *Cancer Epidemiol Biomarkers Prev*. 2007;16:1325–1329.
62. Smith AD, Kim YI, Refsum H. Is folic acid good for everyone? *Am J Clin Nutr*. 2008;87(3):517–533.

Chapter 2

Nutrition Screening and Assessment in Oncology

Pamela Charney, PhD, RD
Andreea Cranganu, RD, LD, CNSD

INTRODUCTION

It has long been known that patients with cancer who experience weight loss tolerate treatment poorly.[1, 2] Poor nutrition status has also been correlated with decreased long-term survival in several tumor types[3, 4] In the 1980s and 1990s, techniques for providing aggressive nutrition support to patients who were unwilling or unable to eat were used with some enthusiasm. Despite this trend, outcomes associated with suboptimal nutrition status did not appear to change, leading to the need to further investigate the role of nutrition and nutrition status in cancer treatment.

There is some indication that the type and amount of nutrition support provided may have been factors in the lack of improvement in treatment outcomes. A large multicenter study published in 1991 investigated the use of preoperative parenteral nutrition (PN) in surgical patients (while the focus was not intended, the majority of patients had gastrointestinal cancer). Study participants who were not malnourished had more complications than those who were malnourished.[5] There is also some indication that energy provided was significantly greater than energy requirements, leading to frequent hyperglycemic events. Although subsequent research has implicated poor glycemic control as an etiologic factor for increased postoperative complications,[6] the results have also highlighted the need to identify more accurately those individuals who might benefit from aggressive nutrition support interventions.

Early attempts at feeding patients with cancer relied on the "more is better" premise. Lacking knowledge regarding the metabolic impact of different tumor types, clinicians thought of the tumor as a "calorie sink" that led to a significant increase in energy expenditure to prevent wasting in the host. Prior to the advent of indirect calorimetry, many nutrition protocols provided nutrition in the range of 150–175% of estimated nutrient requirements. While much remains to be learned about the metabolic impact of different tumor types, it is now known that energy requirements vary greatly depending on the tumor type and stage. Clinicians responsible for assessing the nutritional status of patients with cancer must have an understanding of the potential metabolic impacts of the various tumor types as well as the possible effects of the various types of oncological therapy.

Nutrition screening is the process that identifies patients who might have a nutrition problem or who might be at greater risk for experiencing complications associated with nutrition problems.[7] Nutrition assessment can be defined as collecting and analyzing data about the patient/client to determine whether the individual has a nutrition problem that can be resolved or ameliorated by a nutrition intervention.[8] Individuals with cancer often experience alterations in nutrient intake as well as metabolic abnormalities that affect both their functional status and their quality of life (QOL). Screening is the first step in identifying patients who might require nutrition interventions aimed at improving nutrition status or ameliorating the effects of cancer therapy on nutritional status and QOL. Healthcare professionals caring for patients with cancer must critically analyze the data collected from the assessment process, identify nutrition problems, and implement focused interventions. This chapter defines the nutrition screening and assessment process and examines the tools available for practical application—that is, for providing nutrition care in the oncology setting.

The Nutrition Care Process

The American Dietetic Association (ADA) adopted the Nutrition Care Process (NCP) in 2003 as a framework for dietetics professionals to use to support critical thinking and decision making in a variety of care settings.[9] The NCP consists of four interrelated steps: nutrition assessment, nutrition diagnosis, nutrition intervention, and nutrition monitoring and evaluation. Each step is supported by the International Dietetics and Nutrition Terminology (IDNT), which contains terms that describe the work of dietetics associated with each step.[8] The terminology is specific to dietetics practice and describes the work of the dietetics professional as opposed to another healthcare profession. Although nutrition screening is not considered to be part of the NCP, accurate, timely screening programs are required to identify those patients who require nutrition care.

Following is an example of the nutrition care process for neoplastic disease.[10]

Step One: Nutrition Assessment

MEDICAL/SOCIAL HISTORY

- Diagnoses
- Past medical history
- Sensory limitation(s)
- Medications
- Socioeconomic status/food security
- Support systems
- Education—primary language/literacy

DIETARY ASSESSMENT

- Ability to chew; use and fit of all dentures
- Problems swallowing/changes in saliva production or saliva consistency
- Taste changes
- Nausea, vomiting
- Constipation/diarrhea/normal stool pattern
- Heartburn
- Any other symptoms interfering with the ability to ingest the patient's normal diet
- Ability to consistently purchase adequate amounts of food for daily consumption
- Ability to feed self, cook and prepare meals
- Food allergies, preferences, and method of preparing meals
- Previous food restrictions
- Ethnic, cultural, and religious influences
- Use of alcohol, vitamin, mineral, herbal, or other type of supplements
- Previous nutrition education or nutrition therapy
- Eating pattern: 24-hour food recall, diet history, food frequency

ANTHROPOMETRIC

- Height (measured, recumbent, knee height, or arm span)
- Current weight
- Weight history: usual body weight, recent weight change
- BMI, IBW, %IBW, UBW, %UBW
- Calculation of upper arm muscle area—will need mid-arm circumference and triceps skin fold
- Bioelectrical impedance

BIOCHEMICAL ASSESSMENT

- Serum protein assessment: albumin, prealbumin, retinol-binding protein
- Hematological assessment: hemoglobin, hematocrit, ferritin, MCV, MCHC, MCH, TIBC, platelet count
- White blood cell count, absolute neutrophil count

Step Two: Common Diagnoses

Cancer patients could have any of the following nutritional diagnoses within the NCP:

- Inadequate oral food/beverage intake
- Inadequate fluid intake
- Inadequate bioactive substance intake
- Inadequate vitamin intake
- Hypermetabolism
- Increased nutrient needs
- Swallowing difficulty
- Chewing difficulty
- Altered gastrointestinal function
- Altered nutrition-related laboratory values
- Food-medication interaction
- Involuntary weight loss
- Food, nutrition, nutrition-related knowledge deficit

SAMPLE PES STATEMENT: NI-2.1

Problem: Inadequate oral food/beverage intake
Etiology: Related to mucositis post-radiation
Signs/symptoms: As evidenced by dietary history suggesting intake of less than 50% of estimated needs

Step Three: Sample Intervention

1. Modify texture and consistency of meals, avoiding extremes in temperatures.
2. Increase nutrient-dense foods and initiate oral high-calorie/protein supplements.
3. Encourage initiation of pain medications prior to eating and adequate, appropriate mouth care.

Step Four: Monitoring and Evaluation

1. The patient will consume 50% of estimated energy and protein needs within 48 hours of initiating interventions for mucositis.
2. The patient will be able to meet basic fluid requirements within 24 hours of initiating interventions for mucositis.

Nutritional Implications of Cancer

Cancer can have profound effects on nutritional status. A thorough understanding of the potential impact of the tumor and oncological therapies on host metabolism is essential to ensure a positive response to nutrition interventions. The generic term "cancer" encompasses hundreds of tumor types, each of which has a specific impact on both metabolism and the host's nutrition status. Antineoplastic therapies include surgery, radiation, and chemotherapy; combination therapy may also be indicated, thus making nutrition therapy more complex. For example, a patient who has previously received radiation therapy might subsequently undergo surgery, with the potential for more serious complications from surgery due to radiation enteritis.

Appetite changes leading to weight loss frequently occur prior to cancer diagnosis.[11] In one study, weight loss was strongly associated with decreased appetite in a group of patients with newly diagnosed lung or gastrointestinal (GI) cancers, though tumor burden did not correlate with weight loss or appetite changes.[10] A case-control study found that changes in appetite were strong predictors of pending diagnosis of lung cancer.[12] While the mechanisms for appetite changes are not fully known, clinicians must be aware of the potential for decreased appetite at the time of diagnosis and have treatment strategies at hand.

Metabolic Changes Associated with Cancer

It has long been assumed that all patients diagnosed with cancer experience significant increases in energy expenditure. More recent research utilizing indirect calorimetry, however, has revealed that changes in energy expenditure are more varied and do not occur with all tumor types.[11] Energy expenditure can range from 60% to 150% of expected energy expenditure.[12] Additionally, some patients with elevated energy requirements are able to gain weight, although this weight gain tends to consist of increases in body fat while the person continues to lose lean body mass.[13]

Johnson et al.[14] evaluated the accuracy of predictive equations frequently utilized in estimating resting energy expenditure (REE) during cancer-related weight loss. The study results revealed that weight-loss and weight-stable patients with cancer had similar REEs when adjusted for fat-free mass but were different in terms of the acute-phase response (APR). The APR is believed to be one of many factors that contribute to elevations in the REE in patients with cancer, which in turn could promote weight loss. In addition, the commonly used Harris–Benedict equation (HBE) was in poor agreement with measured REE in both groups and, therefore, was not suitable for REE prediction in a clinical setting.[14]

In another study, Bosaeus et al[15] examined dietary intake, REE, and weight loss in 297 adults primarily with gastrointestinal tumors, considering the relationship between these factors and survival rates. The investigators reported that 48.5% of patients were hypermetabolic, 50% were normometabolic, and 1.4% were hypometabolic. Because dietary intake did not differ between normometabolic and hypermetabolic patients, and because neither tumor type nor gender was related to energy and protein intake, weight loss could not be solely accounted for by diminished intake.[15] These findings suggest that a failure in feedback regulation between dietary intake in relation to energy expenditure may add to the weight loss experienced by many cancer patients.[15] The wide variability in energy expenditure reported thereby contributes to the challenge of accurately predicting energy requirements in this patient population.

Cachexia can be broadly defined as "general ill health, malnutrition, and weight loss, usually associated with chronic disease."[16] More specific definitions of cancer cachexia describe weight loss out of proportion to decreases in energy intake, which are most likely mediated by pro-inflammatory cytokines.[17] The role of inflammatory cytokines and other factors in the development of wasting and cachexia has been of interest. Wasting has been found to correlate with tumor burden and cytokine levels in patients with colorectal cancer, supporting the concept that cytokines are strongly implicated in the development of cancer cachexia.[14]

Unlike starvation, the weight loss experienced by patients with cancer cachexia syndrome cannot be easily reversed solely with increased nutrient provision.[18] In fact, weight loss generally will continue despite increased administration of nutrients.[18] Lymphomas, leukemias, breast cancers, and soft-tissue sarcoma have some of the lowest frequencies of weight loss, while more aggressive lymphomas, colon, prostate, and lung cancers are associated with an approximately 50% incidence of weight loss.[18] The highest incidence and severity is seen in pancreatic and gastric cancer, wherein approximately 85% of patients experience cachexia.[18] The potential consequences of cancer cachexia are outlined in the Table 2.1.[19]

Table 2.1   *Potential Causes of Unintentional Weight Loss in Cancer Patients*

Cause of Weight Loss	Nutritional Consequences
Malignancy	Obstruction/perforation of GI tract Intestinal secretory abnormalities Malabsorption Intestinal dysmotility Fluid/electrolyte abnormalities Anorexia Altered taste Learned food aversion Depression Altered peripheral hormone metabolism: Leptin, ghrelin
Treatment	Chemotherapy, surgery, radiation Other: opioid-induced constipation, GI tract abnormalities associated with fungal, viral, or bacterial infection
Altered metabolism	Tumor-induced alterations in energy expenditure Cori cycling/gluconeogenesis Nitrogen trap Altered fat metabolism Tumor-induced secretion of host mediators Tumor necrosis factor, interleukin-1, interleukin-6, proteolysis-inducing factor

Source: Reprinted from Roberts S, Mattox T. Cancer. In: Gottschlich MM, ed. *The A.S.P.E.N. Nutrition Support Core Curriculum: A Case-Based Approach—The Adult Patient.* Silver Spring, MD: American Society for Parenteral and Enteral Nutrition; 2007:649–675. Used with permission from the American Society for Parenteral and Enteral Nutrition (A.S.P.E.N.). A.S.P.E.N. does not endorse the use of this material in any form other than its entirety.

Metabolic Alterations Associated with Cancer Treatment

Single or combination therapies such as surgery, radiation, chemotherapy, and immunotherapy can produce adverse effects that frequently result in some degree of GI dysfunction.

Surgery is the oldest form of cancer treatment and is an essential tool to diagnose and stage cancer.[19] More than half of all patients with cancer ultimately have cancer-related surgery.[20] Depending on the site and extent of surgery, the body's need for calories, protein, and other nutrients may increase. Malnutrition prior to surgery may prolong recovery owing to poor wound healing or infectious complications. Patients with certain cancers, such as cancers of the head, neck, stomach, and bowel, may be malnourished at diagnosis; therefore, nutrition intervention is often warranted for these individuals prior to surgery.

Nutrition-related side effects may also occur as a result of surgery. Surgical resections and/or excision may result in adverse effects on GI function, depending on the tumor site and extent of the surgery. The following nutrition problems may occur as a result of antineoplastic interventions such as surgery, radiation, chemotherapy, and immunotherapy:

Surgery

- Radical resection of the oropharyngeal area may lead to chewing and swallowing difficulties.
- Esophagectomy may cause gastric stasis, hypochlorhydria, steatorrhea, and diarrhea secondary to vagotomy; early satiety and regurgitation may also result.
- Gastrectomy (partial or total) may cause early satiety, malabsorption, vitamins D and B_{12} deficiency, hypoglycemia, and dumping syndrome.
- Intestinal resection (jejunum or ileum involvement) can lead to maldigestion and malabsorption.

Radiation

Radiation therapy can affect healthy cells that are near the radiation field, leading to a number of side effects. Precisely which side effects arise will depend on the radiation dose, duration, and radiation site. Additionally, nutrition-related impact symptoms may increase if radiation is given in conjunction with another oncologic therapy such as chemotherapy. Radiation to any part of the digestive system is likely to cause nutrition-related side effects, including the following problems:

- Radiation to the oropharyngeal area may cause anorexia, alterations in taste and smell, xerostomia, mucositis, odynophagia, dysphagia, fatigue, osteoradionecrosis, and trismus.
- Radiation to the lower neck and mediastinum can result in esophagitis, dysphagia, odynophagia, esophageal reflux, nausea, or vomiting. Long-term side effects include esophageal fibrosis, stenosis, and necrosis; pulmonary fibrosis, and pneumonitis.
- Radiation to the abdomen or pelvis may cause bowel damage (acute or chronic) accompanied by diarrhea, maldigestion, malabsorption, bloating, abdominal cramps, gas, obstruction, colitis, stricture, ulcerations, or fistulization. Additional side effects include nausea, vomiting, lactose intolerance, hematuria, cystitis, and fatigue.

Chemotherapy

Cytotoxic drugs halt the growth of cancer cells, either through apoptosis or through prevention of cellular differentiation and proliferation. Chemotherapy targets rapidly dividing cells, including those in bone marrow and GI tract; as a consequence, the direct effects of cytotoxic agents can produce nutritional complications. The specific impact of chemotherapy on GI function depends on the chemotherapy agent used, the dose and route of administration, and the length of therapy.[19] The following nutrition-related impact symptoms are commonly observed:

- Anorexia
- Nausea
- Early satiety
- Alterations in olfactory senses
- Vomiting
- Diarrhea or constipation
- Mucositis, stomatitis, and esophagitis
- Xerostomia
- Myelosuppression and infection

Immunotherapy

Immunotherapy (also called biologic therapy or biotherapy) takes advantage of the patient's own immune system to fight cancer. Substances made by the body or synthesized in a laboratory are used to boost or restore the body's natural defenses against cancer.[20] The following nutrition-related side effects are commonly encountered during immunotherapy:

- Fever
- Nausea
- Vomiting
- Anorexia
- Asthenia

If left untreated, the symptoms associated with cancer therapy can lead to weight loss and malnutrition; these problems may then subsequently delay treatment and recovery, and promote poor wound healing and infectious complications. Nutrition interventions (e.g., oral supplements, enteral or parenteral feeding, and modifications in diet consistency) can improve nutrient delivery such that antineoplastic regimens are better tolerated and weight loss is prevented.

Nutrient Requirements

Providing adequate calories is essential to maintain weight and/or prevent weight loss associated with cancer treatment or disease. While indirect calorimetry (IDC) remains the gold standard for determining calorie requirements, energy needs are frequently estimated because IDC is not generally available. The following guidelines are recommended for estimating energy requirements for cancer patients:

- Normometabolic patients: 25–30 kcal/kg/day
- Hypermetabolic or weight gain desired: 30–35 kcal/kg/day*
- Obese patients: 21–25 kcal/kg/day (when weight maintenance is the goal; energy needs may be increased when nutritional status is deteriorating)[19]

The provision of adequate protein is important to prevent or reduce negative nitrogen balance and to meet the increased demands for protein synthesis during and following antineoplastic interventions. Guidelines for protein requirements are as follows:[19]

- Nonstressed: 1–1.5 g/kg/day
- Hypermetabolism or protein-losing enteropathy conditions: 1.5–2.5 g/kg/day

Dehydration is prevalent in many cancer patients, especially those who receive chemotherapy and/or radiation therapy. Chemotherapeutic agents can damage the GI mucosa and cause diarrhea. Also, patients undergoing radiation for head and neck cancer are prone to dehydration owing to their inability to take adequate oral fluids secondary to xerostomia, mucositis, dysgeusia, dysphagia, and odynophagia. High-risk patients should be closely monitored for signs and symptoms of dehydration such as dark, concentrated urine; decreased urine output, dry mouth, acute weight loss, and fatigue. The fluid needs of cancer patients are similar to those of other patient populations without renal disease (30–35 mL/kg/day), although fluid needs may also be greater in the face of increased fluid losses that may occur as a result of vomiting, diarrhea, and fistulas.[10]

---

*More than 35 kcal/kg/day may be required to maintain or promote weight gain in some situations.

Deficiencies of vitamins (especially folate, vitamin C, and retinol) and minerals (magnesium, zinc, copper, and iron) can occur as a result of direct effects of the tumor, effects of cytokines, infectious processes, maldigestion and malabsorption, chemotherapy, radiation, or inadequate food intake.[10] Although adequate micronutrient intake is considered important, specific nutritional guidelines for this population have not been established. The use of a daily multivitamin/mineral supplements with levels not exceeding one to two times the dietary recommended intake values may be beneficial for most patients undergoing chemotherapy and/or radiation therapies.[10]

Nutrition Screening

Regulatory agencies including the Joint Commission on Accreditation of Healthcare Organizations (JCAHO) and the Centers for Medicare and Medicaid Services (CMS) require that nutrition screening be performed in all healthcare settings. Nutrition screening refers to the initial clinical evaluation that is used to identify patients at high risk for malnutrition.[18] Nutrition screening programs should be designed to rapidly and accurately identify those patients who might need a more comprehensive nutrition assessment. Commonly used screening parameters include height, weight, weight change, and change in ability to eat.

Table 2.2 describes the qualities associated with a well-designed nutrition risk screening program. While accurate nutrition screening is a vital support to the NCP, it is not considered part of the NCP because the screen can be conducted by any healthcare professional.

Healthcare clinicians responsible for developing nutrition screening programs should evaluate currently available screening tools before creating new tools. Currently available nutrition screening tools that may be used in a variety of care settings include the Malnutrition Screening Tool (MST), the Malnutrition Universal Screening Tool (MUST), and the Nutrition Risk

Table 2.2 *Qualities Associated with a Well-Designed Nutrition Screening Program*

- Rapid
- Can be conducted by any healthcare professional
- Has acceptable sensitivity, specificity, and positive/negative predictive value
- Cost-effective
- Poses little risk to the person being screened

Screen (NRS). MST is an example of a short screening tool and has been validated in both inpatient and outpatient settings.[18] MUST also consists of a score derived from three items, but it has been found to have a low sensitivity and specificity in oncology patients.[18] Table 2.3 provides a brief description of these screening tools.

Nutrition Assessment

Nutrition assessment can be defined as a method of identifying and evaluating data needed to make decisions about a nutrition-related problem/diagnosis. Nutrition assessment is the first step of the NCP and involves the collection and analysis of data that identify potential nutrition problems. Individuals who have a "positive" screening result should be referred to a registered dietitian (RD) for a comprehensive nutrition assessment. Data gathered in the nutrition assessment are generally clustered into the following groups:

- Nutrition history
- Medical tests, labs, and procedures
- Client history

Table 2.3   *Nutrition Screening Tools*

Tool	*Characteristics*	*Comments*
Malnutrition Screening Tool (MST)	3 items: weight, percentage weight loss, appetite	Validated in oncology patients
Malnutrition Universal Screening Tool (MUST)	3 items: body mass index, percentage weight loss, acute disease effect	Low sensitivity and specificity in oncology patients
Nutrition Risk Index (NRI)	Equation: NRI = 1.519 (serum albumin; g/dL) + 41.7 (current weight/usual weight)	
Mini Nutritional Assessment (MNA)	18 items: Screening (6 questions): food intake, weight loss, mobility stress, body mass index Assessment (12 questions): medical history, eating habits, anthropometric measurements	Validated in the elderly population

Source: Huhmann MB, August DA. Review of American Society for Parenteral and Enteral Nutrition (A.S.P.E.N.) clinical guidelines for nutrition support in cancer patients: Nutrition screening and assessment. *Nutr Clin Pract.* 2008;23:182–188.

- Anthropometric data
- Nutrition-focused physical exam

Review and analysis of these data provides the RD with the information needed to diagnose nutrition problems accurately.

Nutrition History

The nutrition history includes information regarding the types and amounts of foods currently consumed, changes in both quality and quantity of foods eaten, and reported reasons for those changes. Several methods are used to gather information for the nutrition history, including a food record, 24-hour recall, and calorie count. Each is described in Table 2.4.

Table 2.4   *Dietary Assessment Methods*

Tool	*Component*	*Comments*
Food record/food diary	The patient documents his or her dietary intake as it occurs over a specific period of time. Records are kept over a three- or five-day period and should include both weekdays and weekends.	Advantages: data are not totally reliant on patient's memory and may be more accurate. Disadvantages: underreporting and changing of food habits for the recording period. The patient must make a commitment to complete the food record.
24-hour recall	The patient recalls all food and drink that has been consumed in the previous 24-hour period under clinician guidance.	Advantages: short administration time, low cost, low risk for patient. Disadvantages: does not always show typical eating pattern, patients may over or underreport intake, and records may not be accurate because they rely on the patient's memory.
Calorie count	Record of food and beverage intake, mostly used in clinical settings. The RD or RDT calculates nutritional information such as kilocalories and protein content consumed and compares it to the patient's estimated needs.	Disadvantages: inaccurate in most care settings, time-consuming (must wait until complete before determining intervention).

Source: Nelms M, Sucher K, Long S. *Nutrition Therapy and Pathophysiology.* Belmont, CA: Thomson Higher Learning; 2007:101–135, 751–783.

Determination of nutrient intake for hospitalized patients is complicated by a variety of factors: lack of staffing to document intake adequately, difficulty estimating amounts of foods eaten, and inability to determine amounts of snacks or foods consumed from home. For these reasons, the "calorie count" should not be considered an appropriate method to monitor intake of hospitalized patients. Unfortunately, hospitalized patients quite often do not consume enough food to meet their nutrient requirements, thereby making communication with nursing staff and caregivers imperative to determine actual dietary intake.

Depending on the patient population, as much as 40% of foods served in the hospital are not consumed.[21] While oral nutrition supplements are frequently utilized as a first line of nutrition therapy for patients who are not consuming adequate food, some evidence suggests that this intervention might not be appropriate for many patients.[22] Although research shows an increase in energy and protein intake by patients who receive oral supplements as compared to patients who receive standard hospital diets,[15, 23] these studies did not employ additional foods or food preferences for the control groups. Furthermore, several studies have monitored the intake of oral supplements and found significant wastage.[24, 25] Given these caveats, the use of commercially prepared oral supplements over food should not be routinely recommended as an avenue to increase nutrient intake in patients with cancer until other interventions have been explored. The use of dietetic assistants to facilitate feeding was associated with a significant decrease in mortality in elderly hip fracture patients, for example.[26] To date, no research supports the use of assistive personnel at mealtimes for patients with cancer, though the results of the previous study are encouraging.

The importance of obtaining a nutrition history cannot be overstated. Without knowledge about the types and quantities of foods consumed by the patient, the RD cannot accurately diagnose whether nutrition problems exist. It is important not only to determine food intake patterns prior to diagnosis, but also to quantify adequacy of intake and elucidate changes in intake related to the disease and its treatment.

Medical Tests, Labs, and Procedures

In the past, levels of serum hepatic transport proteins (albumin, prealbumin, and transferrin) were commonly cited as "markers of nutrition status." Current knowledge regarding the role of hepatic transport proteins in the acute-phase response (APR), combined with basic understanding of the physiology of starvation, emphasizes the problems with utilizing these markers for assessing nutritional status. During uncomplicated starvation, levels of the serum hepatic proteins are maintained at normal or near-normal levels until fairly late in the process.[18, 19] This lack of specificity of the transport proteins for identifying uncomplicated malnutrition means that patients who have weight loss and poor intake would have false-negative results from a screening or assessment that relied on solely the hepatic transport proteins.

The serum hepatic transport proteins participate in the APR and act as negative acute-phase proteins.[20] As such, their levels often decrease in response to metabolic stress rather than in response to changes in nutrient intake.[27] Patients with cancer are often hypermetabolic as a result of the presence of disease or the oncologic therapies initiated; as a consequence, the use of hepatic transport proteins for assessing nutritional status is problematic and may not accurately reflect nutritional status. When analyzing serum transport proteins, other parameters such as weight history, current medical condition, current nutrient intake, and presence of nutrition-related symptoms should also be critically evaluated to determine nutritional status accurately.

C-reactive protein (CRP) is a nonspecific indicator of inflammation that increases as much as 1,000-fold during an inflammatory event.[10] The levels of acute-phase proteins, including CRP, generally increase concurrently with acute or chronic medical conditions as the levels of serum transport protein levels such as prealbumin or albumin decrease.[10] However, because of the nonspecificity of CRP, and the ability of clinical examination to determine the presence of an inflammatory condition, routine use of CRP in nutrition assessment cannot be recommended.

Client History

The client history includes information about the individual's medical and surgical history, current treatment plans, medications, and socioeconomic data. The patient's medical and surgical history should be thoroughly evaluated to identify factors that may influence the patient's nutritional status or his or her risk for alterations in nutritional status.

Many patients take multiple prescribed and over-the-counter medications and/or dietary supplements. Foods can interact and even interfere with these medications' absorption and effectiveness in different ways. Dietary supplements, including botanicals, can, like conventional medicines, lead to side effects, which may negatively affect oral intake or mimic side effects of conventional cancer therapies.[19] In addition, supplements may interact with conventional medications and cancer therapies and decrease their effectiveness or alter their metabolism.[19] For example, black cohosh—an herb commonly used by breast cancer patients—has been shown to increase doxorubicin and docetaxel cytotoxicity, but to decrease cisplatin cytotoxicity in murine breast cancer cells.[19]

A nonjudgmental approach should be used to inquire whether any supplements are being used during antineoplastic treatments in an effort to help the patient avoid any potential adverse effects. The questions should be specific in regard to what the patient is taking, how much the patient is taking, and whether the supplement is being used in combination with any other agents or drugs.[19] Table 2.5 lists dietary supplements commonly used by cancer patients. The use of dietary supplements is also discussed in greater detail in Chapter 16.

A social history obtains information about an individual's socioeconomic status, housing situation, social support system, access to medical care, activity level, food purchasing and preparation capabilities, and religious practices, as well as involvement in support groups.[28] Understanding of the individual's socioeconomic status should allow the clinician to tailor the patient's nutrition care plan to optimize the chances for success.

Anthropometric Data

Anthropometric data are used to estimate or measure body composition. In some settings, it is possible to measure composition of body compartments via sophisticated techniques such as labeled water or dual-energy x-ray

Table 2.5   *Dietary Supplements Often Used by Cancer Patients*

Astralagus	Kombucha tea
Beta carotene	Iscador (mistletoe)
B vitamins	Laetrile
Cat's claw	Milk thistle (silymarin)
Echinacea	Pau d'arco (lapachol)
Essiac	Pycnogenol
Flaxseed	Selenium
Garlic	Shiitake mushrooms
Ginseng	Soy
Goldenseal	Vitamin A
Grape seed extract	Vitamin C
Green tea	Vitamin E

Source: Roberts S, Mattox T. Cancer. In: Gottschlich MM, ed. *The A.S.P.E.N. Nutrition Support Core Curriculum: A Case-Based Approach—The Adult Patient*. Silver Spring, MD: American Society for Parenteral and Enteral Nutrition; 2007:649–675. Used with permission from the American Society for Parenteral and Enteral Nutrition (A.S.P.E.N.). A.S.P.E.N. does not endorse the use of this material in any form other than its entirety.

absorptiometry (DEXA). These techniques allow the clinician caring for patients with cancer to determine lean body mass (LBM), bone mineral content, and fat mass. In practical terms, as a result of cost and other considerations, most clinicians are limited to estimation of body composition using height, weight, and occasionally bioelectric impedance analysis (BIA). The BIA measures electrical resistance on the basis of lean body mass and body fat composition. Single BIA measures show body cell mass, extracellular tissue, and fat as a percentage of ideal levels, whereas sequential measurements can be used to show body composition changes over time. Because of cost and accessibility issues, the use of BIA is currently limited, and this technology is unavailable in most ambulatory settings.

Other anthropometric measures include skin-fold measurements (to measure subcutaneous fat) and mid-arm muscle circumference (to assess lean body mass). Serial measurements are useful when monitoring weight to determine if fat or lean body mass is being lost or gained.[10] These measurements, while providing useful information, need to be assessed cautiously in cancer patients, because the "norms" on which they are based represent healthy individuals and, therefore, may not have direct applications to the cancer population.[10]

Accurate height and weight measurements at baseline, during treatment, and following treatment are critical for optimal nutritional care. In a busy care setting, it is all too easy to overlook these simple measurements. Care providers often find it easier to estimate height and weight. Of course, the accuracy of such estimations varies depending on the training and experience of the person making the estimation. Bloomfield et al. found that estimates by physicians and nurses heights and weights of patients admitted to intensive care varied significantly from the patients' actual measurements, with greater inaccuracy being observed in weight estimations.[29] Another study found that while estimates of height and weight done by nurses were relatively accurate, the difference between estimated and measured values could be as much as 15 cm and 15 kg.[30]

Nutrition-Focused Physical Exam

As noted earlier, metabolic changes associated with some tumor types may lead to development of cancer cachexia. Cancer cachexia is associated with loss of lean body mass in excess of loss of fat mass. It is entirely possible that a patient might have sufficient adipose tissue to mask the loss of lean body mass, making physical assessment skills vital for early identification of cachexia. Additionally, disease progression often leads to an inability to consume adequate foods with increased consumption of liquids, making treatment of cachexia difficult.[31]

A complete physical assessment should include observation for signs of edema, ascites, temporal lobe wasting, and muscle wasting.[10] The clinician should also assess the gastrointestinal tract to determine whether the patient is having or has a history of anorexia, changes in appetite, nausea and vomiting, diarrhea, constipation, early satiety, mucositis, dysgeusia, or dysphagia. In addition, an oral assessment should be completed to evaluate both the health of the patient's oral cavity, including dentition, and the patient's ability to chew and swallow.

Nutrition Assessment Tools in Common Use

Very few validated tools have been developed to assess nutrition status in patients with cancer. Assessment tools that have been studied include the Subjective Global Assessment (SGA), the Patient-Generated Subjective Global Assessment (PG-SGA; a variation of the SGA that has not been extensively validated), and the Nutrition Risk Index (NRI).

The SGA was initially developed to assess patients for malnutrition by utilizing information that could be easily obtained without the need for laboratory data or other sophisticated equipment. The SGA is also one of the few assessment tools that integrates many of the traditional parameters used in nutritional assessment with current clinical status and functional capacity.[32] Historical information (weight loss, dietary intake, gastrointestinal symptoms, and functional capacity), metabolic demands of the underlying disease, and a nutrition-related physical exam that takes into consideration loss of subcutaneous fat and presence of muscle wasting, edema, and ascites are the key components of the SGA.[33] The SGA relies on the experience and judgment of the clinician to determine whether the patient is well nourished, has moderate/suspected malnutrition, or is severely malnourished. It is considered an efficient and cost-effective avenue for identifying patients at risk of malnutrition. Since its inception, several tools similar to the SGA have evolved but have not been extensively validated.

The PG-SGA was adapted from the SGA specifically for the oncology population (see Figure 2.1).[22] This easy-to-use and inexpensive tool is a scored approach for identifying individuals at nutritional risk and triaging patients for subsequent medical nutritional therapy in a variety of clinical settings. The PG-SGA consists of two sections: a four-question patient-completed section and a section for the healthcare professional. The patient-completed sections provide information about weight history, presence of nutrition-related symptoms, food intake, and activity/functional level. The sections completed by a healthcare professional include an evaluation of metabolic

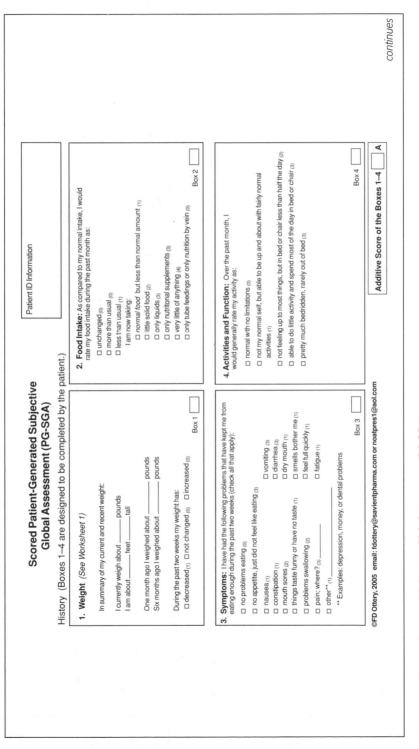

Figure 2.1 *Patient-Generated Subjective Global Assessment (PG-SGA)*
©FD Ottery, 2005.

continues

Scored Patient-Generated Subjective Global Assessment (PG-SGA)

Patient ID Information

History (Boxes 1–4 are designed to be completed by the patient.)

1. Weight *(See Worksheet 1)*

In summary of my current and recent weight:

I currently weigh about _____ pounds
I am about _____ feet _____ tall

One month ago I weighed about _____ pounds
Six months ago I weighed about _____ pounds

During the past two weeks my weight has:
☐ decreased (1) ☐ not changed (0) ☐ increased (0)

Box 1 ☐

2. Food Intake: As compared to my normal intake, I would rate my food intake during the past month as:
☐ unchanged (0)
☐ more than usual (0)
☐ less than usual (1)
I am now taking:
☐ normal food but less than normal amount (1)
☐ little solid food (2)
☐ only liquids (3)
☐ only nutritional supplements (3)
☐ very little of anything (4)
☐ only tube feedings or only nutrition by vein (0)

Box 2 ☐

3. Symptoms: I have had the following problems that have kept me from eating enough during the past two weeks (check all that apply):
☐ no problems eating (0)
☐ no appetite, just did not feel like eating (3)
☐ nausea (1)   ☐ vomiting (3)
☐ constipation (1)   ☐ diarrhea (3)
☐ mouth sores (2)   ☐ dry mouth (1)
☐ things taste funny or have no taste (1)   ☐ smells bother me (1)
☐ problems swallowing (2)   ☐ feel full quickly (1)
☐ pain; where? (3) _____   ☐ fatigue (1)
☐ other** (1) _____
** Examples: depression, money, or dental problems

Box 3 ☐

4. Activities and Function: Over the past month, I would generally rate my activity as:
☐ normal with no limitations (0)
☐ not my normal self, but able to be up and about with fairly normal activities (1)
☐ not feeling up to most things, but in bed or chair less than half the day (2)
☐ able to do little activity and spend most of the day in bed or chair (3)
☐ pretty much bedridden, rarely out of bed (3)

Box 4 ☐

Additive Score of the Boxes 1–4   ☐   A

©FD Ottery, 2005 email: fdottery@savientpharma.com or noatpres1@aol.com

The remainder of this form will be completed by your doctor, nurse, dietitian, or therapist. Thank you.

Scored Patient-Generated Subjective Global Assessment (PG-SGA)

Worksheet 1—Scoring Weight (Wt) Loss

To determine score, use 1 month weight data if available. Use 6 month data only if there is no 1 month weight data. Use points below to score weight change and add one extra point if patient has lost weight during the past 2 wk.

Wt loss in 1 month	Points	Wt loss in 6 months
10% or greater	4	20% or greater
5–9.9%	3	10–19.9%
3–4.9%	2	6–9%
2–2.9%	1	2–5.9%
0–1.9%	0	0–1.9%

Numerical score from Worksheet 1 [ ]

6. Work Sheet 3—Metabolic Demand

Score for metabolic stress is determined by a number of variables known to increase protein & calorie needs. The score is additive so that a patient who has a fever of > 102 degrees (3 points) and is on 10 mg of prednisone chronically (2 points) would have an additive score for this section of 5 points.

Stress	none (0)	low (1)	moderate (2)	high (3)
Fever	no fever	>99 and <101	≥101 and <102	≥102
Fever duration	no fever	<72 hrs	72 hrs	>72 hrs
Corticosteroids	no corticosteroids	low dose (<10mg prednisone equivalents/day)	moderate dose (≥10 and <30mg prednisone equivalents/day)	high dose steroid (≥30mg prednisone equivalents/day)

Numerical score from Worksheet 3 [ ] C

7. Worksheet 4—Physical Exam

Physical exam includes a subjective evaluation of 3 aspects of body composition: fat, muscle, & fluid status. Since this is subjective, each aspect of the exam is rated for degree of deficit. Muscle deficit impacts point score more than fat deficit. Definition of categories: 0 = no deficit, 1+ = mild deficit, 2+ = moderate, 3+ = severe

Muscle Status:

temples (temporalis muscle)	0	1+	2+	3+
clavicles (pectoralis & deltoids)	0	1+	2+	3+
shoulders (deltoids)	0	1+	2+	3+
interosseous muscles	0	1+	2+	3+
scapula (latissimus dorsi, trapezius, deltoids)	0	1+	2+	3+
thigh (quadriceps)	0	1+	2+	3+
calf (gastrocnemius)	0	1+	2+	3+
Global muscle status rating	0	1+	2+	3+

Fat Stores:

orbital fat pads	0	1+	2+	3+
triceps skin fold	0	1+	2+	3+
fat overlying lower ribs	0	1+	2+	3+
Global fat deficit rating	0	1+	2+	3+

Fluid Status:

ankle edema	0	1+	2+	3+
sacral edema	0	1+	2+	3+
ascites	0	1+	2+	3+
Global fluid status rating	0	1+	2+	3+

Numerical score from Worksheet 4 [ ] D

5. Worksheet 2—Disease and its relation to nutritional requirements

Additive Score of the Boxes 1–4 (See Side 1) [ ] A

All relevant diagnoses (specify) _____

One point each:
☐ Cancer ☐ AIDS
☐ Presence of trauma
☐ Pulmonary or cardiac cachexia
☐ Presence of decubitus, open wound, or fistula
☐ Chronic renal insufficiency
☐ Age greater than 65 years

Numerical score from Worksheet 2 [ ] B

Total PG-SGA score
(Total numerical score of A+B+C+D above)

Global PG-SGA rating (A, B, or C) = [ ]
(See triage recommendations below)

Worksheet 5—PG-SGA Global Assessment Categories

Category	Stage A	Stage B	Stage C
Weight	Well nourished OR No loss OR Recent wt gain	Moderately malnourished >5% wt loss in 1 month (or 10% in 6 mos) OR Progressive wt loss	Severely malnourished >5% wt loss in 1 month OR >10% in 6 mos) OR Progressive wt loss
Nutrient intake	No deficit OR Significant recent improvement	Definite decrease in intake	Severe deficit in intake
Nutrition Impact Symptoms	None OR Significant recent improvement allowing adequate intake	Presence of nutrition impact symptoms (PG-SGA Box 3)	Presence of nutrition impact symptoms (PG-SGA Box 3)
Functioning	No deficit OR Recent improvement	Moderate functional deficit OR Recent deterioration	Severe functional deficit OR Recent significant deterioration
Physical Exam	No deficit OR Chronic deficit but recent improvement	Evidence of mild to moderate loss of muscle mass/SQ fat / muscle tone on palpation	Obvious signs of malnutrition (eg, severe loss muscle, SQ tissue, possible edema)

Nutritional Triage Recommendations: Additive score is used to define specific nutritional interventions including patient & family education, symptom management including pharmacologic intervention, and appropriate nutrient intervention (food, nutritional supplements, enteral, or parenteral triage). *First line nutrition intervention includes optimal symptom management.*

Triage based on PG-SGA point score
0–1 No intervention required at this time. Re-assessment on routine and regular basis during treatment.
2–3 Patient & family education by dietitian, nurse, or other clinician with pharmacologic intervention as indicated by symptom survey (Box 3) and lab values as appropriate.
4–8 Requires intervention by dietitian, in conjunction with nurse or physician as indicated by symptoms (Box 3).
≥9 Indicates a critical need for improved symptom management and/or nutrient intervention options.

Clinician Signature _____ RD RN PA MD DO Other _____ Date _____

Figure 2.1 *Patient-Generated Subjective Global Assessment (PG-SGA) continued*

demand, presence of disease and its relationship to nutrition requirements, and elements of the physical examination. The numeric score generated from this information can be used as part of a triage system to determine need for nutrition intervention. The PG-SGA scoring has been found to correlate with readmission within 30 days and mortality in a group of cancer patients.[22] The pros and cons of the PG-SGA are summarized in Table 2.6.

The Mini Nutritional Assessment (MNA; Nestlé Nutrition, Vevey, Switzerland) has been developed to screen and assess for malnutrition in the elderly. This 18-item tool is divided into two sections: screening and assessment.[18] The screening segment contains 6 questions related to food intake, weight loss, mobility, stress, and body mass index.[18] The 12-item assessment focuses on specific medical history and eating habits as well as anthropometric measurements.[18] A total score of less than 17 points indicates malnutrition, whereas a score of 17 to 23.5 indicates risk of malnutrition.[18] There are no intervention guidelines associated with the MNA.

Advantages of the MNA include its inclusion of multiple parameters and established validity in the elderly population. Additionally, the MNA is quick and easy to use. However, this specific tool has not been validated for use in the oncology population.

Nutritional status can quickly deteriorate because of illness and decreased dietary intake. Given that nutritional well-being plays an important role in treatment and recovery from cancer, early screening and intervention for nutritional problems are imperative in the care of patients with cancer.

Table 2.6   *Pros and Cons of the Scored PG-SGA*

Pros	*Cons*
• Allows patient/family participation • Streamlines data collection • Provides a more complete list of nutrition-related symptoms • Parameters are weighted/scored based on nutrition impact • Easier to use; tables and worksheets included on reverse of form • Identifies treatable nutrition-related symptoms • Score can be used to track outcomes • Validated in the oncology setting	• Professional resistance to performing the physical exam • Triage guidelines included • Perception of additional workload • Patients may resist completing more "paperwork" • Patient-generated section relies on patient literacy

Source: Elliott L, Molseed L, McCallum PD, Grant B. *The Clinical Guide to Oncology Nutrition.* 2nd ed. Chicago, IL: American Dietetic Association; 2006:44–53.

Additional Tools

Additional tools used to assess nutritional status include the Activities of Daily Living (ADL) tool, PedsQL Measurement Model, and Karnofsky scores. The ADL assesses routine activities (e.g., eating, bathing, dressing, toileting, walking, continence) that people generally do every day without assistance.[33] It is important to assess the patient's ability to perform ADLs to determine which type of long-term care facility (e.g., nursing home, home care) and coverage (e.g., Medicare, Medicaid, or long-term care insurance) may be needed.[33]

The PedsQL Measurement Model measures health-related quality of life (HRQOL) in healthy children and adolescents as well as in those with acute and chronic health conditions. It integrates generic core scales and disease-specific modules into a single measurement system.[33]

The Karnofsky scores are a subjective measurement used to quantify cancer patients' general well-being. This assessment tool is useful over time, as sequential measurements may be help track the disease process. Scores run from 100 to 0, where 100 indicates good health and 0 equals death.

- 100: normal activity, no complaints or signs of disease
- 90: normal activity, minor symptoms or signs of disease
- 80: normal activity with some effort, some symptoms or signs of disease
- 70: cares for self, not capable of normal activity or work
- 60: requires some help, but capable of handling most personal needs
- 50: requires help and medical care often
- 40: disabled; requires special care and help
- 30: severely disabled; hospitalization indicated but no risk of death
- 20: very ill; requiring admission, supportive measures, or treatment
- 10: moribund; fatal disease process progressing fast
- 0: dead

SUMMARY

There are no studies that directly link the nutrition screening process to improved outcomes in oncology patients, but there is a clear link between screening and identification of nutritional risk.[18] There is also evidence of improved outcomes in severely malnourished patients with nutrition support; therefore, one can draw the conclusion that effective screening and early identification of nutrition risk can affect outcomes.[18]

There are also no data explicitly linking nutrition assessment to outcomes.[18] Nevertheless, nutrition assessment is crucial to designing optimal nutrition intervention to help improve outcomes.

REFERENCES

1. DeWys WD, Begg C, Lavin PT, et al. Prognostic effect of weight loss prior to chemotherapy in cancer patients. *Am J Med*. 1980;69:491–497.
2. Hickman DM, Miller RA, Rombeau JL, Twomey PL, Frey CF. Serum albumin and body weight as predictors of postoperative course in colorectal cancer. *J Parenter Enteral Nutr*. 1980;4(3):314–316.
3. Daly JM, Dudrick SJ, Copeland EM. Evaluation of nutritional indices as prognostic indicators in the cancer patient. *Cancer*. 1979;43:925–931.
4. Stanley KE. Prognostic factors for survival in patients with inoperable lung cancer. *J Natl Cancer Inst*. 1980;65:25.
5. Veterans Affairs Total Parenteral Nutrition Cooperative Study Group. Perioperative total parenteral nutrition in surgical patients. *N Engl J Med*. 1991;325(8):525–532.
6. Van Den Berghe G, Wouters P, Weekers F, et al. Intensive insulin therapy in critically ill patients. *N Engl J Med*. 2001;345(19):1359–1367.
7. Kondrup J, Allison SP, Elia M, Vellas B, Plauth M. ESPEN guidelines for nutrition screening. *Clin Nutr*. 2003;22(4):415–421.
8. American Dietetic Association. *International Dietetics and Nutrition Terminology (IDNT) Reference Manual: Standardized Language for the Nutrition Care Process*. Chicago, IL: Author; 2007.
9. Lacey K, Pritchett E. Nutrition care process and model: ADA adopts road map to quality care and outcomes management. *J Am Diet Assoc*. 2003;103(8):1061–1072.
10. Nelms M, Sucher K, Long S. *Nutrition Therapy and Pathophysiology*. Belmont, CA: Thomson Higher Learning; 2007:101–135, 751–783.
11. Khalid U, Spiro A, Baldwin C, et al. Symptoms and weight loss in patients with gastrointestinal and lung cancer at presentation. *Support Care Cancer*. 2007;15:39–46.
12. Hamilton W, Peters TJ, Round A, Sharp D. What are the clinical features of lung cancer before the diagnosis is made? A population based case-control study. *Thorax*. 2005;60(12):1059–1065.
13. Reeves MR, Battistutta D, Capra S, Bauer J, Davies PSW. Resting energy expenditure in patients with solid tumors undergoing anticancer therapy. *Nutrition*. 2006;22(6):609–615.
14. Johnson G, Sallé A, Lorimier G, et al. Cancer cachexia: Measured and predicted resting energy expenditures for nutritional needs evaluation. *Nutrition*. 2008;24: 443–450.
15. Bosaeus I, Daneryd P, Lundholm K. Dietary intake, resting energy expenditure, weight loss and survival in cancer patients. *J Nutr*. 2002;132(suppl 11):3465S–3466S.
16. Knox LS, Crosby LO, Feurer ID. Energy expenditure in malnourished cancer patients. *Ann Surg*. 1983;197:152–162.
17. Harvie MN, Howell A, Thatcher N, Balidam A, Campbell I. Energy balance in patients with advanced NSCLC, metastatic melanoma and metastatic breast cancer receiving chemotherapy: A longitudinal study. *Br J Cancer*. 2005;92:673–680.
18. Huhmann MB, August DA. Review of American Society for Parenteral and Enteral Nutrition (A.S.P.E.N.) clinical guidelines for nutrition support in cancer patients: Nutrition screening and assessment. *Nutr Clin Pract*. 2008;23:182–188.
19. Gottschlich MM, ed. *The A.S.P.E.N. Nutrition Support Core Curriculum: A Case-Based Approach—The Adult Patient*. Silver Spring, MD: American Society for Parenteral and Enteral Nutrition; 2007:649–675.
20. National Cancer Institute. Effect of cancer treatment on nutrition. http://www .cancer.gov. Accessed May 25, 2005.

21. Barton AD, Beigg CL, Macdonald IA, Allison SP. High food wastage and low nutritional intakes in hospital patients. *Clin Nutr*. 2000;19(6):445–449.

22. Bos C, Benamouzig R, Bruhat A, et al. Nutritional status after short-term dietary supplementation in hospitalized malnourished geriatric patients. *Clin Nutr*. 2001; 20(3):225–233.

23. Fearon KCH, Moses AGW. Cancer cachexia. *Intl J Cardiol*. 2002;85(1):73–81.

24. Gosney M. Are we wasting our money on food supplements in elder care wards? *J Adv Nursing*. 2003;43(3):275–280.

25. Incalzi RA, Gemma A, Capparella O, Cipriani L, Landi F, Carbonin P. Energy intake and in-hospital starvation: A clinically relevant relationship. *Arch Int Med*. 1996;156(4):425–429.

26. Ravasco P, Monteiro-Grillo I, Camilo ME. How relevant are cytokines in colorectal cancer wasting? *Cancer J*. 2007;13(6):392–398.

27. Casati A, Muttini S, Leggieri C, Colombo E, Torri GG. Rapid turnover proteins in critically ill ICU patients: Negative acute phase proteins or nutritional indicators? *Minerva Anesthesiol*. 1998;64(7–8):345–350.

28. Charney P, Malone A. *ADA Pocket Guide to Nutrition Assessment*. Chicago, IL: American Dietetic Association, 2004:23–41.

29. Bloomfield R, Steel E, MacLennan G, Noble DW. Accuracy of weight and height estimation in an intensive care unit: Implications for clinical practice and research. *Crit Care Med*. 2006;34(8):2153–2157.

30. Ferguson M, Capra S, Bauer J, Banks M. Development of a valid and reliable malnutrition screening tool for adult acute hospital patients. *Nutrition*. 1999;15(6):458–464.

31. Ferguson ML. *Determination of the impact of nutrition screening and support on outcomes in adult acute hospital inpatients with malnutrition*. Brisbane, Australia: Center for Public Health Research, Queensland University of Technology; 1998.

32. Baker JP, Detksy AS, Wesson DE, et al. Nutritional assessment: A comparison of clinical judgment and objective measurements. *N Engl J Med*. 1982;306(16):969–972.

33. Elliott L, Molseed L, McCallum PD, Grant B. *The Clinical Guide to Oncology Nutrition*. 2nd ed. Chicago, IL: American Dietetic Association; 2006:44–53.

Chapter 3

Nutrition Support for Oncology Patients

M. Patricia Fuhrman, MS, RD, LD, FADA, CNSD

INTRODUCTION

Cancer is becoming a chronic disease. As a result, treatments for cancer—and especially chemotherapy and radiation therapy—can have both short-term and long-term adverse effects on body systems, such as the gastrointestinal (GI) tract. Nutrition support is adjunctive therapy, rather than curative therapy, for oncology patients. The debate about if and when to initiate nutrition support revolves around the GI tract function, the prognosis of the patient, the experiences of healthcare providers, and the wishes of the patient and family. Patient autonomy should always be the decisive factor when determining the extent of providing nutrition and hydration.[1]

The American Dietetic Association's (ADA) Evidence Analysis Library (EAL) oncology guidelines recommend medical nutrition therapy with individualized nutrition assessment, prescription, and counseling as the first line of nutrition intervention[2] for patients diagnosed with cancer. It is well accepted that nutrition support should not be used routinely in cancer patients, but rather should be reserved for those patients who are unable to meet their nutrient needs orally.[2–4] The provision of home nutrition support in terminally ill cancer patients who are not undergoing active therapy should be limited to those patients who have good functional status with a life expectancy greater than 40 days and supportive caregivers.[4]

Enteral Nutrition

Indications for Enteral Nutrition

Enteral nutrition (EN) is indicated when a patient cannot meet nutrient needs through oral diet and the GI tract is functional. Table 3.1 lists the indications, benefits, contraindications and burdens of enteral and parenteral nutrition.[3, 5, 6]

45

Table 3.1   *Comparison of Enteral and Parenteral Nutrition in Oncology Patients*

	Enteral Nutrition	**Parenteral Nutrition**
Indications	• Functional GI tract • Patient unable to meet needs through oral diet	• GI tract dysfunctional • Patient unable to meet needs through oral diet and/or tube feeding • Severe esophagitis, enteritis, vomiting, and diarrhea • Bowel obstruction • Short bowel syndrome • Severe pancreatitis • Paralytic ileus • GVHD
Benefits	• Less costly • Less invasive • Fewer infectious complications	• Source of nutrition for those unable to meet needs enterally
Contraindications	• GI obstruction • Peritonitis • GI bleeding • Intractable vomiting/ diarrhea • Hemodynamic instability • Inadequate GI perfusion • High-output fistula • Thrombocytopenia • Severe mucositis, esophagitis, rhinitis • Aggressive nutrition support not warranted or desired by patient/family	• Functional GI tract • No IV access • Aggressive nutrition support not warranted or desired by patient/family
Burdens	• Obtaining and maintaining enteral access • GI complications of diarrhea, reflux, vomiting, nausea	• Infectious complications • Cost

GI = gastrointestinal; IV = intravenous; GVHD = graft-versus-host disease.
Sources: A.S.P.E.N. Board of Directors and Clinical Guidelines Task Force. Guidelines for the use of parenteral and enteral nutrition in adult and pediatric patients. *JPEN J Parenter Enteral Nutr.* 2002;26(suppl 1):82SA–85SA; DeChicco RS, Steiger E. Parenteral nutrition in medical or surgical oncology. In: Elliott L, Molseed LL, McCallum PD, eds., *The Clinical Guide to Oncology Nutrition.* 2nd ed. Chicago, IL: American Dietetic Association; 2006:156–164; Robinson CA. Enteral nutrition in adult oncology. In: Elliott L, Molseed LL, McCallum PD, eds., *The Clinical Guide to Oncology Nutrition.* 2nd ed. Chicago, IL: American Dietetic Association; 2006:138–155.

Benefits of Enteral Nutrition

The patients with cancer who appear to benefit the most from enteral nutrition are those with head and neck cancer, esophageal cancer, gastric cancer, and pancreatic cancer.[6] Feeding tube placement should be distal to the tumor and/or surgical site.[6] The ADA EAL states that EN can successfully maintain weight by increasing energy and protein intake in patients with esophageal cancer undergoing chemoradiation and in patients with stage III or IV head and neck cancer receiving intensive radiation therapy.[2] Providing EN and maintaining nutritional status during radiation therapy for head and neck cancer may improve the patient's ability to tolerate the therapy, thereby promoting a better outcome.[2]

Zogbaum et al.[7] retrospectively reviewed 125 cases of head and neck cancer treated with radiation therapy. Seventeen patients who received tube feedings were matched with 17 controls who were not tube-fed. The tube-feeding group missed fewer days of radiation therapy (2.3 days ± 6.6 SD versus 5.5 days ± 4.0 SD; $p < 0.1$) and had less weight loss as measured by BMI (20.64 ± 4.2 to 20.18 ± 4.01 versus 24.32 ± 5.62 to 22.78 ± 5.51; $p = .54$) than the control group. However, enteral nutrition in patients with esophageal cancer has not been shown to improve tolerance to therapy or increase survival.[2]

Enteral nutrition is less expensive than parenteral nutrition and is associated with fewer infectious complications.[8] Its utilization of the GI tract may be one of the major advantages of enteral nutrition in preventing infectious complications, as the GI tract is a major contributor to immunocompetence.

Enteral Nutrition Challenges

Enteral feeding may be problematic in some patients owing to the effects of their tumors and/or the antineoplastic therapies employed. Thrombocytopenia increases the risk of bleeding during tube placement and management. Platelet levels should be greater than 50,000 units/liter and the absolute neutrophil count greater than 1,000 cm² before a feeding tube is placed either endoscopically or surgically.[9]

GI intolerance induced by chemotherapy and radiation therapy can inhibit oral intake and jeopardize tube-feeding success. Patients with mucositis, nausea, vomiting, and diarrhea may tolerate jejunal feedings better than gastric feedings.[3] Feeding tube placement (nasal/orally placed tubes) may be more difficult in patients whose anatomy has been altered as a result of head and neck resection.[10]

Contraindications to Enteral Nutrition

Contraindications to enteral nutrition in oncology patients are similar to those in patients with other diseases and metabolic disorders. Specific contraindications include intestinal obstruction, peritonitis, GI bleeding, intractable vomiting or diarrhea, hemodynamic instability, inadequate GI perfusion, high-output fistulas, and the patient's or family's preference not to pursue enteral feeding.[6] If nutrient and energy needs cannot be met through utilization of the GI tract, a combination of enteral and parenteral nutrition may be required.

Burdens of Enteral Nutrition

Obtaining and maintaining enteral feeding access can be a burden for some patients. If a feeding tube has to be inserted repeatedly, the amount of feeding provided and the patient's comfort are diminished. Burdens of enteral nutrition include adverse effects such as diarrhea, reflux, nausea, and vomiting, which can sometimes outweigh the benefit of using the GI tract for feeding. The emotional burden of stool incontinence and the risk for wound infections in the patient with severe diarrhea can also necessitate discontinuation of enteral feeding. Uncontrolled nausea may negatively impact quality of life for the patient as well.

Enteral Nutrition Access

The least invasive type of enteral access is a nasoenteric feeding tube. Nasoenteric feeding tubes are generally recommended when enteral feedings are required for less than 4 weeks. Such tubes can be placed in several locations, including the stomach, duodenum, or jejunum. When enteral access is required for a longer period of time, the enteral access is typically more permanent, with an ostomy being created, such as a gastrostomy, jejunostomy, percutaneous endoscopic gastrostomy (PEG), percutaneous endoscopic jejunostomy (PEJ), or percutaneous endoscopic gastro-jejunostomy (PEGJ).

Tube type and placement will depend on the location of the cancer and the ability to place the feeding tube distal to the cancer and/or surgical intervention site. Patients with head and neck cancer generally tolerate enteral feedings into the stomach or jejunum; those with esophageal cancer usually have feedings into the stomach or duodenum; those with gastric cancer have feedings into the jejunum; and those with pancreatic cancer have feedings into the jejunum.[6] In any event, each patient must be evaluated individually to determine the optimal enteral feeding access.

Enteral Feeding Formulas

The selection of an enteral nutrition formula depends on the presence of comorbidities, organ function, fluid tolerance, and GI function as well as the length of time for which feedings may be required. In general, it is best to use the most intact enteral formula that meets the patient's nutrient needs and tolerance. The concentration of the formula (measured in kilocalories per milliliter [kcal/mL]) depends on the patient's fluid status and volume tolerance. There is little support in the literature for the use of disease-specific formulas.[11] The use of elemental or semi-elemental formulas should be reserved for those patients with impaired GI digestion and absorption. The addition of modular components to an enteral formula should be avoided because of the risk of formula contamination.

The use of arginine, vitamin E, or antioxidant supplements for patients with breast or oropharyngeal cancers is currently not recommended; consumption of antioxidant vitamins in excess of the upper tolerable limit is also not recommended for patients with lung cancer.[2] Specialty enteral formulas designed for oncology patients contain immuno-enhancing nutrients. Oral consumption of 2 g of eicosapentaenoic acid (EPA) and 1 g of docosahexanoic acid (DHA) per day, for example, has been associated with weight gain in patients with tumor-induced cancer cachexia.[12, 13] In vitro, animal, and epidemiologic studies suggest that EPA may augment the effects of chemotherapeutic agents, and that the ratio of omega-3 (Ω-3) inserted to omega-6 (Ω-6) fatty acids may influence the risk and progression of breast, colon, and prostate cancers.[14] Studies examining the effect of an immuno-enhancing tube feeding formula have yielded inconsistent results when the solutions were provided to patients with gastric cancer.[11] Prospective clinical trials are still needed to determine the role of Ω-3 fatty acids and other immuno-enhancing nutrients in the prevention and treatment of cancer and cancer cachexia.[2, 14] It appears that the use of immuno-enhancing enteral formulas and supplements is not warranted and could even be potentially harmful in this patient population.[4]

Enteral formulas can be administered into the stomach as either a bolus, an intermittent infusion, or a continuous infusion. Small bowel feedings should be continuous. Continuous feeds can be infused over 24 hours or cycled over a shorter time frame depending on patient lifestyle and tolerance.

Complications of Enteral Nutrition

Enteral nutrition is associated with GI, metabolic, septic, and mechanical complications. Nutrition assessment focused on the patient's risk factors related to complications and routine monitoring for potential complications can reduce the incidence and adverse outcomes of complications that do occur.

Potential GI complications include diarrhea, regurgitation, and constipation. Multiple factors contribute to diarrhea, and each must be evaluated separately to determine which treatment should be employed.[15] Diarrhea is often the result of medications. Infection with *Clostridium difficile* is a frequent cause of diarrhea in patients who are treated with antibiotics.

Enteric pathogens should be identified and treated before initiating antidiarrheals to avoid toxic megacolon.[16] Chemotherapeutic drugs and radiation therapy can also result in rapid GI transit. A patient with an impaction could be oozing stool around the impaction.[16] During the process of determining the etiology of the diarrhea, it is important to maintain hydration and electrolyte levels.[15] Fiber-containing formulas may also assist with the management of both diarrhea and constipation. Formulas containing soluble fiber, for example, can help with GI motility as well as provide a source of fuel for the colonocytes with short-chained fatty acids (SFCA).[11]

Regurgitation and subsequent aspiration are always a concern with enteral feeding. To date, no evidence has been gathered that correlates a certain level of gastric residual volume with higher risk of aspiration.[17, 18] Greater than 250 mL of gastric residual volume (GRV) on two consecutive occasions should be investigated for potential problems with poor gastric emptying, however.[19] Elevating the head of the bed 30 to 45 degrees is the only evidence-based recommendation for preventing reflux and the risk of aspiration.[19]

Metabolic complications include refeeding syndrome and dehydration. Patients at the greatest risk of developing refeeding syndrome are those who have had inadequate intake for more than 7 to 10 days and who have lost a significant amount of weight.[6] Starting at a low rate of 20 to 30 mL/h and increasing the amount of the feeding gradually to the infusion goal enables the clinician to monitor the metabolic response and correct any glycemic and electrolyte abnormalities as they occur. For patients with diabetes and glucose intolerance, it is recommended to avoid overfeeding and administer insulin as needed.[11]

A comprehensive nutrition assessment should also include the fluid requirements for all patients to assure adequate fluid intake, to reduce the risk of constipation, and to replace fluids lost, such as from diarrhea or vomiting. Overhydration must also be avoided, especially in patients with renal failure, liver failure, or congestive heart failure. Inadequate fluid intake can contribute to hypernatremia and pre-renal azotemia. Thirst cannot be counted on as a reliable indicator of whether more fluid is needed in elderly individuals and in patients who are unable to communicate. Instead, fluid needs should be estimated using any of several available mathematical formulas, and hydration status then routinely reevaluated based on clinical monitoring.

Mechanical complications may arise related to the feeding tube and equipment used to infuse the formula. Nasoenteric complications include inflammation of the nasal cavity and sinusitis. Sites where gastrostomy, jejunostomy, PEG, PEJ, and PEGJ tubes are placed can become tender and red. Excoriation and infection can also occur. The size of the tube may need to be changed as the patient gains or loses weight or, in the case of children, with growth.

It is imperative to flush the tube routinely with water to maintain patency. Minimal flushes should consist of 20 mL water every 4 hours with a continuous infusion, before and after intermittent and bolus infusions, and before and after medications are delivered.[3] It may be prudent to flush the feeding tube and dilute fluids through the feeding tube with sterile water or saline, particularly in immunocompromised patients and in patients for whom there is concern about the safety of the water supply. Medications should be compatible with feeding tube administration and location of the feeding tube tip.

Home Enteral Nutrition Support

Patients who go home on enteral nutrition should be thoroughly evaluated for appropriateness of the enteral formula, feeding access, and capability of the patient and/or caregiver(s) to manage the therapy. It is imperative to teach patients how to prepare formula and manage their feeding access properly so that they know how to avoid the risk of contamination. A study by Thompson et al. examined the coping skills of patients receiving home enteral nutrition.[20] In this study, patients who were successful at coping with the nutrition system accepted personal responsibility for life's conditions, took charge of their own well-being, sought and accepted support from others, optimized their independence, and focused on the positive aspects of their lives. Given these considerations, the authors remind clinicians to work with their home enteral nutrition patients to facilitate these coping skills.

Parenteral Nutrition

Indications for Parenteral Nutrition

Parenteral nutrition (PN) should be reserved for patients who are unable to tolerate any or sufficient nutrient needs through the GI tract. Indications for PN may include severe esophagitis, enteritis, vomiting, and diarrhea, as well as bowel obstruction and short bowel syndrome. Other indications may include severe pancreatitis, paralytic ileus, and graft-versus-host disease (GVHD) involving the GI tract.[5] PN should not be used unless there is an impediment to oral intake of nutrients and/or digestion or absorption of nutrients after consumption. The ADA EAL states that routine use of PN is not recommended for patients with esophageal cancer who are receiving chemoradiation therapy (CRT).[2] To reiterate, PN should be reserved for only those patients who are unable to meet their nutritional needs through the GI tract.

Benefits of Parenteral Nutrition

Parenteral nutrition is a life-saving therapy for patients who are unable to tolerate enteral nutrition. The goal of providing parenteral nutrition is to meet nutrient needs until the patient can resume oral intake or tube feeding. Some patients will remain dependent on parenteral nutrition for the rest of their lives. Careful management can reduce the risk of complications during both short-term and long-term therapy.

Contraindications to Parenteral Nutrition

If the gut works adequately to meet the patient's nutritional needs, parenteral nutrition should not be used. Likewise, PN may be contraindicated when the patient has no intravenous (IV) access. It may also be inappropriate to start or to continue PN when aggressive nutrition support is not warranted or if it is not desired by the patient and his or her family. Communication between the patient, family, and clinicians is necessary to determine the goals of feeding and to clarify the expectations for nutrition support.[21]

Burdens of Parenteral Nutrition

PN is not indicated when the burdens of providing PN outweigh the benefits—for example, when the patient's prognosis is extremely poor. Although PN is not a curative therapy for oncology patients, it can help sustain them nutritionally during curative and palliative therapy when they cannot meet their nutrient needs via the GI tract. As the end of life approaches, the patient and family must evaluate the burdens and benefits of this nutritional therapy. Laboratory monitoring, preparation and infusion issues, and risk of infection from the IV catheter must all be considered. If the patient is seeking hospice care, it may not be possible to continue PN after hospice admission.[21]

Access for Parenteral Nutrition

Central IV access is required for PN. Like enteral access, parenteral access can be either temporary or permanent. Temporary access involves a direct puncture into a central vein, such as the internal jugular, subclavian, or femoral vein. Permanent central access is achieved either through a tunneled catheter, an indwelling port, or a peripherally inserted central catheter (PICC).

Peripheral parenteral nutrition (PPN) does not require access to a central vein but rather is delivered through the small veins in the hand and distal arm or via a peripherally inserted catheter (PIC). The tip of a PIC is generally placed in a deep peripheral vein. This means of access should not be confused with a PICC, which has its tip in the superior vena cava or right atrium. PPN is generally not used because of the volume required to dilute the formula for peripheral infusion and its large lipid load for adequate energy. For best tolerance, the osmolality should be less than 600 to 900 mOsm/L.[22]

Parenteral Nutrition Components and Formulations

Parenteral formulations can contain dextrose, lipids, amino acids, multivitamins, trace elements, electrolytes, water, and compatible medications (Table 3.2). These components may be combined in one bag, referred to as a total nutrient admixture or 3-in-1, or lipids can be infused separately in conjunction with a 2-in-1 (dextrose and amino acids along with micronutrients and medications).

Macronutrients include dextrose, lipids, and amino acids. A minimum of 100 to 150 g/day dextrose is appropriate, with an upper limit of 4 mg/kg/min in the critically ill patient and an upper limit of 7 mg/kg/min in the stable patient.[23] Lipids provide an additional source of energy that can help reduce the dextrose load. Intravenous delivery of lipids limited to 0.11 g/kg/h has not been associated with adverse effects.[24] Minimizing the lipid amount to approximately 1 g/kg or less than 30% of the individual's total kilocalories per day has not been associated with complications.[23, 25] Although no consensus has been reached regarding how much lipids should be given, it is prudent to limit the amount provided to avoid potential complications. If a patient does not receive lipids for greater than 2 weeks, a minimum of 10% of the total caloric provision from lipids should be administered to prevent essential fatty acid deficiency (EFAD).[5]

Micronutrients include vitamins, trace elements, and electrolytes. Vitamins and trace elements should be added to the PN solution on a daily basis.[26] If the patient is on anticoagulation therapy, it is important to be aware of the vitamin K content of the multivitamin preparation and to adjust the anticoagulation therapy accordingly. Multivitamin preparations are available without vitamin K, though these solutions should not be used routinely. By contrast, trace element preparations containing zinc, chromium, copper, manganese, and selenium are recommended for routine use.[27] Copper and

Table 3.2   *Standard PN Composition of PN Solution for Adults*

Component	Recommendations
Amino acids	10–20% total estimated or measured energy needs Adjust based on organ function and metabolic stress
Dextrose	Consider all sources of dextrose (IVF, medications) Initiate with 100–200 g/day 4 mg/kg/min maximum in critically ill 7 mg/kg/min maximum in stable patients Maintain normal glucose levels
Lipids	Include propofol infusion in lipid sources Lipid should be less than 1 g/kg or 20–30% of total kilocalories Limit lipids with serum TG levels > 400 mg/dL
Fluid	Volume depends on patient tolerance/requirements

Electrolytes

Amounts depend on patient tolerance. Higher requirements may occur with refeeding syndrome and GI losses; decreased requirements occur with organ failure.

Sodium	1–2 mEq/kg
Potassium	1–2 mEq/kg
Phosphorus	20–40 mMol/day
Calcium	10–15 mEq/day
Magnesium	8–20 mEq/day
Chloride and acetate	Proportions vary depending on acid–base status

Vitamins

A	3,300 IU
D	200 IU
E	10 IU
K*	150 mcg
Thiamin	6 mg
Riboflavin	3.6 mg
Niacin	40 mg
Pyridoxine	6 mg
Cyanocobalamin	5 mcg
Folacin	600 mcg

(continues)

Table 3.2 *Standard PN Composition of PN Solution for Adults*, Continued

Component	Recommendations
Pantothenic acid	15 mg
Biotin	60 mcg
Ascorbic acid	200 mg
Trace Elements	
Increased needs may occur with large GI losses.	
Zinc	2.5–5 mg
Copper	0.3–0.5 mg
Chromium	10–15 mg
Manganese	20–100 mcg
Selenium	40–120 mcg
Medications	
Check with the pharmacist to verify compatibility and doses based on patient's comorbidities and metabolic needs.	

*Multivitamin preparation available without vitamin K.
GI = gastrointestinal; IVF = intravenous fluids; TG = triglyceride.
Sources: A.S.P.E.N. Board of Directors and Clinical Guidelines Task Force. Guidelines for the use of parenteral and enteral nutrition in adult and pediatric patients. *JPEN J Parenter Enteral Nutr.* 2002;26(suppl 1):82SA–85SA; Sacks GS, Mayhew S, Johnson D. Parenteral nutrition implementation and management. In: Merritt R, ed. *The A.S.P.E.N. Nutrition Support Practice Manual.* 2nd ed. Silver Spring, MD: American Society for Parenteral and Enteral Nutrition; 2005:108–117; Lenssen P, Bruemmer BA, Bowden RA, Gooley T, Aker SN, Mattson D. Intravenous lipid dose and incidence of bacteremia and fungemia in patients undergoing bone marrow transplantation. *Am J Clin Nutr.* 1998;67:927–933; McMahon MM. Management of parenteral nutrition in acutely ill patients with hyperglycemia. *Nutr Clin Pract.* 2004;19:120–128; Lipkin AC, Lessen P, Dickson BJ. Nutrition issues in hematopoietic stem cell transplantation: State of the art. *Nutr Clin Pract.* 2005;20:423–439.

manganese may be omitted when a patient develops hyperbilirubinemia. In such a case, the patient should be monitored closely because copper deficiencies can lead to pancytopenia over time.[28] Electrolytes are added daily in amounts based on laboratory values and the patient's current condition. GI and urinary losses as well as organ function should be considered in determining electrolyte content of the PN.[5] Although electrolytes are listed as individual minerals, they are added to the PN as salts; for example, sodium can be provided as sodium chloride, sodium acetate, and sodium phosphate.

Water can be added to the PN solution for patients who need additional fluid and to dilute a peripheral solution to achieve the osmolality compatible with this route of infusion. It may also be necessary to concentrate the PN formula by using the most concentrated source of dextrose (70%), lipids (30%), and amino acids (20%). In any event, fluid status and sources of other IV fluids should be regularly assessed with PN administration.

Medications commonly added to PN include regular insulin, heparin, and famotidine.[5] It is not recommended to use PN as a drug delivery method. Always confirm drug and PN compatibility with the pharmacist.

Infusion of parenteral nutrition can be either continuous or cycled. Most infusions begin as continuous and then are converted to a cycle schedule as indicated by patient activities or in anticipation of discharge home on PN. When cycling PN, it is recommended to taper the infusion for 1 to 2 hours when starting and stopping the infusion. Some debate has arisen over whether it is necessary to taper PN infusions before stopping the infusion,[29, 30] but the potential risk of rebound hypoglycemia can be avoided by tapering.

Complications of Parenteral Nutrition

Concern about the potential complications associated with PN often prompts clinicians to use it only as a last resort. As a result, they sometimes wait past the point when maximum benefit could be realized before initiating this type of nutritional therapy. Careful management and monitoring, however, can reduce the risk of complications.

Metabolic Complications

Ensuring glycemic control in which blood sugars remain within normal levels improves outcomes in critically ill patients.[31] Glucose levels of 80 to 120 mg/dL in critically ill patients and 100 to 150 mg/dL in non-critically ill patients have been recommended.[32] Initiating PN with 150 to 200 g dextrose can enable the clinician to monitor glycemic response and maintain glucose levels within acceptable ranges. When blood glucose levels are within an acceptable range, the PN dextrose content can be increased.

A general rule of thumb for adding insulin to PN in patients with a history of diabetes or insulin resistance or currently with hyperglycemia is to provide 0.1 unit of regular insulin for each 1 g of dextrose.[32] Additional insulin needs can be covered by using an insulin sliding scale. A portion (generally one half or two thirds) or all of the amount of sliding-scale insulin required during a 24-hour period can be added to the next bag of PN.

Hypoglycemia can occur with abrupt disruption of PN or overzealous addition of insulin to PN. If PN is abruptly interrupted, a 10% dextrose solution should be given for an hour. Hypoglycemia can also be treated with oral carbohydrate or by giving an ampule of 50% dextrose intravenously. A PN bag that contains more insulin than necessary and that results in hypo-glycemia should be discontinued.[5]

Refeeding syndrome occurs more often with PN than EN because PN is often started at the goal rate rather than implementing a gradual increase in the infusion rate over a few days, as happens with EN. In patients at risk, it is prudent to start PN with 150 to 200 mg/day of dextrose and to monitor glucose levels as well as potassium, phosphorus, and magnesium. Correct the patient's serum glucose and replace electrolytes before increasing the dextrose content.[5]

For patients on long-term home PN, there is a valid concern about PN-associated liver disease. In one study, a reduction in severe liver dysfunction in home parenteral nutrition patients was seen with a modest provision of kilocalories (approximately 25 kcal/kg), generous protein (approximately 1.45 g/kg), and a lipid infusion rate of 0.28 g/kg per day.[33] Note, however, that this study involved a heterogeneous group of patients requiring home PN; only a small percentage had an underlying diagnosis of cancer.

Infectious Complications

Poor glycemic control contributes to both mortality and morbidity (including infectious complications) in critically ill patients receiving PN.[19, 31] Glycemic control should be maintained to reduce the risk of infection in immunosuppressed oncology patients. Using sterile technique in catheter placement and catheter care can also reduce the risk of infectious complications.

Lipids containing Ω-6 fatty acids can affect the reticuloendothelial system adversely when they are given in large doses over short periods of time.[34] When given judiciously—for example, as 30% of total kilocalories or less—no adverse effects from providing lipids have been noted.[25]

Gastrointestinal Complications

Gastrointestinal complications of PN result from the lack of GI stimulation when the GI tract cannot be utilized. These complications can include GI atrophy, bacterial overgrowth, and bacterial translocation. Liver disease and metabolic bone disease are also associated with PN. Prevention and management of these complications includes using the GI tract as much as feasible, even if trickle feeds are all that the patient can tolerate. To date, researchers have not determined the amount of enteral stimulation required to maintain GI integrity. Other recommendations are to avoid overfeeding, control hyperglycemia, and provide micronutrients daily.

Special Considerations for Nutrition Support

Cancer Cachexia

The symptoms of cancer cachexia are the essence of malnutrition: anorexia, fatigue, inadequate nutrient and energy intake, weight loss, and wasting of muscle and fat mass. Current theories regarding the etiology of cancer cachexia center on the effects of a cytokine cascade and hormones on metabolism.[4, 35] As yet, the specific mediators have not been defined, making it problematic to determine the optimal therapeutic approach for treatment.[36] Cancer cachexia is not reversed with adequate nutrient intake. Interventions should treat the symptoms of anorexia, nausea, vomiting, and mucous membrane inflammation.[4, 35] Alternative therapies such as acupuncture, guided imagery, hypnosis, and music therapy have also been used to stimulate appetite.[35] Unfortunately, effective therapy is complex because the etiology of symptoms is multifactorial.

Hematopoietic Cell Transplantation

PN was historically part of the standard of care for patients undergoing a bone marrow transplant. However, the combination of autologous transplants, new medications, peripheral stem cell harvesting, and less toxic conditioning regimens have eliminated the need for routine use of PN in this patient population.[37]

If nutrition support is required to compensate for poor intake, EN should be considered in patients whose inadequate intake is expected to continue for longer than one week.[9] Patients who may tolerate EN include those who receive non-myeloablative therapy; have chronic GVHD; suffer neurological complications that impede swallowing, or are on mechanical ventilation; and in those patients whose appetite does not improve after engraftment.[9]

Inability to use the GI tract due to severe GI toxicity from the conditioning regimen and severe intestinal GVHD may necessitate the implementation of PN in malnourished patients until oral intake can be resumed.[3, 38] There continues to be insufficient evidence to recommend PN supplemented with glutamine in patients following hematopoietic cell transplantation (HCT).[3] While PN has not been found to affect either the length of hospital stay or mortality in breast cancer patients undergoing autologous HCT, an increased risk of infectious complications does exist.[2] PN should be reserved for those HCT patients who are unable to meet their nutrient and energy requirements by oral diet or tube feeding.

PN has been shown to maintain nutritional status and restore hematopoietic function in patients undergoing HCT.[39] In one study, 35 patients undergoing

HCT received either PN ($n = 19$) or an oral diet ($n = 16$).[39] The criteria for providing PN included oral intake of less than 50% of estimated nutrient needs over 2 days. Patients on PN were encouraged to eat what was tolerated; if their oral intake exceeded 50% of their nutrient needs, the PN was gradually tapered off over 1 to 2 days. The PN was given for an average of 9.4 days and provided 25–30 kcal/kg, including 20–30% of total kilocalories as lipids and 1–1.5 g protein/kg per day. There was no difference in development of malnutrition or hematopoietic recovery between the groups, demonstrating the safety of PN in patients who are assessed to require nutrition support during HCT.

Feeding the Tumor

Tumor growth increases when patients are aggressively fed, but a difference in overall clinical outcome has not been shown in patients who are aggressively fed versus those who are not aggressively fed.[40] A study in patients with metastatic melanoma and renal cell carcinoma ($n = 37$) showed a 50% decrease in complete and partial responses to chemotherapy when it was given concurrently with PN for 14 days.[41] In terms of nutrients, the patients on PN received 25 kcal/kg, whereas the patients on oral diet received only 2.5 kcal/kg. Tumor progression was found to occur 17% faster in the PN group, but there was no difference in overall survival between the two groups.[41] In contrast, in another study, a group of GI cancer patients given PN and chemotherapy preoperatively demonstrated an improved nutritional status without an increase in the proliferation of tumor cells and did not have an increase in postoperative complications.[42]

Despite the conflicting results of studies evaluating the use of nutrition support in oncology patients, it is more important to address the clinical needs of the patient, rather than the pathology, when making determinations about nutritional needs.[40, 43, 44] Feeding the patient may result in more rapid growth of the tumor, but starving the patient can result in debilitation while the tumor continues to thrive. PN should not be avoided in malnourished patients who are unable to tolerate sufficient nutrients and energy delivered via the GI tract.

Home Parenteral Nutrition Support

Some patients may require home parenteral nutrition (HPN). Home nutrition support is appropriate for a patient who has a safe home environment and supportive and capable caregiver(s). One study of patients with cancer who were receiving HPN showed that the quality of life was improved and nutritional status was preserved for patients on PN for more than 3 months.[45]

In another study, involving 17 HPN patients with inoperable malignant bowel obstruction, researchers examined the efficacy of HPN as rated by both patients and their physicians.[46] The mean survival rate for the patients was 53 days. In this study, 14 (82%) patients and their families rated HPN as beneficial or highly beneficial. The clinicians managing the care of the patients agreed with 11 of these patient ratings. The 3 patients with whom the clinicians did not agree were patients whose duration of therapy was less than 25 days. Patients who survived 40 days or longer and had a committed and supportive family benefited from palliative HPN with few complications. It appears that delaying the initiation of PN could result in less benefit for patients who require it.

Palliative Care

Palliative care is the bridge from curative therapy to hospice care.[21] The goal of palliative care is to decrease suffering and provide comfort when a cure is no longer feasible or being pursued. The aggressiveness of the palliative therapies provided will depend on the prognosis and personal wishes of the patient and family. Nutrition support can provide hydration and reduce nutrient deprivation, thereby improving the quality of life for some patients. Nutrition support and hydration decisions should be based on effective communication between clinicians, patients, and families, with the ultimate decision being based on the wishes of the patient and family.[47]

SUMMARY

Nutrition support with enteral and parenteral nutrition should be considered only when the patient is unable to meet his or her nutrient needs through the oral diet. Tube feeding should be the first choice for nutrition support whenever feasible. Parenteral nutrition should be used when the enteral route—either by oral diet or by tube feeding—cannot be used or is insufficient to meet the patient's nutrient and energy needs. Careful monitoring and management is essential for effective nutrition support in the oncology patient.

REFERENCES

1. Position of the American Dietetic Association: Ethical and legal issues in nutrition, hydration, and feeding. *J Am Diet Assoc.* 2002;102:716–726.
2. Oncology guideline. ADA Evidence Analysis Library. http://www.adaevidence library.com. Accessed September 1, 2007.
3. A.S.P.E.N. Board of Directors and Clinical Guidelines Task Force. Guidelines for the use of parenteral and enteral nutrition in adult and pediatric patients. *JPEN J Parenter Enteral Nutr.* 2002;26(1S):82SA–85SA.

4. August DA. Nutrition and cancer: Where are we going? *Top Clin Nutr.* 2003; 18(4):268–279.

5. DeChicco RS, Steiger E. Parenteral nutrition in medical or surgical oncology. In: Elliott L, Molseed LL, McCallum PD, eds. *The Clinical Guide to Oncology Nutrition.* 2nd ed. Chicago, IL: American Dietetic Association, 2006;156–164.

6. Robinson CA. Enteral nutrition in adult oncology. In: Elliott L, Molseed LL, McCallum PD, eds. *The Clinical Guide to Oncology Nutrition.* 2nd ed. Chicago, IL: American Dietetic Association ed. *The* 2006:138–155.

7. Zogbaum AT, Fitz P, Duffy VB. Tube feeding may improve adherence to radiation treatment schedule in head and neck cancer: An outcomes study. *Top Clin Nutr.* 2004;19(2):95–106.

8. Braunschweig C, Levy P, Sheenan PM, Wang X. Enteral compared with parenteral nutrition: A meta-analysis. *Am J Clin Nutr.* 2001;74:534–542.

9. Charuhas PM, Lipkin A, Lessen P, McMillen K. Hematopoietic stem cell transplantation. In: Merritt R, ed. *The A.S.P.E.N. Nutrition Support Practice Manual.* 2nd ed. Silver Spring, MD: American Society for Parenteral and Enteral Nutrition; 2005:187–199.

10. Trujillo EB, Bergerson SL, Graf JC, Michael M. Cancer. In: Merritt R, ed. *The A.S.P.E.N. Nutrition Support Practice Manual.* 2nd ed. Silver Spring, MD: American Society for Parenteral and Enteral Nutrition; 2005:150–170.

11. Marian M, Carlson SJ. Enteral formulations. In: Merritt R, ed. *The A.S.P.E.N. Nutrition Support Practice Manual.* 2nd ed. Silver Spring, MD: American Society for Parenteral and Enteral Nutrition; 2005:63–75.

12. Barber MD, Fearon KC, Tisdale MJ, McMillan DC, Ross JA. Effect of a fish oil-enriched nutritional supplement on metabolic mediators in patients with pancreatic cancer and cachexia. *Nutr Cancer.* 2001;40:118–124.

13. Fearon KCH, von Meyenfeldt MF, Moses AGW, et al. Effect of a protein- and energy-dense Ω-3 fatty acid enriched oral supplement on loss of weight and lean tissue in cancer cachexia: A randomized double blind trial. *Gut.* 2003;52:1479–1486.

14. Lee S, Gura KM, Kim S, Arsenault DA, Bistrian BR, Pruder M. Current clinical applications of Ω-6 and Ω-3 fatty acids. *Nutr Clin Pract.* 2006;21:323–341.

15. Fuhrman MP. Diarrhea and tube feeding. *Nutr Clin Pract.* 1999;14:83–84.

16. Lord L, Harrington M. Enteral nutrition implementation and management. In: Merritt R, ed. *The A.S.P.E.N. Nutrition Support Practice Manual.* 2nd ed. Silver Spring, MD: American Society for Parenteral and Enteral Nutrition; 2005:76–89.

17. McClave SA, DeMeo MT. Proceedings of the North American summit on aspiration in the critically ill patient. *J Parenter Enteral Nutr.* 2002;26(suppl):S1–S85.

18. McClave SA, Lukan JK, Stefater JA, et al. Poor validity of residual volumes as a marker for risk of aspiration in critically ill patients. *Crit Care Med.* 2005;33:324–330.

19. Critical illness guideline. ADA Evidence Analysis Library. http://www.ada evidencelibrary.com. Accessed September 1, 2007.

20. Thompson CW, Durrant L, Barusch A, Olson L. Fostering coping skills and resilience in home enteral nutrition (HEN) consumers. *Nutr Clin Pract.* 2006; 21:557–565.

21. Fuhrman MP, Herrmann VM. Bridging the continuum: Nutrition support in palliative and hospice care. *Nutr Clin Pract.* 2006;21:134–141.

22. Krzywada EA, Edmiston CE. Parenteral nutrition access and infusion equipment. In: Merritt R, ed. *The A.S.P.E.N. Nutrition Support Practice Manual.* 2nd ed. Silver Spring, MD: American Society for Parenteral and Enteral Nutrition; 2005:90–96.

23. Sacks GS, Mayhew S, Johnson D. Parenteral nutrition implementation and management. In: Merritt R, ed. *The A.S.P.E.N. Nutrition Support Practice Manual.* 2nd ed. Silver Spring, MD: American Society for Parenteral and Enteral Nutrition; 2005:108–117.

24. Klein S, Miles JM. Metabolic effects of long-chain and medium-chain triglyceride emulsions in humans. *JPEN J Parenter Enteral Nutr.* 1994;18:396–397.

25. Lenssen P, Bruemmer BA, Bowden RA, Gooley T, Aker SN, Mattson D. Intravenous lipid dose and incidence of bacteremia and fungemia in patients undergoing bone marrow transplantation. *Am J Clin Nutr.* 1998;67:927–933.

26. Berger MM, Shenkin A. Vitamins and trace elements: Practical aspects of supplementation. *Nutrition.* 2006;22:952–955.

27. Mirtallo J, Canada T, Johnson D, et al. Task Force for the Revision of Safe Practices for Parenteral Nutrition. Safe practices for parenteral nutrition. *JPEN J Parenter Enteral Nutr.* 2004;28(suppl):S52–S57.

28. Fuhrman MP, Herrmann VM, Masidonski P, et al. Pancytopenia after removal of copper from total parenteral nutrition. *JPEN J Parenter Enteral Nutr.* 2000;24:361–366.

29. Krzywda EA, Andris DA, Whipple JK, et al. Glucose response to abrupt initiation and discontinuation of total parenteral nutrition. *JPEN J Parenter Enteral Nutr.* 1993;17:64–67.

30. Eisenberg PG, Gianino S, Clutter WE, et al. Abrupt discontinuation of cycled parenteral nutrition is safe. *Dis Colon Rectum.* 1995;38:933–939.

31. van den Berghe G, Wouters P, Weekers F, et al. Intensive insulin therapy in critically ill patients. *N Engl J Med.* 2001;345:1359–1367.

32. McMahon MM. Management of parenteral nutrition in acutely ill patients with hyperglycemia. *Nutr Clin Pract.* 2004;19:120–128.

33. Salvino R, Ghanta R, Seidner DL, Mascha E, Xu Y, Steiger E. Liver failure is uncommon in adults receiving long-term parenteral nutrition. *JPEN J Parenter Enteral Nutr.* 2006;30:202–208.

34. Seidner DL, Mascioli EA, Istfan NW, et al. Effects of long-chain triglyceride emulsions on reticuloendothelial system function in humans. *JPEN J Parenter Enteral Nutr.* 1989;13:614–619.

35. Finley JP. Management of cancer cachexia. *AACN Clin Issues ADV Pract Acute Crit Care.* 2000;11(4):590–603.

36. Argiles JM, Meijsing SH, Pallares-Trujillo J, Guiraro X, Lopez-Soriano FJ. Cancer cachexia: A therapeutic approach. *Med Res Rev.* 2001;21:83–101.

37. Lipkin AC, Lessen P, Dickson BJ. Nutrition issues in hematopoietic stem cell transplantation: State of the art. *Nutr Clin Pract.* 2005;20:423–439.

38. Torino J. Parenteral nutrition in adult hematopoietic stem cell transplantation: The evolution of clinical practice. *Support Line.* 2006;28(6):3–9.

39. Skop A, Kolarzyk E, Skotnicki AB. Importance of parenteral nutrition in patients undergoing hemopoietic stem cell transplantation procedures in the autologous system. *JPEN J Parenter Enteral Nutr.* 2005;29(4):241–247.

40. Canada T. Clinical dilemma in cancer: Is tumor growth during nutrition support significant? *Nutr Clin Pract.* 2002;17:246–248.

41. Samlowski WE, Wiebke G, McMurray M, et al. Effects of TPN during high-dose interleukin-2 treatment for metastatic cancer. *J Immunol.* 1998;21:65–74.

42. Jin D, Phillips M, Byles J. Effects of parenteral nutrition support and chemotherapy on the phasic composition of tumor cells in gastrointestinal cancer. *JPEN J Parenter Enteral Nutr.* 1999;23:237–241.

43. Bozzetti F. Home total parenteral nutrition in incurable cancer patients: A therapy, a basic humane care or something in between? *Clin Nutr.* 2003;22:109–111.
44. Bozzetti F, Gavazzi C, Mariani L, Crippa F. Glucose-based total parenteral nutrition does not stimulate glucose uptake by human tumors. *Clin Nutr.* 2004;23:417–421.
45. Bozzetti F, Cozzaglio L, Biganzoli E, et al. Quality of life and length of survival in advanced cancer patients on home parenteral nutrition. *Clin Nutr.* 2002;21:281–288.
46. August DA, Thorn D, Fisher RL, et al. Home parenteral nutrition for patients with inoperable malignant bowel obstruction. *JPEN J Parenter Enteral Nutr.* 1991;15 (3):323–327.
47. Casarett D, Kapo J, Caplan A. Appropriate use of artificial nutrition and hydration: Fundamental principles and recommendations. *N Engl J Med.* 2005;353:2605–2612.

Chapter 4

Medical and Radiation Oncology

Carole Havrila, RD, CSO
Paul W. Read, MD, PhD
David Mack, MD

INTRODUCTION

An estimated 1,437,000 people will be diagnosed with cancer and 565,000 people will die of cancer in the United States in 2008. Cancer is second only to heart disease as the cause of death in the United States, accounting for one-fourth of all deaths in this country. Men have a 50% chance of developing cancer during their lifetime and women have a 33% chance, with half of all cancer diagnoses involving breast, prostate, lung, or colon cancer. With earlier detection and more advanced treatments, two-thirds of all cancer patients will live at least 5 years.[1]

Cancer treatments have become increasingly more complicated over the past two decades, with many patients being treated with combinations of surgery, chemotherapy, and radiation in a multidisciplinary approach requiring coordination of care among many healthcare professionals. Newer chemotherapy drugs hold the promise of reduced toxicity and target novel cancer pathways, offering new hope to cancer patients. Advancements in radiation therapy planning and delivery have reduced acute and late toxicity by reducing the dose delivered to normal adjacent tissues.

This chapter reviews the basics of chemotherapy and radiation therapy and outlines the role of nutrition and the registered dietitian in the care of cancer patients in modern cancer centers.

Background

With the evolution of multicellular life from less complex ancestors, cancer became possible. Early life forms were likely similar to extant simple bacteria.

Their growth and division were limited only by their food sources and the need to avoid toxic concentrations of their own wastes. More than a billion years after the emergence of primitive bacterial cells, nucleated cells appeared in the fossil record, although their original forms may have been closer to those of the bacteria.[2] Some lineages of nucleated cells found survival advantages in forming colonial assemblies for part or all of their life cycles; from these lineages, true multicellular organisms likely developed.

The cells composing a multicellular organism needed to develop an entire repertoire of molecular machinery to interact and communicate with one another, derived from precursors used by their unicellular ancestors. Adhesion molecules were modified from less specialized precursors, as were surface, cytoplasmic, and nuclear receptors. Signal transduction pathways that relayed, amplified, or attenuated signals from the external environment to the cell's interior became more complex, allowing for a host of graduated responses to external stimuli or the lack thereof. The genome of cells grew in complexity, and new methods of controlling and regulating cellular division and gene expression evolved, allowing for the new organisms to radiate beyond the niches occupied by their unicellular cousins.

With multicellularity came the need for the individual cells within an organism to regulate their growth, division, and gene expression in response to both the external environment and signals from adjoining and distant cells. Multicellularity allowed cells the potential to differentiate into increasingly specialized forms, then to form tissues and organs—and even obligated them to commit a form of cellular suicide in response to the proper signals for the benefit of the survival of the organism. When the ancient control systems regulating the cells of a multicellular organism go significantly awry, cancer is the result.

A brief overview of cellular information flow is necessary to understand how malignancy can arise and the conceptual framework for its therapy. Deoxyribonucleic acid (DNA) is the material encoding genetic information in all living cells. DNA exists as immensely long sequences of purine bases—adenine (A) and guanine (G)—and pyrimidine bases—thymine (T) and cytosine (C). Each base is linked to a sugar (deoxyribose) and phosphate backbone. By convention, the linkage of a base with a sugar molecule is called a nucleoside (e.g., adenine + sugar = adenosine; similarly for guanosine, thymidine, and cytidine). The phosphorylation of a nucleoside yields a nucleotide (e.g., adenosine monophosphate—AMP, diphosphate—ADP, or triphosphate—ATP). Each sequence of DNA has a complementary sequence coupled to it through hydrogen bonds acting across paired bases: Adenine associates with thymine, and cytosine associates with guanine. From the sequence of one strand, the sequence of its complementary partner can be determined easily, as shown in Figure 4.1.

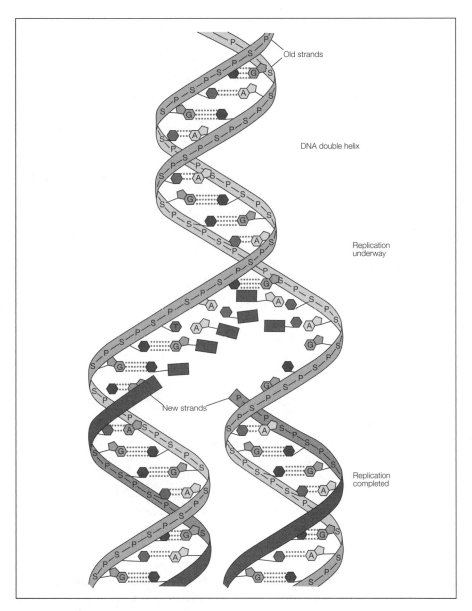

Figure 4.1 *Deoxyribonucleic Acid Strand*

As complementary sequences associate, they spontaneously wind into the famous double helix described by Watson and Crick, which earned them the Nobel Prize. More than 3 billion bases in the DNA sequence code for a human being. These bases are packaged into 23 pairs of chromosomes carried within the nucleus of almost every one of the 60 trillion cells in the body, with each instruction set encoding an estimated 25,000 to 30,000 genes.

Even though almost every human cell carries the entire instruction set to build a human being, vast stretches of DNA are quiescent and inactive. Some DNA is tightly coiled around small proteins, known as histones, silencing it; other stretches are modified by methylation of cytosine bases as a silencing mechanism. Only the DNA that is necessary for each cell's particular function is normally transcriptionally active. A common set of instructions is necessary for any nucleated cell: to synthesize proteins involved in energy utilization, intracellular transport, membrane synthesis, and destruction of damaged structures. Other instructions tell the cell to become a certain subtype—for example, colonic epithelial, breast ductal, or cardiac muscle. Certain cells are multipotent; that is, they are able to differentiate into multiple types. For example, a hematopoietic stem cell is able to differentiate into an array of cells to reconstitute the blood-forming tissues and immune system.

Transcriptionally active DNA is loosely packaged within the nucleus to allow access for transcription proteins. Thus information encoded in the DNA can be transcribed into short stretches of messenger ribonucleic acid (mRNA), which then translocates to the cell's cytoplasm, where it is translated into proteins the cell requires to function. An entire repertoire of additional proteins, nucleic acids, and organelles is necessary for this process: gene enhancers, gene promoters, initiation factors, transcription factors, RNA polymerases, topoisomerases, free RNA bases, transfer RNAs, and ribosomes, just to start. Genes can be constitutively activated (i.e., always "on" and being used to synthesize RNA and then protein), or they can be switched on or off depending on the needs of the cell.

There are also times when cells must die for the benefit of the organism as a whole. For example, during a certain period in utero, a fetus's eyelids are fused shut and its fingers are webbed. These states would impose a selective disadvantage to a newborn infant. Particular instructions expressed in development cause those extraneous cells to die off—a controlled, energy-requiring process called *apoptosis*—at the right time to allow for the proper human form to develop. Besides regulating development, apoptosis can occur as a result of a cell's failing to replicate properly, in response to other external "death signals," or when certain thresholds of cellular damage are exceeded, especially damage to DNA. Repair enzymes constantly scan the genome, excising mismatches in DNA bases and correcting them, replacing missing bases that have spontaneously hydrolyzed off the sugar–phosphate backbone, and repairing single- and double-stranded breaks. The process is not perfect, however, and mistakes occur, which is part of why cancer is usually (but not always) a disease of aging, and probably part of why aging itself occurs. Maintaining the fidelity of a sequence of 3 billion bases over decades of life and use requires a great deal of cellular effort.

When a cell is ready to divide, as dictated by its environment and genetic program, it normally does so in a controlled fashion (Figures 4.2 and 4.3). First, the cell moves from a relatively quiescent state called G_0, to a growth phase, G_1, in which it enlarges its contents and synthetic pool of raw materials (e.g., amino acids, ATP) and synthesizes the replication machinery. It then moves to S (for *synthesis*) phase, where its DNA is replicated with the aid of DNA polymerases and ligases (enzymes that link stretches of DNA), to phase G_2, preparatory to mitosis, the actual phase where division occurs. Mitosis occurs in the familiar five-stage pattern:

1. *Prophase:* the condensation of loosely organized DNA into discrete chromosomes.
2. *Metaphase:* where chromosomes line up in the center of the cell, attached to a microtubule spindle apparatus that will separate them.
3. *Anaphase:* where the chromosomes are pulled to opposite poles of the dividing cell.
4. *Telophase:* where the daughter cells' DNA starts to decondense and new nuclear envelopes form around them.
5. *Cytokinesis:* where the cells finally separate and become independent entities.

As with protein synthesis, this process is tightly regulated at checkpoints during G_1, allowing entry into the S phase, and at G_2, allowing entry into

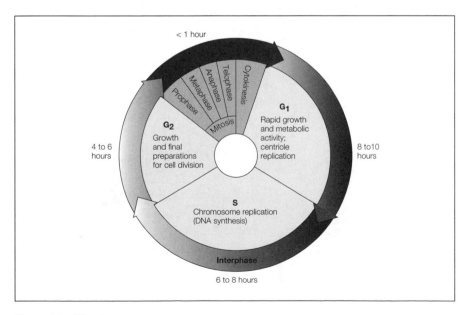

Figure 4.2 *Mitosis*

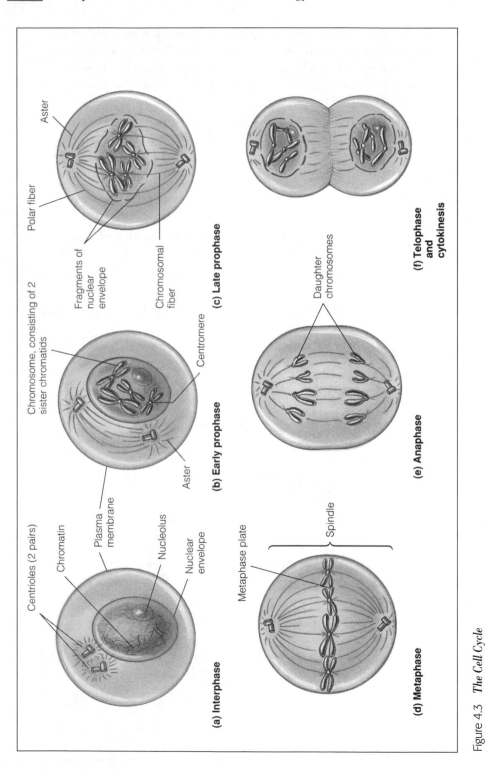

Figure 4.3   *The Cell Cycle*

mitosis. Failure to progress through these checkpoints, or through mitosis, normally triggers apoptosis.

Not surprisingly given the complexity of the cell, both genetic errors and dysregulation may occur. When a cell acquires a threshold amount of genetic damage, it has the potential to become cancerous. The amount of damage can be as small as a single gene, as happens with chronic myelogenous leukemia, but is usually much larger. The cell may become semiautonomous, with growth and replication pathways fixed in the "on" position, and the cell becoming increasingly unresponsive to external signals that would normally halt its division, cell-cycle checkpoints, and apoptotic signals telling it to die. Note that this condition may not be frankly malignant—malignancy is a continuum, not a binary condition—but the same genetic damage that allows for release from normal growth restraints also tends to result in increasing genetic instability with each cellular replication.

Over time, the premalignant cell can give rise to a family of closely related subclones, each competing for resources to outgrow its competitors. Eventually—and this may take many decades—one or more subclones may gain a growth advantage over their neighbors and acquire first the ability to avoid immune surveillance and elimination, then the ability to grow through tissue compartments otherwise limiting them from access to surrounding structures, then the ability to recruit blood vessels to bring oxygen and nutrients and take away wastes, and finally the ability to metastasize—that is, to send forth cells in the circulation and lymphatic system to implant themselves in other tissues to grow. This is cancer.

Fundamentally, then, cancer is a collection of genetic diseases. Scientists and physicians have made great strides in understanding and treating some of these diseases, whereas other diseases have proved very resistant to all forms of therapy to date. Surgery, radiation, and chemotherapy deployed in different combinations have been the mainstays of treatment for decades, supplemented by (for some diseases) hormonal therapy, immunotherapy with monoclonal antibodies, and, most recently, rationally designed small-molecule inhibitors of the signaling pathways driving a cancer's growth.

Cancers are characterized according to their organ of origin (e.g., lung, colon, breast), and their treatment and prognosis are guided by the degree of advancement of disease at discovery, categorized into stages. Stages are usually defined based on a combination of tumor size, nodal involvement, and presence or absence of metastases—the so-called TNM classification system. For the example of breast cancer, a T1 tumor is 2 centimeters or less and does not involve the skin or chest wall; a T2 tumor is greater than 2 centimeters and not more than 5 centimeters and does not involve the previous structures. N1 disease is present in fewer than four nodes, N2 in four to nine nodes, and so on. Metastases are either absent (M0) or present (M1). Various

TNM combinations are empirically grouped together, based on large data sets that correlate to the prognosis of the disease: Stage I breast cancer is T1N0M0; stage II can be T0N1M0, T1N1M0, T2N0M0, T2N1M0, or T3N0M0. Unsurprisingly, the aforementioned five stage II breast cancers are not identical diseases—what is it about a particular T1 tumor that allows it to spread to lymph nodes at a small size, and why don't all T3 tumors do so? A great deal of research is directed toward unraveling the genetic basis for a particular cancer's behavior and propensity to recur after definitive treatment.

As a general principle of solid malignancies, stage I disease is localized and often curable by some form of surgery alone: Examples include a stage I melanoma or a stage I colon cancer. Depending on the tumor type, adjuvant therapy might be deployed, which is therapy designed to increase the chances for cure after the primary surgical treatment. For example, small breast cancers often are treated with lumpectomy alone, with consideration given to using an individualized combination of chemotherapy, immunotherapy, radiation, and endocrine therapy afterward, depending on the size of the cancer, the receptors it expresses, the desire the patient has to retain the breast, and the age and health of the patient.

Stage II and III disease usually involve tumors that have grown larger than a certain size or have approached or invaded adjacent structures or have spread to nearby lymph nodes—the specifics depend on the cancer type. The prognosis for stage II and III disease is increasingly poorer than that for stage I, and aggressive adjuvant therapy is often used to give the patient the best chance for long-term disease-free survival after surgery.

Stage IV disease is usually metastatic; in other words, the cancer—regardless of the primary tumor size or nodal involvement—has succeeded in seeding itself in other organs or outside of lymph nodes in the vicinity of the primary tumor. Stage IV cancer is usually not treated surgically for cure, as undetectable micrometastatic disease generally coexists with radiologically apparent metastases. Instead, its treatment normally involves some combination of chemotherapy and radiation (with immunotherapy and/or hormonal therapy if the cancer is susceptible) delivered with palliative intent, so as to improve survival or to reduce symptoms. Many exceptions to this general system exist, however: Stage IV testicular cancer is usually highly curable, and other stage IV cancers can occasionally be treated with good results, especially if a long time has passed between treatment of the primary malignancy and the appearance of a distant metastasis.

The staging system is somewhat different for the hematologic malignancies that originate in lymphoid tissue or bone marrow and have immediate access to the circulatory system. These conditions tend to be (but are not always) disseminated diseases at the outset, as opposed to solid tumors. Also, their treatment is rarely surgical; rather chemotherapy, immunotherapy, and radiation are deployed for cure or to relieve symptoms (refer to Chapter 12).

Overview of Radiation Oncology

Radiation therapy is the clinical subspecialty in which cancer is treated with high-energy photons or particles. These photons and particles deposit energy into the patient's tissues, resulting in biochemical reactions that cause cell injury or cell death.[3,4] Radiation oncologists prescribe radiation to patients in units of energy per unit mass called a gray (Gy; 1 gray = 1 joule/kilogram body weight). Radiation therapy has been used for more than a century to treat cancer[5] and is a critical component in curative protocols for many patients with diverse diagnoses.[6] It is also widely used as a palliative measure for patients with advanced cancer symptoms such as pain, luminal obstruction, and bleeding. Radiation causes characteristic side effects depending on which tissues are being irradiated,[7] and these iatrogenic toxicities can significantly affect the nutritional status of patients.

Historical Development of Radiation Therapy as a Major Cancer Treatment

X-rays were first generated by electricity in the laboratory of Roentgen in 1895.[8] Two years later, in 1897, a case using x-rays to treat a skin lesion was reported at the Vienna Medical Society.[5] In 1898, Becquerel and the Curies discovered radioactivity,[9] which is the ability of natural elements to emit energy in the form of gamma rays or particles. The potential biologic consequences of gamma rays were discovered accidentally when Becquerel left a container with 200 mg of radium in his vest pocket for 6 hours and subsequently developed a chest wall ulcer, which took several weeks to heal.[5] Physicians soon thereafter purified and concentrated radium and implanted it adjacent to tumors in patients to treat head and neck, gynecologic, and breast malignancies with high local radiation doses.[10] This regimen ushered in the practice of brachytherapy, which is described in greater detail later in this chapter. Although x-rays and gamma rays come from different sources—they are created from electrical devices and natural radioactive material, respectively—both are highly energetic photons with identical properties. Both sources of photon radiation are currently used in the treatment of cancers in radiation therapy departments.

In the 1920s, x-ray units were built to treat cancer patients with photon energies of as much as 100–200 kilovolts.[10] This effort marked the beginning of external beam radiation, also known as teletherapy. Due to complex physics, higher-energy photon beams penetrate more deeply into tissues and deliver a lower relative skin dose exposure than do low-energy photons. The early treatment units resulted in very high skin dose exposures, causing skin erythma (redness) and moist desquamation (blistering). These side effects limited the tolerable total radiation dose deliverable to deep-seated tumors in the chest, abdomen, and pelvis and, therefore, the effectiveness of radiation treatments.

In an effort to improve the efficacy and reduce the toxicity of radiation therapy, higher-energy photon beams were required to reduce the skin dose exposure and allow for higher doses of radiation to be delivered to tumors. Cobalt-60 was concentrated to have a very high activity, and the first megavoltage (MeV) teletherapy units were built in the 1950s.[5] The cobalt units used large quantities of high-activity cobalt-60, which reliably produced a clinically stable high-dose rate beam with photon energies of approximately 1.25 MeV. They dramatically reduced the skin dose for patients, allowing curative doses of radiation to be delivered to tumors deep within the body. These units are still routinely used in many countries around the world owing to their dependability and clinical utility—indeed, few other medical devices can claim a 60-year lifespan with relatively few major changes.

In the 1950s and 1960s, the first linear accelerators were built to deliver megavoltage radiation beams with even higher photon energy capabilities as well as a new clinical option, the electron beam.[5] Electrons travel into tissues to an energy-specific distance and then deliver essentially no dose to tissues that are deeper within the body, with a rapid dose fall-off from 100% to 0% dose over a span of 1–8 centimeters.[11] When used properly, linear accelerators can be extremely useful for high-dose treatment of superficial tumors such as head and neck cancers, breast cancers, and skin cancers while sparing deeper tissues.[12] During the 1950s and 1960s time period, which included the Cold War, both the United States and the Soviet Union performed a tremendous amount of scientific research to study the biologic effects of radiation. Since the 1980s, most cancer patients in the United States have been treated with linear accelerators, which are now capable of producing photon energies in the range of 6–18 MeV photons.

Radiation therapy has advanced to the point of providing wide-scale proton particle beam units, a technology being pioneered at major universities with large cancer centers.[13] Proton therapy is unique because of the ability of the proton to penetrate deeply into tissues with relatively little dose being delivered to entrance tissues; instead, it delivers its dose over the narrow distance range where the tumor lies without any dose being delivered beyond that point. Therefore, proton beam treatments result in less radiation to adjacent organs and hold the promise of less treatment-related toxicity compared to treatments delivered with photons.

Radiation Biology: Biologic Effects of Radiation

The physical interaction of photons with biologic tissues lasts less than a nanosecond and results in the photon either being absorbed and depositing energy in the tissue, or passing straight through the patient without interaction or energy delivery to the tissues.[8] When high-energy photons are absorbed by atoms in cells, they cause electrons to be knocked out of their atomic orbits and to move, a process called ionization. These highly energetic moving electrons cause DNA damage.[7] With this treatment method, the physical interaction of radiation with biologic material is converted into biochemistry capable of killing tumor cells and potentially injuring normal tissues. The basic biologic rationale for treating tumors with radiation is that tumor cells are less capable of repairing DNA injury and are preferentially killed compared to normal cells.[7] The physics and biochemistry of this interaction are completed in less than a millisecond, well before the patient gets off the treatment table.

The subsequent biologic consequences of the radiation-induced biochemical reactions on adjacent organs, or treatment-related toxicities, depend on the total dose of radiation, the type of tissue or organ irradiated, and the volume of tissue treated.[7] The side effects are divided into acute and late toxicities, based on when they develop. Acute toxicities generally occur during the course of treatment or shortly thereafter, resolve within three months of completing treatment, and are related to temporary depletion of stem cells resulting in mucosal injury as well as congestion of the microvasculature resulting in edema (swelling) and erythema.[7] Late toxicities occur three or more months after the completion of treatment and are generally related to reduced blood flow secondary to radiation damage to the microvasculature and to reduced numbers of stem cells that are normally present for regenerating the mucosa and skin and for healing injured tissue. Both of these conditions predispose patients to infection and ulceration and can lead to serious late complications involving heavily irradiated tissues. Radiation can also result in secondary cancers in the irradiated tissues, which can develop years or even decades after treatment.

In general, the risk of acute and late radiation toxicity increases with higher daily doses of radiation. To minimize this risk, radiation treatments are usually divided into many smaller daily treatments, a strategy called fractionated radiation therapy. Curative treatments are usually given on a daily basis Monday through Friday over 3–8 weeks (depending on the total dose of radiation to be delivered), with a daily fractionated dose of 1.8–2.0 Gy being delivered with each treatment. Each radiation treatment generally takes 10–15 minutes per day.

Medications can be given to patients either to protect normal tissues from the effects of radiation (radiation protectors) or to make the radiation more effective at killing cancers (radiation sensitizers), thereby resulting in improved eradication of tumors. Currently the only FDA-approved radiation protector is amifostine, which has been shown to reduce radiation injury to the salivary glands.[14] Many chemotherapy agents are used as radiation sensitizers. In fact, the combination of concurrent chemotherapy with radiation (given at the same time), called chemoradiation, is considered the standard of care for many brain tumors, head and neck cancers, lung cancers, gastrointestinal cancers, and cervical cancer.[6] For other tumors, such as breast cancer and lymphomas, chemotherapy and radiation are given sequentially (one and then the other) instead of concurrently.[6] The improvement in local control provided by combining chemotherapy and radiation generally comes at the cost of increased toxicity for patients compared to treatment with radiation alone.

Modern Radiation Delivery Techniques

Radiation can be delivered to patients in one of three basic ways: teletherapy, brachytherapy, or radioactive nucleotides.

The vast majority of patients are treated with teletherapy—that is, the use of external beam units. With teletherapy, external beams of radiation are generated either by large amounts of cobalt-60 that create the beam via radioactivity, or by photons that are electrically generated via a linear accelerator. Protons are generated in a cyclotron or synchrotron. In this method of treatment, the beam is created outside the patient and then is targeted to travel into the patient and hit the tumor. The radiation beam can be collimated or focused for various medical purposes. Wide beams are used to treat large-volume tumors or even for total body irradiation (TBI) prior to hematopoietic cell transplantation. Very narrow radiation beams can be used to treat small, sub-centimeter-sized tumors in the body; with this approach, one to five high-precision ablative treatments are delivered, called stereotactic radiosurgery.[15]

Modern photon beam linear accelerators are built with arrays of paired multi-leaf collimators consisting of thin 3- to 10-mm tungsten blocks that can be independently moved to block portions of the radiation beam. These blocks are used to create customized radiation treatments for individual patients. Intensity-modulated radiation therapy (IMRT) utilizes many different multi-leaf collimator positions and beam entry angles calculated by sophisticated radiation treatment planning software to deliver highly focused or conformal radiation treatments. With this approach, the high radiation doses conform to the tumor-containing tissues and adjacent normal tissues are spared, thereby minimizing toxicity.

Modern linear accelerators are also equipped with fluoroscopic or CT scan capabilities built into the treatment units. This capability allows daily imaging prior to each treatment so as to ensure accurate treatment delivery, a process known as image-guided radiation therapy (IGRT). Tumors in the lung and abdomen, for example, move secondary to breathing. Some treatment units are capable of tracking or synchronizing the radiation beam delivery with patient breathing to ensure the accurate treatment of a moving tumor with the least amount of adjacent normal tissue being irradiated. This process is called respiratory gated radiation therapy.

Brachytherapy is the second way to deliver radiation therapy. It involves physically implanting sources of high radioactivity into patients' tissues or body cavities via seeds, plastic catheters, and various applicators; these sources then deliver high doses of radiation to adjacent tumors, with the radiation dose rapidly falling off with distance from the source. Frequently the placement of seeds or applicators is performed in the operating room as a surgical procedure. Brachytherapy is further characterized by the dose rate, with low-dose-rate (LDR) implants treating patients for hours or days and high-dose-rate (HDR) implants treating patients for just a few minutes. Some brachytherapy implants involve the permanent placement of radioactive seeds into patients, such as prostate seed implants. Other brachytherapy implants involve the temporary placement of radioactive sources into plastic catheters or applicators, with all radioactive sources being removed upon completion of treatment.

The third method of delivering radiation to patients is to treat them with oral or intravenous unsealed radioactive nucleotides. Examples include oral administration of iodine-131 for thyroid cancer, intravenous administration of radioactive-labeled monoclonal antibodies to treat lymphoma (Bexxar® and Zevalin®), and use of radioactive microspheres infused into the livers of patients with tumors (TheraSpheres® or SIR-Spheres®). Radionuclide administration can occur in a radiation therapy department or in the nuclear medicine and interventional radiology divisions of radiology departments.

Radiation Therapy Department Personnel

Radiation oncology departments include a diverse group of healthcare personnel working together as a team. These personnel may include radiation oncologists, oncology nurses, radiation therapists, medical physicists, dosimetrists, clerical staff, social workers, and registered dietitians (RD).

A radiation oncologist is a physician specializing in the treatment of cancers with radiation. He or she is ultimately responsible for the safety and welfare of the patients. In addition to prescribing the dose of radiation and the tumor volumes in the patient to be treated, the radiation oncologist is responsible for: ensuring that adjacent critical organs do not receive excessive radiation, managing treatment-related toxicities, evaluating tumor response to treatment, and coordinating patient care with other oncology specialists.

Oncology nurses perform initial and weekly patient assessment; identify issues such as patient malnutrition, social problems, or psychiatric problems that may interfere with treatment; and help coordinate consultations with appropriate healthcare professionals to facilitate optimal care. They also assist in brachytherapy procedures, give medications and infusions, and maintain code carts and departmental medications.

Radiation therapists are specially trained to assist in the treatment planning simulation process and administration of daily radiation treatments. Medical physicists ensure that treatment units and brachytherapy sources are properly calibrated and maintained; they also commission all new equipment and review all treatment planning calculations to verify their accuracy prior to treatment. Dosimetrists run the treatment planning software and work with physicians to create individualized radiation treatment plans based on the prescribed dose to the tumor volume and the dose constraints to adjacent critical organs. The clerical staff is involved in scheduling, processing insurance preauthorization, and maintaining departmental charts. Social workers help solve complex social problems such as transportation difficulties, childcare requirements, requirements for local temporary housing, lack of insurance requiring application for Medicaid and/or disability benefits, and, in general, they work to mitigate the potential negative impacts of these issues on patient care.

Registered dietitians meet with patients initially, and in an ideal setting, they perform weekly follow-up assessments. The RD assesses the patient's nutritional status, changes in the patient's caloric requirements, the need for tube feeding, and refeeding risks. He or she frequently works with the social worker to obtain nutritional supplementation if patients cannot afford to pay for these products.

Radiation Oncology Work Flow

The patient care process for most cancer patients undergoing radiation therapy is a fairly standard one. Patients undergoing radiation therapy are first registered by the clerical staff and then undergo a consultation including an initial assessment by the oncology nurse and a complete history and physical by the radiation oncologist. In general, patients are seen in the radiation oncology department, although hospitalized patients may be seen in consultation in their hospital rooms. Social workers and RDs may then be asked to see patients for assessments.

If it is determined that the patient would benefit from external beam radiation therapy, the patient is scheduled to undergo a treatment planning simulation. This procedure generally consists of a special CT scan performed by the radiation therapists and radiation oncologists in which personalized immobilization equipment is used to ensure reproducible daily treatment setup. It is called simulation because the patient immobilization and positioning simulate how the patient will be treated on the actual treatment unit. In the simulation, the physician uses a laser to place marks or tattoos on the patient or marks the immobilization equipment to guide daily patient alignment prior to treatment. PET, CT, or MRI scans may also be used for treatment planning simulation.

Following simulation, the patient goes home, and the physician digitally contours or draws the target volumes for radiation treatment and the adjacent critical organs on the simulation scan, prescribes a target tumor dose, and places constraints or limits for the maximum radiation dose to be received by adjacent critical organs. The dosimetrist then uses this contoured treatment planning CT scan and the tumor prescription and adjacent organ dose constraints to create an individualized treatment plan for each patient. The physician approves the dosimetrist's plan if it meets all the required criteria, and the medical physicist checks the plan for accuracy and performs all necessary quality assurance tests to ensure safe delivery of the plan. The plan is then imported into the treatment unit software, and the radiation therapist subsequently uses this information for daily patient treatment. In total, this radiation planning process generally takes three to five days.

Modern treatment units have imaging capabilities that are used by radiation therapists and physicians to ensure that the patient setup maintains millimeter accuracy on a daily basis. Special consideration must be given to pediatric patients, such as construction of specialized immobilization equipment or even the need for daily anesthesia, to make treatment possible for small children and infants. During the treatment course, the patient is seen at least once a week for toxicity assessment and management and assessment of tumor response by the physicians and nurses. Ideally, a RD also sees the patient weekly to assess his or her nutritional status and the need for intervention with supplementation or enteral feedings. Following completion of the course of radiation, the patient is followed by the healthcare team to manage the acute and then late treatment-related toxicities, for evaluation of tumor response, and for surveillance of tumor recurrence.

Radiation therapy may be given with the intention of curing patients of their cancer and is frequently combined with surgical resection and/or chemotherapy. In contrast, palliative radiation is used to reduce symptoms such as bleeding, obstruction, or pain, with the twin goals of minimizing distressing symptoms and improving quality of life. Curative treatment courses frequently last three to eight weeks, whereas palliative treatment courses last one to two weeks.

Standard curative external beam radiation prescriptions for common tumors have been developed based on the optimal dose to cure a given tumor and the dose limitations of adjacent organs. Table 4.1 lists common tumors, standard external beam radiation prescription doses, and treatment durations, and identifies whether concurrent chemotherapy is administered for the most commonly treated adult tumors.

Overview of Medical Oncology

Physicians have attempted to treat cancers with pharmacologic agents for millennia, almost entirely without success until the last century.[16-18] Early successes in the prevention and treatment of bacterial diseases in the nineteenth century led researches to hypothesize that malignancies could be treated with chemical compounds as well. During World War I, young men

Table 4.1 *Frequently Used Radiation or Chemoradiation Treatment Regimens for Common Adult Malignancies*

Cancer Primary Site	Common Prescribed Dose (Gy)	External Beam Treatment Duration	Concurrent Chemotherapy
Breast	60–66 Gy	6 weeks	No
Prostate	72–78 Gy or brachytherapy implant	7–8 weeks 5 weeks	No (hormonal—yes)
Lung	60–74 Gy	6–7.5 weeks	Yes
Head and neck	60–72 Gy	6–7 weeks	Yes
Gastrointestinal	50–56 Gy	5–6 weeks	Yes
Gynecologic	45–50 Gy + brachytherapy implant	5 weeks	Yes
Brain	50–60 Gy	5–6 weeks	Yes
Sarcoma	60–74 Gy	6–7.5 weeks	No
Lymphoma	30–50 Gy	3–5 weeks	No

Source: Treatment recommendations data from *National Comprehensive Cancer Network clinical practice guidelines in oncology.* © 2008 National Comprehensive Cancer Network, Inc. http://www.nccn.org.

exposed to mustard agents (named for their odor) were sometimes found to have a paucity of normal bone marrow cells at autopsy.[18] In the early 1940s, Gilman and Philips conducted studies of nitrogen mustard derivatives in patients with lymphoma. Their work was spurred by a 1943 German air attack on U.S. ships—one of which was loaded with mustard agents—at the port of Bari, Italy, which injured hundreds of seamen, soldiers, and civilians who were exposed to the gas, and caused the deaths of dozens of people. The survivors were found to develop lymphoid and myeloid bone marrow suppression.

Gilman and Philips' work was classified at the time it was being conducted, as was the release of chemical weapons in Italy. Nevertheless, the line of research they began led to a publication in 1946 by Goodman and colleagues containing the first description of the use of recognizably modern chemotherapy in humans.[19] This work was quickly followed by breakthroughs in treating certain leukemias with the antifolate agent methotrexate, and the first cure of a cancer (choriocarcinoma) with this compound. The growth of knowledge in molecular biology over subsequent decades has led to increasingly effective and less toxic interference with different cellular processes using chemotherapy.

Traditional cytotoxic chemotherapy agents can be categorized by the mechanisms used to interrupt cell division and cause cell death (see Table 4.2). Classical alkylators include mechlorethamine, cyclophosphamide, and ifosfamide, all of which are descendants of the original mustard agents. These compounds bind directly to DNA, either causing cross-links across complementary strands or within the same strand, and resulting in irreparable damage and preventing the proper unwinding of DNA during replication or gene expression. Chemically unrelated compounds with similar mechanisms of action include the platinum agents. The first platinum agent was *cis*-diaminodichloroplatinum (CDDP), also known as cisplatin, which is used frequently to treat lung cancer. Its cousins, oxaliplatin and carboplatin, are often used in combination with other agents to treat colorectal cancer and lung cancer, respectively.[20]

Nucleoside analogs are compounds that chemically resemble the constituent bases of DNA or RNA. The prototypes of this class of compounds are 6-mercaptopurine, which is used to treat certain types of leukemia, and 5-fluorouracil (5-FU), which was synthesized more than 50 years ago as an analog of uracil; uracil is an RNA base and a substrate for thymidine synthesis. A relatively new compound, capecitabine, is an oral agent that is converted to 5-FU within the body; it is increasingly being used to replace infusional 5-FU. Other pyrimidine nucleoside analogs include gemcitabine and cytarabine. Purine nucleoside analogs commonly used in cancer therapy include fludarabine, 2-chlorodeoxyadenine (2-COA), and pentostatin. These compounds work against cancer cells in different ways. For example, they

Table 4.2   *Representative Types of Chemotherapeutic Agents in Common Use*

Class	Examples	Mechanisms of Action
Alkylators	Cyclophosphamide, ifosfamide, platinum agents	Bind directly to DNA, resulting in irreparable damage and preventing the proper unwinding of DNA during replication or gene expression
Nucleoside analogs	5-Fluorouracil, capecitabine, gemcitabine, cytarabine, fludarabine, 2-CDA, pentostatin	Become incorporated into a growing DNA sequence, causing chain termination and triggering apoptosis; alternatively, inhibit enzymes involved in DNA and/or RNA synthesis
Topoisomerase inhibitors	Etoposide, topotecan, irinotecan	Interfere with enzymes involved in uncoiling DNA to allow for replication and gene expression
Microtubule inhibitors	Paclitaxel, docetaxel, vinorelbine, vinblastine	Prevent assembly or disassembly of microtubules necessary for mitosis
Multifunctional	Daunorubicin, idarubicin, doxorubicin	Free radical generators; physically interfere with DNA replication; topoisomerase inhibition
Tyrosine kinase inhibitors	Imatinib, erlotinib, sunitinib, sorafenib	Bind to proteins involved in cellular signaling
Monoclonal antibodies	Rituximab, bevacizumab, cetuximab	Bind to proteins involved in cellular signaling, activate the immune system against target cells

become integrated into a growing DNA sequence, causing chain termination and triggering apoptosis. Some also competitively inhibit enzymes involved in DNA or RNA synthesis, arresting the cell's ability to replicate or produce needed proteins from messenger RNA.[20]

In contrast to chemotherapeutic agents that inflict direct damage on DNA, the topoisomerase inhibitors block enzymes involved in DNA uncoiling. As an illustration of this principle, picture a double helix that is fixed on both ends. Pulling on the strands in the middle to uncoil and separate them, as must occur during DNA replication or gene expression, increases coiling both upstream and downstream of the separation point; it also increases tension on the strands. Topoisomerases are enzymes that induce single- or double-stranded breaks in DNA upstream and downstream of an uncoiled region, allow the strands to rotate to relieve the tension, and then anneal the break. Not surprisingly, compounds have been developed to interfere with these enzymes. Etoposide (used to treat testicular and lung cancer), topotecan (used for lung and ovarian cancer), and irinotecan (used in lung cancer) are all topoisomerase inhibitors that are commonly used as chemotherapeutic agents.[20]

Other compounds have multiple functions. For example, the anthracycline antibiotics, which include doxorubicin and epirubicin (often used to treat breast cancer), are derived from natural antibacterial compounds. These compounds posses topoisomerase-inhibiting activity, but also interact directly with DNA to hinder its replication; in addition, they are free radical generators of other DNA-damaging species.[20]

A wide array of agents has been developed to interfere with cytoplasmic processes outside the cell's nucleus, including the taxanes paclitaxel and docetaxel. Taxanes bind to and stabilize microtubules, and prevent the dynamic changes necessary for the spindle apparatus to accurately separate chromosomes during mitosis, inducing mitotic arrest and apoptosis. The taxanes' cousins, vinca alkaloids (e.g., vincristine, vinblastine, and vinorelbine), have the opposite effect: They prevent the synthesis of microtubules from tubulin monomers, with similar catastrophic effects on cellular division.[20]

Besides the development of new cytotoxic agents, another major advance in treating malignancies over the last decades has been the combination of agents with different mechanisms of action and non-overlapping toxicities to minimize the chances for cancer cells developing resistance to treatment. This approach led to curative regimens for Hodgkin's lymphoma and childhood acute lymphoblastic leukemia in the 1960s. With rare exceptions, modern chemotherapy regimens deployed for cure rely on two or more agents for maximum effectiveness.[20]

Traditional cytotoxic chemotherapy acts on the replicative machinery of a cell. Other cellular processes have now been sufficiently characterized to allow for the development of agents to disrupt them. The prototype for these compounds is imatinib, which was developed to treat chronic myelogenous leukemia (CML). The genetic defect in CML arises from a translocation between chromosomes 9 and 22, giving rise to an abnormal stretch of DNA called the Philadelphia chromosome. A particular gene product of the Philadelphia chromosome is the chimeric protein BCR-ABL. BCR-ABL is the fusion product of two genes, *bcr* and *abl*, which normally do not interact. The fusion protein is constitutively active and drives the cell containing it to replicate without end, giving rise to CML. If CML is left untreated, additional genetic errors accumulate over the course of several years, and the disease moves first to an accelerated phase, then an acute leukemic phase that is usually rapidly fatal. Imatinib binds to the BCR-ABL protein, preventing its activity and causing the death of the cell by means of a still-unclear process.[21] An entire cohort of agents targeted against specific cellular proteins involved in intracellular signaling has been developed since imatinib, and these drugs are becoming increasingly important in treating cancer.

Monoclonal antibody-based therapy against cell-surface proteins is another area under development. Monoclonal antibodies work in a variety of ways. Some trigger the immune system to destroy the malignant cells by antibody-dependent cellular cytotoxicity (ADCC), which recruits natural killer cells and macrophages to the tumor. Others cause the deposition of complement proteins (complement-dependent cytotoxicity [CDC], a form of innate immunity), which leads to the death of the targeted cell. Still other monoclonal antibodies indirectly downregulate the cell's growth by activating or inhibiting signaling pathways, possibly potentiating the effectiveness of cytotoxic chemotherapy. The prototypic monoclonal antibody agents are rituximab and trastuzumab. Rituximab is directed against the protein CD20, which is expressed on normal B lymphocytes as well as on the B cells of malignant disorders. Trastuzumab works against HER-2, a cell-surface protein that is expressed on certain breast cancers and portends very aggressive behavior of the cancer. The use of trastuzumab has dramatically improved the treatment of this type of breast cancer, providing approximately a 50% relative reduction in the relapse risk after local treatment and chemotherapy. Another extremely promising agent of this type is bevacizumab, which is an antibody to circulating vascular endothelial growth factor (VEGF). Bevacizumab binds to VEGF, clearing it from the circulation and decreasing the rate at which a malignancy can recruit new blood vessels to supply its growth needs.[22]

Not surprisingly, other classes of agents are in use or in development for cancer therapy. Examples include histone deacetylase inhibitors and hypomethylating agents, which alter genetic expression directly, by activating genes that have aberrantly become silenced during the process of carcinogenesis.[23, 24]

The complexity of modern cancer therapy reflects both the difficulty and the advances in treating the heterogeneous collection of diseases lumped together as cancer. A full review of all the types of pharmaceutical agents now being deployed or being developed to work against malignancies is beyond the scope or purpose of this text. Nevertheless, the growing number of agents active against cancer is testament to the progress that has been made over the last 60 years.

Oncologists are often asked why it is so difficult in many cases to treat or cure advanced malignancy, especially when compared to other superficially similar conditions, such as infectious diseases. The answer is that the rogue cells of cancer arose from normal cells around them, and the differences between the cancerous cells and healthy ones are not enormous. Both cancerous cells and healthy cells make use of the same cellular processes to survive, grow, and replicate, and most of our current therapies are limited by the toxicity to normal cells, and thus to the organism as a whole. Bacteria, in contrast, have been evolving apart from humans for billions of years, and their cellular machinery is much more vulnerable to our treatments—not only because it is less complex and redundant than our own cellular machinery, but also because it is evolutionarily divergent, allowing us to develop agents that are extremely toxic to bacterial processes yet relatively innocuous to the human body.

The final goal of chemotherapy is to cure cancers at any stage with a minimum of toxicity—or better still, to prevent them from occurring in the first place. Until this goal can be achieved, an interim step that many scientists and oncologists are working toward is to convert advanced cancers into manageable chronic diseases. Toward that end, the medical oncologist has a number of increasingly effective tools at his or her disposal. Cytotoxic chemotherapies have been used for decades and are still being developed, but as the understanding of cellular processes evolves, the ability to exploit the differences between malignant and healthy cells will advance as well.

Nutritional Implications of Medical and Radiation Oncology

Advancements in cancer therapies achieved over the past two decades have led to better treatment outcomes and improved survival rates for many cancers.[25] However, side effects associated with cancer treatments continue to afflict patients during these treatments and beyond. Many side effects are nutrition related and should be managed as soon as possible. Today, many patients receive treatments with combined radiation and chemotherapy, and such treatments can cause significant weight loss in as many as 70% of patients.[26]

Regardless of cancer diagnosis, unintentional weight loss of more than 5% predicts a poor prognosis even after adjusting for performance status.[27] It is well accepted that malnourished patients with cancer are more likely to have infections and treatment toxicities with associated increases in healthcare costs and decreases in treatment response.[28] Today, quality of life is paramount as more patients are being treated, but not necessarily with the goal of obtaining a cure. Because malnutrition can significantly influence response to treatment, it should be the goal of all RDs working with cancer patients to provide tailored nutritional interventions throughout cancer treatment and into survivorship to maximize quality of life. Other clinicians should screen and refer patients at nutritional risk to the RD for individualized care.

Nutritional Implications of Radiation Therapy

Radiation therapy is widely used to treat a number of malignancies, including those affecting the lung, head and neck, brain, cervix, prostate, gastrointestinal tract, and breast. As mentioned earlier in this chapter, high-dose radiation is delivered via radiotherapy, brachytherapy, or radiopharmaceutical therapy. Radiation therapy is given in precise, fractionated doses to the site of disease. Despite this narrowing of the scope of therapy, radiation affects healthy tissue, in addition to cancer cells, in the targeted treatment field it is given. Radiation to any part of the gastrointestinal tract or pelvic area, for example, leaves a patient vulnerable to nutrition-related side effects (see Table 4.3).[29]

Radiation to the cervix, colon/rectum, stomach, and pancreas can lead to side effects of nausea, vomiting, and diarrhea. Medically, diarrhea is typically managed with antidiarrheal medicines such as Imodium® (loperamide hydrochloride) and Lomotil® (diphenoxylate/atropine). Bulk-forming agents such as psyllium (Metamucil®) and the amino acid glutamine may also be used alongside these medications.[30] According to the American Dietetic Association's (ADA) *Oncology Evidence Analysis* guidelines, glutamine has not been proven effective to reduce radiation-associated diarrhea, and its usage warrants further study. In addition, limiting dietary fiber, lactose, and spicy foods is sometimes helpful to decrease symptoms of bloating, cramping, and diarrhea. In some patients, radiation enteritis can develop as an early (developing within two to three weeks of treatment) or late (several weeks, months, or years after the end of treatment) side effect. In severe cases, malabsorption of nutrients and severe fluid losses can occur. In those

Table 4.3 *Acute Nutrition-Related Side Effects of Radiation*[29, 31]

Area in Which Radiation is Applied	*Nutrition-Related Side Effects*
Central nervous system	Fatigue, hyperglycemia associated with steroids
Head/neck/thorax	Mucositis, stomatitis, thick saliva, xerostomia, loss of taste, altered taste, dysphagia, odynophagia, esophagitis, nausea and vomiting, fatigue
Abdomen/pelvis	Nausea, vomiting, diarrhea, gas, malabsorption, lactose intolerance, fatigue

Sources: Unsal D, Mentes B, Akmansu M, et al. Evaluation of nutritional status in cancer patients receiving radiotherapy: A prospective study. *Am J Clin Oncol.* 2006;29:183–188; Chencharick JD, Mossman KL. Nutritional consequences of the radiotherapy of head and neck cancer. *Cancer.* 1983;51:811–815.

patients who develop severe enteritis, the use of nutrition support is often warranted to treat severe weight loss and vitamin/mineral deficiencies.[29]

Cancers of the head and neck and thorax treated with radiation therapy are associated with many nutritional challenges.[31] Many patients have tumors that physically prevent eating or limit intake, and many patients have a history of heavy alcohol and tobacco abuse, which further compromises nutritional status prior to treatment. Given that radiation fields involve rapidly dividing tissues, this population may experience significant mucositis, stomatitis, xerostomia, thick saliva, altered taste and smell, dysphagia, and nausea and vomiting. The incidence of malnutrition in this population is common, with as many as 57% of patients with head and neck cancer experiencing weight loss before starting radiation.[32]

Today, multimodality (radiation therapy and concurrent chemotherapy) treatment is being used more often for these malignancies. The increased toxicities associated with such therapy can cause significant weight loss, which can in turn lead to frequent treatment interruptions, hospital or emergency room admissions for hydration and nutritional support, and, most importantly, decreased treatment response.[26] Many cancer centers routinely place percutaneous gastrostomy tubes in patients who receive concurrent chemotherapy and radiation. Such early and aggressive nutrition intervention has been shown to decrease weight loss and deterioration of nutritional status in these patients.[26]

Most side effects associated with radiation therapy are acute, beginning around the second to third week into the course of radiation treatment, and then declining two to three weeks after the completion of treatment. Regardless of the body area being treated with radiation therapy, universal side effects include fatigue, loss of appetite, and skin changes. Some side effects become chronic, such as with radiation enteritis or osteonecrosis, and may last weeks to months beyond the completion of treatment.[33]

Nutritional Implications of Chemotherapy

More than 90 chemotherapy agents are used to treat a variety of cancers.[34] Chemotherapy agents are classified based on their mechanism of action and are administered either intravenously or in the form of an oral drug. Chemotherapy treatments may take minutes or hours. Certain chemotherapy agents have more toxic effects on kidney and liver function owing to their elimination or metabolism pathways. These regimens require aggressive hydration and hospital admission to carefully monitor vital signs and deliver intravenous fluids along with the chemotherapy. Chemotherapy can be given as one single agent or a combination of agents, depending on the type of cancer. Chemotherapy given concurrently with radiation is the standard

of care for a variety of cancers. Patients receiving such treatments experience more severe side effects and, therefore, must be considered at high
nutritional risk.[34]

Because chemotherapy is a systemic treatment, it affects the entire body.
As a consequence, it has the potential to cause more side effects than radiation therapy or surgery alone.[34, 35] The side effects associated with chemotherapy typically depend on the specific treatment regimen, including the dose
of medication(s), the length of planned treatment, and the patient's stage of
disease and health status. Normal gastrointestinal function may be affected
by damage to the cells lining the digestive tract, leading to nausea, vomiting,
diarrhea, and altered gastric motility. Chemotherapy drugs are graded for
their emetogenic potential, and a variety of medicines are used to mitigate
treatment-related nausea and vomiting, including Compazine® (prochlorper-
azine) , Emend® (aprepitant), and Zofran® (ondansetron).[36, 37]

When faced with gastrointestinal side effects, patients benefit from education on low-fat, bland foods that are easily digested. Dry toast, broth-based
soups, fresh fruit, and Popsicles are some examples of foods that are better
tolerated during periods of nausea and vomiting. Small, frequent snacks are
encouraged, rather than the typical three meals per day, as many patients are
overwhelmed at the sight of food and become anorexic. Oftentimes, patients
benefit from being given a written meal schedule including meal/snack
times, sample foods, and amounts needed. Some may benefit from setting a
kitchen timer or a watch alarm to sound when the next snack time approaches. Patients with anorexia or little caregiver support find this strategy particularly helpful. Providing information on daily calorie requirements
is often too intense for the patient, whereas giving patients approximate
amounts of foods to be eaten, 6–8 times daily, is more realistic and helpful
for obtaining adequate calories. If counseling interventions alone are not
helpful, appetite stimulants should be considered. Patients must also be
counseled on appropriate fluid intake to prevent dehydration.[34, 36]

It is crucial to reassess patients often to assure adequate control of nausea and vomiting with nutrition and medication interventions. Weight loss
can be significant in patients who follow the correct dietary modifications,
yet do not receive adequate medical management of symptoms. Regular
weight checks at each chemotherapy or oncologist appointment are needed
to document progressive weight loss. In some cases, the doses of chemotherapy drugs may be reduced or the drugs changed if the toxicity of nausea and
vomiting is severe.[36, 37]

Myelosuppression is another significant side effect of many chemotherapy
drugs. Decreases in the number of white blood cells, red blood cells, and
platelets leave patients at higher risk for infections, anemia, and bleeding.[36]
In most cases, blood cell counts return to normal approximately 21–24 days

after chemotherapy. Severe neutropenia, however, increases a patient's susceptibility to life-threatening infection.[34, 36] The oncology RD should counsel patients and caregivers on the importance of cooking meats well, avoiding foods past their expiration date, and washing fruits and vegetables thoroughly during this time period. Dietitians must monitor patients for diet adequacy as some patients—being fearful of infection—may limit their food intake unnecessarily. Anemia associated with chemotherapy may be treated with erythropoietic factors to improve red cell return to the bone marrow.[36] Oncology RDs are frequently asked if there are particular foods or dietary supplements that can hasten the return of bone marrow cells. Patients need to be encouraged to consume adequate calories and protein to facilitate recovery of their bone marrow cells. Any patient with inadequate intake will suffer immune dysfunction, and this will impair recovery of the bone marrow post chemotherapy. Due to limited evidence-based research for many dietary supplements, use of these supplements is typically discouraged for this purpose.[37]

Altered taste is another common side effect of chemotherapy, and is associated most commonly with treatment consisting of cisplatin, carboplatin, cyclophosphamide (Cytoxan®), doxorubicin (Adriamycin®), 5-fluorouracil (5-FU), and methotrexate.[34-36] The use of antifungal medicines for treatment-induced thrush worsens alterations in the sense of taste, as do some antidepressants and analgesics.[37] Attention to meticulous mouth care (brushing, flossing, mouth wash or baking soda rinses) is often helpful to reduce offending tastes. Also, using plastic utensils is often effective to reduce the "metallic" taste many patients report with platinum-based chemotherapies.[36] Ongoing and aggressive counseling is necessary to recommend less offending foods and liquids. For some patients, using a straw with liquids is helpful to limit exposure of the liquid on the tongue. Others complain that the altered taste is more pronounced after swallowing. Patients must be encouraged to persevere in finding less offensive foods to maintain caloric intake. Many patients must have a feeding tube placed to avoid severe weight loss.

Table 4.4 provides a summary of recommendations for managing nutrition-related side effects of chemotherapy.

The side effect of cancer treatment universally reported by patients is fatigue.[34, 35] For some, this fatigue is debilitating and unrelenting. After ruling out anemia and other possible causes such as pain and depression, RDs can assess their patients' diets for adequate calories, protein, and fluid, and provide appropriate counseling.[34, 35]

Ongoing nutritional intervention throughout cancer diagnosis and treatment can prevent or decrease complications and the severity of side effects.[38] Maintaining good nutritional status and a healthy weight during treatment increases the likelihood of successful treatment completion. Indeed, the identification of nutritional problems and implementation of interventions for

Table 4.4 *Nutritional Management of Treatment-Related Symptoms*

Side Effect	Strategy
Nausea/vomiting/poor appetite	Clear liquids taken in small amounts; high-carbohydrate foods such as fruit and Popsicles. Set meal patterns/schedules to provide 6–8 small meals/snacks daily.
Thickened saliva	Seltzer and tonic waters, papaya nectar may help thin secretions; increased fluid intake; Consider guaifenesin (Mucinex®).
Diarrhea	Avoid high-fat foods; avoid dairy if it worsens diarrhea. Eat bananas. Consider soluble fiber supplements such as Benefiber®.
Weight loss	Eat smaller, frequent scheduled meals with nutrient-dense foods. Use calorie/protein supplements.
Neutropenia	Encourage safe food preparation/handling/cooking to avoid food-borne infections. Ensure adequate calorie/protein intake to support weight maintenance.
Altered taste	Provide regular dental care (brushing/flossing), and use baking soda/water rinses. Use plastic eating utensils if metallic taste is bothersome. Use sugar-free mints/candies or gum; use sauces/marinades on meats; try colder foods versus warm foods; use straws with liquids.
Fatigue	Assure adequate calorie, protein, and fluid intake; engage in activity as tolerated.

Sources: Byron J. Nutrition implications of chemotherapy. In: Elliott L, Molseed LL, McCallum PD, Grant B, eds., *The Clinical Guide to Oncology Nutrition.* 2nd ed. Chicago, IL: American Dietetic Association; 2006:72–87; Fishman M, Mrozek-Orlowski M, eds., *Cancer Chemotherapy Guidelines and Recommendations for Practice.* 2nd ed. Pittsburgh, PA: Oncology Nursing Press; 1999; Camp-Sorrell D. Chemotherapy: Toxicity management. In: Yarbro, MH, Frogge MH, Goodman M, et al, eds., *Cancer Nursing: Principles and Practice.* 5th ed. Sudbury, MA: Jones and Bartlett; 2000:412–455.

nutrition-related symptoms have been shown to stabilize or reverse weight loss in patients with cancer.[39] If a patient is unable to tolerate therapy due to side effects, the intent of treatment, whether curative or palliative, is compromised. The goals of nutritional care for all patients receiving chemotherapy or radiation therapy should include preserving lean body mass, preventing or reversing any known deficiencies, minimizing nutrition-related side effects, improving tolerance to treatment, protecting immune function, and maximizing quality of life.[40]

Patients receiving chemotherapy and radiation therapy should be screened for nutritional risk as soon as possible after their initial diagnosis (see Table 4.5). Those deemed to be at nutritional risk must be assessed and

Table 4.5 *Nutritional Screening and Assessment Parameters*

Anthropometrics	Laboratory Values
Weight	Albumin
Height	Complete blood count
Body mass index (BMI)	Serum electrolytes, creatinine, blood urea nitrogen
Recent weight changes	Liver function tests
Usual body weight	Micronutrient levels
Patient History	**Physical Findings**
Diet history	Muscle and fat stores
Pertinent medical history	Oral health
Medicine/supplement usage	Skin appearance
Gastrointestinal symptoms	

Sources: Blackburn GL, Bistrian BR, Maini BS, et al. Nutritional and metabolic assessment of the hospitalized patient. *J Parenter Enteral Nutr.* 1977;1:11–22; McCallum PD. Nutrition screening and assessment in oncology. In: Elliott L, Molseed LL, McCallum PD, Grant B, eds., *The Clinical Guide to Oncology Nutrition.* 2nd ed. Chicago, IL: American Dietetic Association, 2006:44–53.

followed throughout treatment according to their needs.[41] Screening includes reviewing a patient's height, weight, any recent weight loss or gain in relation to usual body weight, current dietary intake, labs, and any significant nutrition-related symptoms. Nutrition assessment then assigns a level of nutritional risk reflecting the patient's nutrient needs and the plan to manage the problem or improve symptoms.

Currently, a number of tools are available to help the oncology RD assess patients.[41] These include institution-specific guidelines, Subjective Global Assessment (SGA) and the Patient-Generated Subjective Global Assessment (PG-SGA).[42, 43] The PG-SGA is a validated tool for use in the oncology population that allows the RD to measure nutritional status and then to track changes in status, based on nutritional intervention, over a short period of time.[42, 43] The form consists of one part to be completed by the patient or caretaker, including questions related to weight history, recent eating patterns, nutrition-related symptoms, and functional status. After the patient or caretaker fills out the form, the RD or other member of the healthcare team evaluates the patient for weight loss, disease status, and metabolic stress. Next, a nutrition-related physical exam is performed looking for visible nutritional deficiencies, and the need for nutritional involvement is quantified by assigning a score to the patient. Patients deemed at significant nutritional risk are counseled and monitored closely throughout treatment and into recovery.

A system such as the PG-SGA requires a multidisciplinary commitment to the nutritional care of patients. In the face of today's nursing shortage, many clinics have difficulty implementing such a thorough screening tool. In some cases, the oncology RD must identify patients at nutritional risk via his or her own screening methods and institution-specific criteria. This can be accomplished by attending patient rounds and tumor boards, or being available during certain clinic times to identify patients at nutritional risk.

Determining the nutritional needs of patients receiving chemotherapy and/or radiation therapy can be done using a variety of methods.[44] Most RDs are quite familiar with the Harris–Benedict equation (HBE),[45] which uses a patient's height, weight, age, and sex to determine resting energy expenditure. Activity or stress/injury factors are also integrated into this equation to give the final tally of calories needed daily. Compared to indirect calorimetry, HBE often overestimates calorie needs for many patients.[46] Of note, one study found that HBE underestimated the resting energy expenditure of patients with head and neck cancer receiving radiation therapy when compared to indirect calorimetry.[47]

Although indirect calorimetry is a well-established method of determining energy needs of patients, it requires the use of equipment that is more often used and housed in the inpatient/critical care setting. Many cancer centers do not have access to this equipment. Recent studies have validated the use of Mifflin–St. Joer formula to more accurately assess the energy expenditure of healthy outpatients,[48] but this formula has not yet been validated in oncology patients or acutely ill individuals.

In the end, dietitians must use clinical judgment when assessing the calorie needs of cancer patients. And, because calorie needs can and do change throughout the course of therapy, it is important to track weights in relation to caloric intake to assess whether goals are being met or need to be changed. Current treatment intensity, the patient's general health, and performance status at the start of treatment should be considered when estimating calorie and protein needs.

It is a common misconception that all patients with cancer have increased calorie needs. Studies have shown this is not the case: Only some 30% of cancer patients actually have increased needs.[44, 49] Some data support increased calorie needs in patients with cancers of the head and neck.[47] Weekly weights and careful record keeping of calories eaten by the patient are necessary to accurately determine the level of calorie support needed by the patient. Because patients are typically quite fatigued and suffering treatment-related side effects, family members and friends are often enlisted to help with this process. In one study conducted within the head and neck cancer population receiving radiotherapy, patients reported increased intake with the support and encouragement of family.[50]

Nutrition counseling has been shown to improve nutritional status and quality of life significantly in patients with head and neck and gastrointestinal cancers.[51] Individual counseling may be the most effective nutrition intervention to affect nutritional status. This type of interaction involves giving patient-specific information to help the individual manage nutrition-related symptoms. Some studies have indicated that intensive nutrition counseling can significantly improve dietary intake in patients receiving radiation therapy.[52] Other studies have shown that medical nutrition therapy can improve calorie/protein intake, help maintain weight, and increase quality of life.[53]

To be effective, nutrition counseling must be thorough and frequent. For example, patients receiving combined chemotherapy and radiation for cancer of the head and neck can lose weight rapidly when symptoms of mucositis and dysphagia begin, which typically occur by the second week of treatment. Ideally, the RD should counsel the patient on the need for aggressive nutritional intake prior to the onset of the side effects. Weekly follow-up visits are crucial for managing side effects as they develop. The oncology RD must identify nutrient-dense foods that the patient will and can eat, and then provide specific information about the recommended amounts to eat daily. This process involves lengthy discussions regarding food preferences, identification of tolerances, and clear instructions regarding serving sizes and types of foods to buy and eat. Patient-specific meal patterns can illustrate the types and amounts of foods needed to meet nutritional needs, in conjunction with the medical management of pain, nausea, and other side effects. Weekly weights and symptom assessments will help to identify problems that affect patient intake. Food records kept by patients may be evaluated to determine whether patients are meeting their estimated nutritional needs.

Nutrition Support During Oncologic Therapies

Ideally, patients undergoing treatment for cancer will meet their nutritional needs via oral intake. The oral route is physiologically superior and should be maintained as long as possible.[38] Recommending modified textures, fortifying calories in liquids and soft solids, and spacing out eating times are important management tips to help patients complete treatment with minimal nutritional compromise. Liquid medical food supplements are widely used today to boost calorie and protein intake. These flavored supplements, which often replace some or most of a meal's calories and protein content, can minimize large weight losses. This, in turn, is helpful in preventing treatment interruptions.[38, 39] Modular carbohydrate, protein, and fat products are also available and can be added to a variety of common foods to boost caloric, protein, or fat intake. While patients should always be encouraged to maintain some level of oral intake of foods, many become reliant on the use of supplements as a significant source of calories and protein during treatment.

Simply telling patients to drink a nutritional supplement is rarely enough. Patients are more likely to meet their nutritional needs if they are given a number of cans or supplements to consume daily. This type of education also makes patients more accountable in the management of their care.

Although many patients are willing to use nutritional supplements early on, taste fatigue and aversion after prolonged use of these products are quite common.[38] The nutritional supplements typically used by cancer patients are flavored milk-type supplements (although most are lactose-free). Juice-type calorie/protein-fortified medical food supplements are available as well. Given that the side effects associated with radiation continue one to two weeks after completion of treatment, ongoing follow-up after treatment ends is important to assure continued attention to adequate nutrition. Weight monitoring and symptom tracking are often useful in adjusting supplement requirements post treatment.

Despite the widespread availability and relatively modest cost of nutritional supplements, many patients are unable to afford them. Generic formulas, which are nutritionally comparable to the brand-name products, are available and less expensive. It is vital that the entire multidisciplinary team, but especially the social worker, be prepared to assist with issues that can affect intake and ultimately nutritional status, such as ability to purchase nutritional supplements. The oncology RD can also provide patients with recipes for homemade supplements. These mixtures are frequently better tolerated if patients have caregiver support or the energy to prepare drinks, shakes, or fortified foods.

Patients receiving radiation and/or chemotherapy—and especially those being treated for cancers of the head and neck, thorax, and gastrointestinal tract—may require nutritional support beyond what medical food supplements and food can provide. Tumor-related symptoms, increased metabolic needs, and the inability to meet nutritional needs orally are all indications for nutrition support.[54] The use of nutrition support in individuals with cancer is still the subject of debate, with some researchers suggesting that it may have detrimental effects on outcomes and length of life. However, when used appropriately, enteral and parenteral nutrition support have been shown to be an effective way to nourish cancer patients who cannot maintain adequate oral intake.[54, 55] Malnourished cancer patients may benefit from nutrition support by achieving increased energy, strength, activity level, and weight gain.[54] Patients with cancers (especially those of the head and neck) that are treated with radiation alone or with chemoradiation often develop significant mucositis, taste changes, thickened saliva, nausea, and vomiting that preclude oral intake as a sole source of nutrient intake. Prophylactic percutaneous endoscopic gastrostomy (PEG) tube placement before treatment begins is becoming more accepted when the toxicity of treatment is expected to be severe.[25, 31] Patients with cancer who may benefit from nutrition support include those with recent significant weight loss (more than 10% usual body weight within the previous 6 months), those unable to eat or drink for more than 5 days, and those with known malabsorption, small bowel obstruction, or fistulas affected by oral intake.[47]

Enteral nutrition is the preferred nutrition support route, as it is the most physiologic. Feeding into the gut maintains the integrity of the gastrointestinal tract, thereby avoiding the risk of bacterial translocation.[38] The translocation of bacteria into the systemic circulation can lead to sepsis, organ failure, and death.[56] PEG tubes are often used in patients receiving cancer treatment when the expected duration of use is greater than 2 weeks. PEG tubes have a larger diameter than nasogastric tubes, so they allow for easier passage of tube feeding products as well as medications. PEG tubes also reduce the risk of aspiration compared to nasogastric tubes.[55]

The primary oncologist should present the option of feeding tube placement as part of a patient's overall treatment plan. The psychological effects of PEG tubes are variable and not well studied; however, they may include depression, stress, and change in lifestyle.[50] Early discussion with the patient and caregivers at the time of diagnosis and education regarding the indi-cations for the tube, expected length of use, and benefits of aggressive nutritional intervention are helpful to reduce anxiety related to these tubes. Often, patients have fears based on past experiences with family members or friends, and education and reassurance may be helpful in overcoming their trepidation. It is this author's experience that feeding tubes placed in patients who are undergoing treatment are less effective owing to an increased rate of complications, more pain associated with the procedure, and less tolerance to tube feedings after placement. Patients who undergo gastrostomy tube placement prior to head and neck radiation treatment, by contrast, lose less weight during the treatment course and have increased quality of life.[26, 57]

Enteral formulas are typically infused via a bolus method by syringe (over 10–30 minutes) or through a continuous feeding pump. Although enteral nutrition is not risk free, it is considered to be safer than parenteral feeding.[58] Patients can usually tolerate standard polymeric formulas, either isocaloric (1 cal/mL) or calorically dense (2 cal/mL) for those with volume intolerances. Carbohydrates are usually the major calorie source, with whey or casein supplying the protein content. Fat is typically provided via vegetable oils or triglycerides.

Specialty formulas are available, but their benefits and drawbacks should be weighed carefully relative to standard formulas. Many are difficult to obtain through local pharmacies or home health companies, and they are usually quite expensive compared to standard formulas. Immuno-enhanced enteral feeding (formulas with added omega-3 fatty acids, arginine, and nucleotides) may decrease postoperative complications from gastrointestinal surgeries when given preoperatively to very malnourished cancer patients.[24] Currently, there is limited support for tube feeding (and oral) products formulated for cancer patients and enriched with eicosopentanoic acid (EPA). While some research has shown that EPA can be an effective modulator of cancer cachexia, this relationship has not been proven in larger, well-designed studies.[59]

Parenteral nutrition (PN) delivers nutrients directly into the circulation via a central vein or a peripheral vein. PN may be necessary in a select population of cancer patients receiving treatment, including those with gut dysfunction receiving aggressive treatment, short bowel syndrome, intractable nausea and vomiting with enteral feedings, bowel obstruction, or enterocutaneous fistulas requiring bowel rest. Contraindications for PN include a functional gut, poor prognosis, or nutritional support that is needed for less than five days.

PN carries more risk than enteral feedings. Because it is administered via vein, there is a higher risk of infection with both peripheral and central parenteral nutrition support. Most patients requiring PN are weaned off and transitioned back to an oral diet as soon as possible.

The use of PN in patients with cancer is controversial. Some studies support the use of preoperative PN in malnourished patients with gastrointestinal cancer.[38, 60] Those receiving such nutrition support develop fewer surgical complications and infection and have decreased mortality.[38, 60] Other studies have shown contradictory results, likely due to small sample sizes, variations in the patient populations studied, and differences in treatment plans.[60] Despite the inconsistent results, the risks of overfeeding associated with PN have been identified and new practice recommendations made.[60] It appears that PN during chemotherapy is most appropriate for those patients with significant weight loss and malnutrition who are responding to the prescribed treatment.[60] Limited studies are available on PN use during radiation therapy; the ones that have been published do not show any survival benefit or reduction in treatment toxicity with this type of nutritional therapy.[60] Patients with radiation enteritis may require bowel rest, and a course of PN may be warranted in such cases to prevent nutritional decline.

Clearly, the advantages and disadvantages of PN should be considered carefully before such treatment is undertaken in cancer patients. The American Society for Parenteral and Enteral Nutrition and the American Dietetic Association Oncology Evidence Analysis Library provide guidelines for appropriate use of PN in this population to help guide the oncology RD and other clinicians.

SUMMARY

Chemotherapy and radiation therapy are key components in the care of many patients with cancer who cannot be treated by surgery alone. Advances in these cancer treatments continue to emerge, yet these therapies still cause significant toxicities that negatively affect many patients. Because this population has unique nutritional needs, early and ongoing intervention by a RD is essential to assist in the multidisciplinary care of these patients. The oncology RD provides individualized counseling to patients and families, and helps guide other members of the healthcare team regarding the nutritional status of those treated. This type of nutritional counseling can improve both quality of life and outcomes in patients with cancer. This chapter should equip healthcare professionals working with oncology patients with a better understanding of both radiation and chemotherapy principles, and assist them in understanding the nutrition screening, assessment, and counseling processes. Ultimately, the goal is to provide cancer patients with the best nutritional care centered on evidence-based practice.

REFERENCES

1. American Cancer Society. *Cancer Facts and Figures, 2008*. Atlanta, GA: Author; 2008.
2. Knoll, AH. The early evolution of eukaryotes: A geological perspective. *Science*. 1992;256:622–627.
3. Puck TT, Markus PI. Action of x-rays on mammalian cells. *J Exp Med*. 1956;103: 653–666.
4. Spear FG. On some biological effects of radiation. *Br J Radiology*. 1958;31:114–124.
5. Cox JD. *Moss's Radiation Oncology: Rationale, Techniques, Results*. 7th ed. St. Louis, MO: Mosby; 1994.
6. National Comprehensive Cancer Network, Inc. The National Comprehensive Cancer Network clinical practice guidelines in oncology. 2008. http://www.nccn.org.
7. Hall EJ, Giaccia AJ. *Radiobiology for the Radiologist*. 6th ed. Philadelphia, PA: Lippincott Williams and Wilkins; 2006.
8. Roentgen WC. On a new kind of rays (preliminary communication). Translation of a paper read before the Physi-kalische-medicinischen Gesellschaft of Wursburg December 12, 1895. *Br J Radiol*. 1931;4:32.
9. Curie P, Curie P, Bemont G. Sur une nouvelle substance fortement radioactive continue dans la pechblende. *Compt Rend Acad Sci (Paris)*. 1898;127:1215–1217.
10. Perez CA, Brady LW. *Principles and Practice of Radiation Oncology*. 2nd ed. Philadelphia, PA: J.B. Lippincott; 1992.
11. Khan FM. *The Physics of Radiation Therapy*. Baltimore, MD: Lippincott Williams and Wilkins; 1984.
12. Tapley N. *Clinical Applications of the Electron Beam*. New York, NY: John Wiley and Sons; 1976.

13. Lodge M, Pijls-Johannesma M, Stirk L, et al. A systematic literature review of the clinical and cost effectiveness of hadron therapy in cancer. *Radiother Oncol.* 2007;83(2):110–122.

14. Brizel DM, Wasserman TH, Henke M, et al. Phase III randomized trial of amifostine as a radioprotector in head and neck cancer. *J Clin Oncol.* 2000;18:3339–3345.

15. Kavanagh BD, Timmerman RD. *Stereotactic Body Radiation Therapy.* Philadelphia, PA: Lippincott Williams and Wilkins; 2005.

16. Hadju SI. 2000 years of chemotherapy of tumors. *Cancer.* 2005;103(6):1097–1102.

17. Kardinal CG. Cancer chemotherapy: Historical aspects and future considerations. *Postgraduate Medicine.* 1985;77:165–174.

18. Papac RJ. Origins of cancer chemotherapy. *Yale J Biol Med.* 2001;74:391–398.

19. Goodman LS, Wintrobe MM, Dameshek W, et al. Nitrogen mustard therapy. Use of methyl-bis(beta-chloroethyl)amine hydrochloride and tris(beta-chloroethyl) amine hydrochloride for Hodgkin's disease, lymphosarcoma, leukemia and certain allied and miscellaneous disorders. *JAMA.* 1946;132:126–132.

20. Chu EC, DeVita VT. *Physicians' Cancer Chemotherapy Drug Manual 2006.* Sudbury, MA: Jones and Bartlett; 2006.

21. Goldman JM, Melo JV. Chronic myeloid leukemia: Advances in biology and new approaches to treatment. *N Engl J Med.* 2003;349:1451–1464.

22. Dalle S, Thieblemont C, Thomas L, Dumontet C. Monoclonal antibodies in clinical oncology. *Anticancer Agents Med Chem.* 2008;8:523–532.

23. Shankar S, Srivastava RK. Histone deacetylase inhibitors: Mechanisms and clinical significance in cancer: HDAC inhibitor-induced apoptosis. *Adv Exp Med Biol.* 2008;615:261–298.

24. Allen A. Epigenetic alterations and cancer: New targets for therapy. *IDrugs.* 2007;10:709–712.

25. Rowland JH, Hewitt M, Ganz PA. Cancer survivorship: A new challenge in delivering quality cancer care. *J Clin Oncol.* 2006;24:5101–5104.

26. Lee, JH, Machtay M, Unger LD, et al. Prophylactic gastrostomy tubes in patients undergoing intensive irradiation for cancer of the head and neck. *Arch Otolaryngol Head Neck Surg.* 1998;124:871–875.

27. Blackburn GL, Bistrian BR, Maini BS, et al. Nutritional and metabolic assessment of the hospitalized patient. *J Parenter Enteral Nutr.* 1977;1:11–22.

28. Nitenburg G, Raynard B. Nutritional support of the cancer patient: Issues and dilemmas. *Crit Rev Oncol-Hematol.* 2000;34:137–168.

29. Unsal D, Mentes B, Akmansu M, et al. Evaluation of nutritional status in cancer patients receiving radiotherapy: A prospective study. *Am J Clin Oncol.* 2006;29: 183–188.

30. Von Roenn JH. Pharmacological management of nutrition impact symptoms associated with cancer. In: Elliott L, Molseed LL, McCallum PD, Grant B, eds. *The Clinical Guide to Oncology Nutrition.* 2nd ed. Chicago, IL: American Dietetic Association; 2006:165-179.

31. Chencharick JD, Mossman KL. Nutritional consequences of the radiotherapy of head and neck cancer. *Cancer.* 1983;51:811–815.

32. Lees J. Incidence of weight loss in head and neck cancer patients on commencing radiotherapy treatment at a regional oncology center. *Eur J Cancer Care.* 1999;8: 133–136.

33. Beaver ME, Matheny KE, Roberts DB, Myers JN. Predictors of weight loss during radiation therapy. *Otolaryngol Head Neck Surg.* 2001;125:645–648.

34. Byron J. Nutrition implications of chemotherapy. In: Elliott L, Molseed LL, McCallum PD, Grant B, eds. *The Clinical Guide to Oncology Nutrition.* 2nd ed. Chicago, IL: American Dietetic Association; 2006:72–87.

35. Fishman M, Mrozek-Orlowski M, eds. *Cancer Chemotherapy Guidelines and Recommendations for Practice.* 2nd ed. Pittsburgh, PA: Oncology Nursing Press; 1999.

36. Camp-Sorrell D. Chemotherapy: Toxicity management. In: Yarbro, MH, Frogge MH, Goodman M, et al, eds. *Cancer nursing: Principles and Practice.* 5th ed. Sudbury, MA: Jones and Bartlett; 2000:412–455.

37. Doyle C, Kushi L, Byers T, et al. Nutrition and physical activity during and after cancer treatment: An American Cancer Society guide for informed choices. *CA Cancer J Clin.* 2006;56:323–353.

38. Rivandeneira DE, Evoy D, Fahey TJ, et al. Nutritional support of the cancer patient. *CA Cancer J Clin.* 1998;48:69–80.

39. Whitman MM. The starving patient: Supportive care for people with cancer. *Clin J Oncol Nurs.* 2000;4:121–125.

40. Dempsey DT, Mullen JL, Buzby GP. The link between nutritional status and clinical outcome: Can nutritional intervention modify it? *Am J Clin Nutr.* 1988;47 (suppl 2):352–356.

41. McCallum PD. Nutrition screening and assessment in oncology. In: Elliott L, Molseed LL, McCallum PD, Grant B, eds., *The Clinical Guide to Oncology Nutrition.* 2nd ed. Chicago, IL: American Dietetic Association; 2006:44–53.

42. Ottery FD. Definition of standardized nutritional assessment and interventional pathways in oncology. *Nutrition.* 1996;12(suppl 1): S15–S19.

43. Bauer J, Capra S, Ferguson M. Use of the scored Patient-Generated Subjective Global Assessment (PG-SGA) as a nutrition assessment tool in patients with cancer. *Eur J Clin Nutr.* 2002;56:779–785.

44. Hurst JD, Gallagher AL. Energy, macronutrient, and fluid requirements. In: Elliott L, Molseed LL, McCallum PD, Grant B, eds. *The Clinical Guide to Oncology Nutrition.* 2nd ed. Chicago, IL: American Dietetic Association; 2006:54–71.

45. Harris JA, Benedict FG. *Biometric studies of basal metabolism in men* (Publication 270). Washington, DC: Carnegie Institute of Washington; 1919.

46. Frankenfield DC, Rowe WA, Smith JS, Cooney RN. Validation of several established equations for resting metabolic rate in obese and non obese people. *J Am Diet Assoc.* 2003;103:1152–1159.

47. Garcia-Peris P, Lozano MA, Velasco C, et al. Prospective study of resting energy expenditure changes in head and neck cancer patients treated with chemoradiotherapy measured by indirect calorimetry. *Nutrition.* 2005;21:1107–1112.

48. Mifflin MD, St. Joer ST, Hill LA, et al. A new predictive equation for resting energy expenditure in healthy individuals. *Am J Clin Nutr.* 1990;51:241–247.

49. Knox LS, Crosby LO, Feurer ID, et al. Energy expenditure in malnourished cancer patients. *Ann Surg.* 1983;197:152–162.

50. Larsson M, Hedelin B, Athlin E. Lived experiences of eating problems for patients with head and neck cancer during radiotherapy. *J Clin Nurs.* 2003;12:562–570.

51. Isenring EA, Capra S, Bauer JD. Nutrition intervention is beneficial in oncology outpatients receiving radiotherapy to the gastrointestinal or head and neck area. *Br J Cancer.* 2004;91:447–452.

52. Isenring EA, Bauer JD, Capra S. Nutrition support using the American Dietetic Association medical nutrition therapy protocol for radiation oncology patients improves dietary intake compared with standard practice. *J Am Diet Assoc.* 2007; 107:404–412.

53. American Dietetic Association. Evidence-based nutrition practice guideline on oncology. http://www.adaevidencelibrary.com/template.cfm?template=guide_summary&key=1751. Published October 2007. Accessed December 21, 2008.

54. Capra S, Bauer J, Davidson W, Ash S. Nutritional therapy for cancer-induced weight loss. *Nutr Clin Practice.* 2002;17:210–213.

55. Wong PW, Enriquez A, Barrera R. Nutritional support in critically ill patients with cancer. *Crit Care Clin.* 2001;17:743–767.

56. Alexander WJ. Bacterial translocation during enteral and parenteral nutrition. *Proc Nutr Soc.* 1998;57:389–393.

57. Nguyen NP, North D, Smith HJ, et al. Safety and effectiveness of prophylactic gastrostomy tubes for head and neck cancer patients undergoing chemoradiation. *Surg Oncol.* 2006;15:199–203.

58. Robinson CA. Enteral nutrition in adult oncology. In: Elliott L, Molseed LL, McCallum PD, Grant B, eds. *The Clinical Guide to Oncology Nutrition.* 2nd ed. Chicago, IL: American Dietetic Association; 2006:138–155.

59. Jatoi A, Loprinzi CL, Rowland K, et al. An eicosapentanoic acid supplement versus megastrol acetate versus both for patients with cancer associated wasting: A North Central Cancer Treatment Group and National Cancer Institute of Canada collaborative effort. *J Clin Oncol.* 2004;22:2469–2476.

60. Chan S, Blackburn GL. Total parenteral nutrition in cancer patients. Orthomolecular oncology. http://www.canceraction.org.gg/tpn/htm. Accessed December 21, 2008.

Chapter 5

Surgical Oncology

Maureen B. Huhmann, DCN, RD, CSO
David August, MD

INTRODUCTION

Malnutrition is a significant contributor to surgical morbidity and mortality in cancer patients.[1] The role of nutrition support therapy (NST)—either enteral or parenteral—in the prevention and treatment of the malnutrition in surgical oncology patients has been explored in depth.[2–5] This research has elucidated both benefits and risks to these therapeutic interventions. This chapter discusses the role of NST in cancer patients undergoing primarily gastrointestinal (GI) surgery and the evidence on which it is based.

Consequences of Malnutrition

Malnutrition is defined as "any disorder of nutrition status, including disorders resulting from deficiency of nutrient intake, impaired nutrient metabolism, or overnutrition."[6] The prevalence of weight loss in oncology patients ranges from 31% to 100%, depending on tumor site, stage, and treatment (Table 5.1).[2, 7–10] Minimal weight loss, in the range of 5%, is associated with increased mortality and poor prognosis for a patients with a variety of tumor types.[7] Multiple factors contribute to the weight loss observed in cancer patients, including complications arising from the tumor itself, such as obstruction or tumor-induced anorexia; treatment-induced complications such as gastrointestinal (GI) symptoms, fatigue, or loss of anatomy; and psychological stress.[11–15]

Cancer cachexia is another common cause of weight loss in this patient population. Cancer cachexia syndrome (CCS) is characterized by progressive, involuntary weight loss that often presents as host tissue wasting, anorexia, skeletal muscle atrophy, anergy, fatigue, anemia, and hypoalbuminemia. This syndrome is potentially life-threatening; it is caused by physiologic and metabolic derangements[16, 17] that lead to depletion of energy

Table 5.1   *Incidence of Weight Loss or Malnutrition in Adult Cancer Patients by Primary Tumor Site*

Site of Cancer	Bozetti[1]*	DeWys et al.[2]†	Hammerlid et al.[3]*	Others
Acute non-lymphocytic leukemia		39%		
Breast	9%[4]–36%[5]	36%		
Bronchial carcinoma	66%[5]			
Colon	54%[4]	54%		
Colorectal	60%[6,7]			
Diffuse lymphoma	55%[8]			
Esophagus	79%[5]		100%	85%[9]†
Gastric	83%[2]	83–87%		44%[9]†
General cancer population	60%[10]–63%[11]			
Head and neck	72%[12]			57%[13]*
Larynx			40%	
Lung (all types)	50%[4]			
Lung (non-small cell)		61%		
Lung (small cell)	60%[4]	57%		
Lung (squamous cell)	36%[4]			
Neuroblastoma	56%[14]			
Non-Hodgkin's lymphoma (favorable)		31%		
Non-Hodgkin's lymphoma (unfavorable)		48%		
Oral cavity			63%	41%[15]†
Pancreas	83%[2]	83%		
Prostate	56%[4]	56%		
Rectum	40%[5]			
Sarcoma	39%[4]–66%[16]	40%		
Sinus			30%	
Skin			50%	
Testicular	25%[17]			

*Results described as "malnutrition."
†Results described as "weight loss" of any amount.

(continues)

Table 5.1 *Incidence of Weight Loss or Malnutrition in Adult Cancer Patients by Primary Tumor Site, Continued*

Data Sources
1. Bozzetti F. Rationale and indications for preoperative feeding of malnourished surgical cancer patients. *Nutrition.* 2002;18(11–12):953–959.
2. DeWys WD, Begg C, Lavin PT, et al. Prognostic effect of weight loss prior to chemotherapy in cancer patients: Eastern Cooperative Oncology Group. *Am J Med.* 1980;69(4):491–497.
3. Hammerlid E, Wirblad B, Sandin C, et al. Malnutrition and food intake in relation to quality of life in head and neck cancer patients. *Head Neck.* 1998;20(6):540–548.
4. Issell BF, Valdivieso M, Zaren HA, et al. Protection against chemotherapy toxicity by IV hyperalimentation. *Cancer Treat Rep.* 1978;62(8):1139–1143.
5. Bashir Y, Graham TR, Torrance A, Gibson GJ, Corris PA. Nutritional state of patients with lung cancer undergoing thoracotomy. *Thorax.* 1990;45(3):183–186.
6. Nixon DW, Lawson DH, Kutner MH, et al. Effect of total parenteral nutrition on survival in advanced colon cancer. *Cancer Detect Prev.* 1981;4(1–4):421–427.
7. Nixon DW, Moffitt S, Lawson DH, et al. Total parenteral nutrition as an adjunct to chemotherapy of metastatic colorectal cancer. *Cancer Treat Rep.* 1981;65(suppl 5):121–128.
8. Popp MB, Fisher RI, Wesley R, Aamodt R, Brennan MF. A prospective randomized study of adjuvant parenteral nutrition in the treatment of advanced diffuse lymphoma: Influence on survival. *Surgery.* 1981;90(2):195–203.
9. Haugstvedt TK, Viste A, Eide GE, Soreide O. Factors related to and consequences of weight loss in patients with stomach cancer: The Norwegian multicenter experience. Norwegian Stomach Cancer Trial. *Cancer.* 1991;67(3):722–729.
10. Bozzetti F, Migliavacca S, Scotti A, et al. Impact of cancer, type, site, stage and treatment on the nutritional status of patients. *Ann Surg.* 1982;196(2):170–179.
11. Tan YS, Nambiar R, Yo SL. Prevalence of protein calorie malnutrition in general surgical patients. *Ann Acad Med Singapore.* 1992;21(3):334–338.
12. Goodwin WJ Jr, Torres J. The value of the Prognostic Nutritional Index in the management of patients with advanced carcinoma of the head and neck. *Head Neck Surg.* 1984;6(5):932–937.
13. Linn BS, Robinson DS, Klimas NG. Effects of age and nutritional status on surgical outcomes in head and neck cancer. *Ann Surg.* 1988;207(3):267–273.
14. Rickard KA, Loghmani ES, Grosfeld JL, et al. Short- and long-term effectiveness of enteral and parenteral nutrition in reversing or preventing protein-energy malnutrition in advanced neuroblastoma: A prospective randomized study. *Cancer.* 1985;56(12):2881–2897.
15. Nguyen TV, Yueh B. Weight loss predicts mortality after recurrent oral cavity and oropharyngeal carcinomas. *Cancer.* 2002;95(3):553–562.
16. Shamberger RC, Brennan MF, Goodgame JT Jr, et al. A prospective, randomized study of adjuvant parenteral nutrition in the treatment of sarcomas: Results of metabolic and survival studies. *Surgery.* 1984;96(1):1–13.
17. Samuels ML, Selig DE, Ogden S, Grant C, Brown B. IV hyperalimentation and chemotherapy for stage III testicular cancer: A randomized study. *Cancer Treat Rep.* 1981;65(7–8):615–627.

and protein stores in cancer patients.[18] In contrast to starvation, CCS results in the loss of both adipose and skeletal muscle mass, while visceral muscle mass is preserved and hepatic mass increases.[19] Also unlike starvation, the weight loss associated with CCS generally cannot be reversed with increases in nutrient intake alone,[20] and it continues despite increased administration of nutrients.[19] Appetite stimulants are only minimally effective for treatment of CCS.[19] Whereas starvation elicits a conservation response in the host, CCS is characterized by increased cycling (synthesis and catabolism) of a variety of metabolic intermediaries, including amino acids, fatty acids, and carbohydrates.[21, 22]

Although there is no universally accepted model that adequately explains the etiology of CCS in all patients,[23] CCS is caused in part by pro-inflammatory cytokines such as tumor necrosis factor, interferon-γ, and interleukin-1 and -6. Tumor-produced substances such as proteolysis-inducing factor, lipid-mobilizing factor, and mitochondria-uncoupling proteins 1, 2, and 3 also affect nutrient metabolism.[24]

Diagnosis of CCS and the promotion of nutritional adequacy are essential in surgical patients with cancer. Indeed, the presence of malnutrition has important consequences for recovery following surgery. For example, preoperative malnutrition is highly correlated with postoperative morbidity.[25] Suboptimal intake of nutrients produces changes in intermediary metabolism, tissue function, and body composition.[26] In addition, major surgery itself is linked with deterioration in nutrition status,[25] as major surgical procedures are associated with a higher incidence of complications, longer hospital stays, prolonged anorexia, and protein calorie malnutrition.[25, 27]

Nutrition Assessment

Oncology-related nutritional issues are best addressed within the context of the Nutrition Care Process (NCP). In 2003, the American Dietetic Association published a description of a model of the NCP,[28] which provides a framework for the critical analysis and decision-making process regarding medical nutrition therapy. As illustrated in Figure 5.1, this process contains four steps: nutrition assessment, nutrition diagnosis, nutrition intervention, and nutrition monitoring and evaluation.[28]

Nutrition Screening

It is difficult to define and measure nutrition status in cancer patients. Many markers utilized for assessing nutrition status (e.g., serum albumin, total lymphocyte count, immune competence, anthropometric changes, body composition) may also be affected by the severity of the underlying cancer. Differentiation of the effects of malnutrition from the effects of disease severity is problematic.

Nevertheless, several parameters have been explored as indicators of nutrition status. Hypoalbuminemia is associated with increased surgical mortality and morbidity, especially that related to sepsis and poor healing.[1] Unfortunately, the interaction between malnutrition and the acute-phase

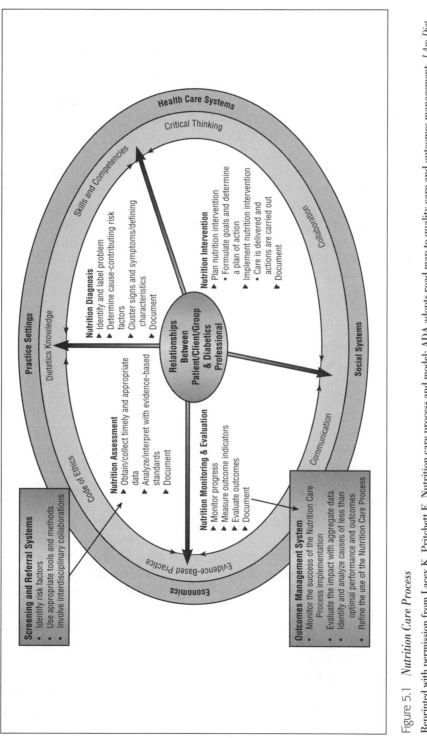

Figure 5.1 *Nutrition Care Process*

Reprinted with permission from Lacey K, Pritchett E. Nutrition care process and model: ADA adopts road map to quality care and outcomes management. *J Am Diet Assoc.* 2003;103(8):1061–1072.

response proteins limits the use of nutrition indicators such as albumin and prealbumin for specifically assessing nutrition status. Weight loss, another suggested indicator, can also be an unreliable indicator of nutritional status in cancer patients owing to fluid shifts and the presence of edema. It has been suggested that neither albumin nor weight loss in isolation is a specific predictor of complications,[29] although both are strong predictors within multivariable models. Many formulae have been developed to predict the impact of nutrition status related to morbidity and mortality in surgical patients; the predictive value of these formulae varies (Table 5.2).[27]

Nutrition screening, as a precursor step to identify those patients who should undergo a more formal nutrition assessment, facilitates the early recognition of malnutrition.[28] The American Society for Parenteral and Enteral Nutrition (A.S.P.E.N.) and the American Dietetic Association (ADA) recommend that all cancer patients undergo nutrition screening as a component of their initial evaluation.[6, 30] The purpose of such screening is to identify quickly those individuals who are at risk for nutritional deterioration as well as those individuals who are malnourished. An effective screening process utilizes both objective and subjective data that can be obtained quickly.[30] In this process, individual objective measures, such as a single laboratory parameter or current weight, are not specific enough to indicate nutrition risk.[31] Instead, multiple objective measures must be combined with subjective measures related to nutrition.[30] To facilitate routine screening of all patients, nutrition screening tools should also be easy to use, cost-effective, valid, reliable, and sensitive.[6]

Several nutrition screening tools have been used in the cancer population to identify those patients who are at greatest risk for developing nutritional problems. The Patient-Generated Subjective Global Assessment (PG-SGA)[32] is a modification of an earlier screening tool called the Subjective Global Assessment (SGA)[33]. It is broken into two sections: a patient-completed section, which includes data regarding weight history, symptoms, dietary intake, and activity level; and a section completed by the healthcare professional, which evaluates metabolic demand, considers disease in relation to nutritional requirements, and incorporates a physical assessment (Table 5.3). A numeric score is calculated by adding the points obtained in both of the two sections. A score of 4–8 requires an intervention by a dietitian, and a score greater than 9 indicates the need for improved symptom management. A SGA score of mild, moderate, or severe malnutrition is assigned based on this overall assessment. The numeric scores generated in this way can be used as a triage system to initiate a formal nutrition assessment leading to intervention and to guide follow-up care.[34, 35] The PG-SGA numeric score, when repeated at subsequent time points, is also useful for identifying small improvements or deteriorations in nutrition status.[36]

Table 5.2   *Nutritional Assessment Formulae/Methods in Gastrointestinal Surgery*

	History/Uses	Formula
Subjective Global Assessment (SGA)[1]	• Validated in a number of diverse patient populations[1]	Utilizes physical assessment, weight change, change in intake, GI symptoms, and functional capacity to assign a score: SGA-A: well nourished SGA-B: moderately malnourished SGA-C: severely malnourished
Prognostic Nutritional Index (PNI)[2]	• Validated prospectively • Calculates percentage risk of an operative complication occurring in an individual • Can distinguish patients at low risk for nutrition-related complications (<10%) from those at high risk (>50%)	Percentage risk of complication = 158 − 16.6(serum albumin; g/dL) − 0.78(TSF; mm) − 0.20(serum transferrin; g/dL) −5.8 (delayed hypersensitivity reaction)
Nutrition Risk Index (NRI)[3, 4]	• Used to stratify nutrition risk in the Veterans Affairs Total Parenteral Nutrition Cooperative Study Group trial of perioperative PN • Classifies individuals as either well nourished or malnourished	NRI = 1.519(serum albumin; g/dL) + 41.7(current weight/usual weight)
Hospital Prognostic Index (HPI)[5]	• Identifies high-risk patients and evaluates the efficacy of hospital therapy	HPI = 0.91(serum albumin; g/dL) − 1.0(delayed hypersensitivity reaction) − 1.44(sepsis rating) + 0.98(diagnosis rating) − 1.09

TSF: triceps skin fold.
Delayed hypersensitivity reaction: 0 = nonreactive, 1 = 5-mm induration, 2 = >5-mm induration.
PN: total parenteral nutrition.
Sepsis rating: 1 = present, 2 = absent.
Diagnosis rating: 1 = cancer present, 2 = cancer not present.

Data Sources
1. Detsky AS, McLaughlin JR, Baker JP, et al. What is subjective global assessment of nutritional status? *JPEN J Parenter Enteral Nutr*. 1987;11(1):8–13.
2. Buzby GP, Mullen JL, Matthews DC, Hobbs CL, Rosato EF. Prognostic Nutritional Index in gastrointestinal surgery. *Am J Surg*. 1980;139(1):160–167.
3. Veterans Affairs Total Parenteral Nutrition Cooperative Study Group. Perioperative total parenteral nutrition in surgical patients. *N Engl J Med*. 1991;325(8):525–532.
4. Franch-Arcas G. The meaning of hypoalbuminaemia in clinical practice. *Clin Nutr*. 2001;20(3):265–269.
5. Harvey KB, Moldawer LL, Bistrian BR, Blackburn GL. Biological measures for the formulation of a hospital prognostic index. *Am J Clin Nutr*. 1981;34(10):2013–2022.

Table Source: Adapted with permission from August DA, Huhmann MB. Nutritional care of cancer patients. In: Norton J, Barie P, Bollinger R, et al., eds. *Surgery: Basic Science and Clinical Evidence*. 2nd ed. New York, NY: Springer; 2008:2123–2150.

Table 5.3   *Patient-Generated Subjective Global Assessment*

Section	Components
Patient-completed section	Weight history Symptoms Food intake Activity level
Healthcare professional–completed section	Metabolic demand Diagnosis and comorbidities Physical examination
Scoring	Each question is assigned a numeric score. • Score 2–3: Patient and family education • Score 4–8: Intervention by dietitian • Score > 9: Improved symptom management and/or nutrient intervention

Source: Ottery FD. Definition of standardized nutritional assessment and interventional pathways in oncology. *Nutrition.* 1996;12(1)(suppl):S15–S19.

The Nestlé Mini Nutritional Assessment (MNA), an 18-item screening tool commonly used in older adult patients, was developed by Guigoz with Nestlé Nutritional Corporation.[37] This tool can be broken into two main components: screening and assessment. The six-item screen takes approximately three minutes to complete and includes questions related to changes in food intake, weight loss, mobility, stress, and body mass index (BMI). If the score is 11 or less, the healthcare practitioner should complete the assessment section of the MNA.[37] The assessment component includes specific medical history and eating habits as well as some anthropometric measurements. Empirical evidence on the use of this instrument in the cancer population is limited, making it an area of focus for research.

Several abbreviated nutrition screening tools have also been developed. The Malnutrition Screening Tool (MST) is a short nutrition screening tool that is rarely used in the United States. This three-item tool utilizes data on weight history and appetite to predict nutrition risk. The MST has been validated in both hospitalized non-oncology patients[38] and oncology patients receiving radiation therapy.[39] Another short tool, the Malnutrition Universal Screening Tool (MUST), also utilizes a score derived from three items.[40] However, the MUST has been found to be unsuitable for use in an oncology population because of its low sensitivity and specificity.[41]

The Nutrition Risk Assessment (NRA) tool, developed in 1999 by the American Dietetic Association and the Consultant Dietitians in Health Care Facilities Practice Group, is widely used in U.S. long-term care facilities.[42] It utilizes data collected for the Minimum Data Set (MDS), a government-mandated screening and assessment form for Medicare- and Medicaid-certified long-term care facilities.[43] A randomized, prospective trial is currently under way to assess the validity of this tool in nursing home residents.[42] As yet, the NRA has not been validated in a population of cancer patients.

Nutrition Assessment

Nutrition screening is of little benefit if it is not followed by a formal, systematic nutrition assessment and development of a clearly outlined plan for intervention and reassessment in those patients whose screen demonstrates risk. Nutrition assessment is a thorough evaluation that assimilates data obtained from the medical history, dietary history, physical examination, anthropometric measurements, and laboratory data.[30] A comprehensive assessment of nutritional status typically integrates a review of anthropometrics with data on disease and clinical status to evaluate their effects on the patient's metabolism and nutrient need.[6] In addition, an appraisal of disease- and treatment-related symptoms is necessary to plan nutrition interventions. This step is especially important in surgical patients, as preoperative planning in the oncology patient for postoperative feeding can help to prevent feeding delays and other nutrition-related complications.

Nutrition Diagnosis

The process of nutrition assessment results in a nutrition diagnosis. The nutrition diagnosis identifies the actual occurrence of, the risk of occurrence of, or the potential for developing a nutrition-related problem.[28] The nutrition assessment includes evaluation of the etiology and signs and symptoms of nutrition problems, which in turn directs the selection of an appropriate nutrition intervention.[28]

The ADA has developed standardized nomenclature to use for determining nutrition diagnoses.[44] An example of a nutrition diagnostic term frequently utilized in cancer patients is "involuntary weight loss," which is defined as "decrease in body weight that is not planned or desired."[45]

Nutrition Intervention

Nutrition intervention refers to the specific activities required to address and correct the nutrition diagnosis.[28] The nutrition intervention is designed, planned, and implemented with the intent of improving the patient's nutrition status.[28] Planning of the intervention requires the input of all disciplines involved in the care of the patient.

Nutrition Monitoring and Evaluation

The goals of the intervention must be documented and reevaluated frequently.[28] The intervention must be patient-specific and accommodate the patient's comfort and wishes.[28, 34] Although they vary between and among patients, common nutrition goals for surgical patients include symptom management, weight maintenance, and preservation of functional status and body composition.[34] Attaining these goals often requires modulation of dietary components, the addition of oral nutritional supplements, or provision of enteral or parenteral nutrition (NST). Figure 5.2 illustrates the recommendations for nutrition intervention in cancer patients undergoing surgery.

Nutrition Support Therapy in Surgical Patients

In 2002, A.S.P.E.N. published guidelines for the use of specialized nutrition support (SNS) in hospitalized patients. These guidelines are currently being updated. The guidelines provide evidence-based direction regarding the use of enteral nutrition (EN) and parenteral nutrition (PN) support (Table 5.4). This section discusses the historical use as well as the current recommendations for use of EN and PN in surgical oncology patients.

The use of EN in surgical oncology patients has been explored in depth.[2, 46] Although EN is associated with improvements in nitrogen balance in patients with cancer, improvements in weight gain have been more inconsistent.[2] PN has also been associated with improvements in nitrogen balance, and PN appears to support weight gain more consistently.[2] However, this weight gain reportedly consists of primarily fat.[47] While PN may improve patient comfort and sense of well-being, it has little impact on the physiologic effects of malnutrition.[2, 48] Because of the underlying metabolic abnormalities induced by CCS, SNS appears to have fewer benefits in cancer patients than in noncancer patients.[6] Neither EN nor PN in cancer patients has beneficial effects on serum proteins, such as albumin, when administered for 7–49 days.[2, 46]

The use of SNS in cancer patients has been approached with caution in the past, reflecting concerns that provision of nutrients might stimulate tumor growth and metastasis. Murine models indicate that PN provision in excess of energy requirements more than doubles the rate of tumor growth.[49-51] Some human data on this issue are also available. For example, a study of malnourished gastric cancer patients receiving PN indicated no increase in tumor proliferation.[52] Conversely, an increase in tumor cell proliferation and protein synthesis was observed in head and neck and colorectal

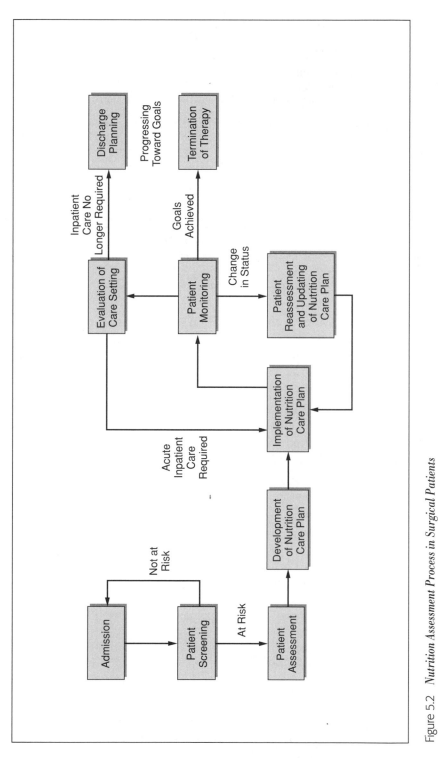

Figure 5.2 *Nutrition Assessment Process in Surgical Patients*

Reprinted with permission from A.S.P.E.N. Standards for Nutrition Support: Hospitalized Patients. Nutrition in Clinical Practice.1995;10:208-219.

Table 5.4   *Route of Nutrition Administration*

Route	Risks/Benefits
Enteral	Requires functioning GI tract Reduced cost Better maintenance of gut integrity; prevention of bacterial translocation Earlier return of bowel function postoperatively Reduced infection rate Shorter length of stay
Parenteral	Should be avoided with functioning GI tract Invasive therapy Increased cost Increased risk of infection Decreased incidence of gastrointestinal upset (i.e., nausea, diarrhea)

Source: Reprinted with permission from Huhmann M, August D. General gastrointestinal and vascular surgery. In: Marian M., Russell M., Shikora S, eds. *Clinical Nutrition for Surgical Patients.* Sudbury, MA: Jones and Bartlett; 2007:99–128.

cancer patients receiving PN. It is unlikely that this effect is of clinical significance, although it often comes up as an issue in clinical practice.[53-55]

The American Gastroenterological Association[56] and A.S.P.E.N.[6] hold similar positions on the use of PN in oncology patients. According to these organizations, the use of SNS for patients with cancer should generally be reserved for those circumstances when a patient is moderately or severely malnourished; and in whom active therapy is planned to treat the underlying malignancy; and who is unlikely to be able to meet his or her nutritional requirements orally for more than 7–10 days.[6] PN should not *routinely* be administered to patients undergoing cancer chemotherapy or radiation therapy. Instead, PN is appropriate only in malnourished patients who are anticipated to be unable to ingest and/or absorb adequate nutrients for a prolonged period of time, defined as greater than 7–10 days.[6] This type of nutrition is considered aggressive because its invasive nature. Aggressive nutrition support such as PN should be avoided in most cases if a patient's life expectancy is less than 40–60 days.[6] If maintenance of fluid balance in a patient with a life expectancy of less than 40 days is desired, hydration therapy with intravenous fluids is recommended rather than PN.[6]

Perioperative Nutrition Support

Studies in the 1980s and 1990s indicated reduced morbidity and mortality with perioperative PN supplementation in cancer patients, especially those with GI malignancies.[57] Viewed in retrospect, these studies had serious design flaws (e.g., the inclusion of heterogeneous populations, variable and likely suboptimal macronutrient provision, and inadequate sample sizes).[58] More recent studies of routine (e.g., not guided by nutrition risk and the results of a formal nutrition assessment) perioperative PN, primarily in GI cancer patients, indicate increased incidence of infection in patients receiving PN, with no improvements in survival being noted.[46, 59, 60] The limited data in significantly malnourished GI cancer patients also indicate no benefit of perioperative PN over EN, but do indicate a benefit over standard isotonic fluids.[46, 59, 60] In any event, the use of PN in cancer patients is not without risk, including increased infection rate, increased surgical complication rate, and increased cost.[59, 61–63]

Enteral administration of nutrients postoperatively is generally acknowledged to be the initial intervention of choice in surgical patients[64] because it is theoretically more physiologic, may be associated with fewer complications, and is less expensive.[65] Studies confirm that EN has advantages over PN. For example, an early meta-analysis suggested that EN has cost benefits relative to PN.[66] Subsequent meta-analyses have confirmed this economic advantage and also indicated a decreased risk of infection associated with EN in comparison to PN.[6, 67] Studies also indicate decreased intestinal permeability and a lower incidence of hyperglycemia in comparison to PN.[6] Enteral nutrition is generally well tolerated postoperatively, with gastrointestinal side effects including diarrhea and vomiting that can usually be corrected with temporary decreases in the enteral formula infusion rate.[58] Table 5.5 summarizes the studies utilizing nutrition support therapy for surgical cancer patients.

Immunonutrition

The use of enteral and parenteral formulas supplemented with macronutrients and micronutrients intended to preserve or improve immune function has increased in the last two decades. Multiple studies have investigated the use of "immunonutrition" and its effects on outcomes in GI cancer patients. Meta-analyses have demonstrated improved outcomes (reductions in morbidity and mortality) with the use of immunonutrition perioperatively in patients undergoing major GI cancer resections.[5] Immune-enhancing nutrients that have been explored include omega-3 fatty acids (Ω-3), glutamine (GLN), arginine (ARG), nucleic acids, and combinations of these nutrients.

Glutamine (GLN), which is the most abundant amino acid in the human body, is an important substrate for rapidly proliferating cells such as lymphocytes, macrophages, enterocytes, fibroblasts, and renal epithelium.[4, 68] Although several studies have investigated the use of GLN in the prevention or treatment of chemotherapy-induced side effects such as diarrhea and neuropathy,[69–73] few studies have examined GLN as a "single agent" in surgical

Table 5.5 *Studies of the Use of Nutrition Support Therapy in Surgical Cancer Patients*

Issue	Studies (Patients)	Findings
Preoperative NST	4 (449)	Improved morbidity and mortality[1-4]
Perioperative NST	8 (1,659)	Improved morbidity[3, 4] and mortality[1, 2, 5-8]
Immune-enhancing formulae	ARG, RNA, Ω-3 FA: 9 (1,281)	Improved immune parameters[6-8] and clinical outcomes[9-11]
	ARG, Ω-3 FA: 1 (200)	Improved immune parameters and gut profusion[9-16]
	ARG: 2 (139)	Improved GI function[17]
	GLN: 1 (28)	Improved immune parameters[18]
Enteral nutrition versus parenteral nutrition	11 (1,742)	Few differences in morbidity[19] or mortality[20-24] EN preserved gut integrity[2, 20, 21, 23] and immune markers[24-26] Better glycemic management[7, 22, 27, 28] with EN

ARG = arginine; RNA = ribonucleic acid; Ω-3 FA = omega-3 fatty acids; GLN = glutamine.

Data Sources
1. Muller JM, Keller HW, Brenner U, Walter M, Holzmuller W. Indications and effects of preoperative parenteral nutrition. *World J Surg*. 1986;10(1):53–63.
2. Meijerink WJ, von Meyenfeldt MF, Rouflart MM, Soeters PB. Efficacy of perioperative nutritional support. *Lancet*. 1992;340(8812):187–188.
3. Foschi D, Cavagna G, Callioni F, Morandi E, Rovati V. Hyperalimentation of jaundiced patients on percutaneous transhepatic biliary drainage. *Br J Surg*. 1986;73(9):716–719.
4. Muller JM, Brenner U, Dienst C, Pichlmaier H. Preoperative parenteral feeding in patients with gastrointestinal carcinoma. *Lancet*. 1982;1(8263):68–71.
5. Snyder-Ramos SA, Seintsch H, Bottiger BW, Motsch J, Martin E, Bauer M. Patient satisfaction and information gain after the preanesthetic visit: A comparison of face-to-face interview, brochure, and video. *Anesth Analg*. 2005;100(6):1753–1758.
6. Asilioglu K, Celik SS. The effect of preoperative education on anxiety of open cardiac surgery patients. *Patient Educ Couns*. 2004;53(1):65–70.
7. Bozzetti F, Braga M, Gianotti L, Gavazzi C, Mariani L. Postoperative enteral versus parenteral nutrition in malnourished patients with gastrointestinal cancer: A randomised multicentre trial. *Lancet*. 2001;358(9292):1487–1492.
8. Wu GH, Liu ZH, Wu ZH, Wu ZG. Perioperative artificial nutrition in malnourished gastrointestinal cancer patients. *World J Gastroenterol*. 2006;12(15):2441–2444.
9. Daly JM, Lieberman MD, Goldfine J, et al. Enteral nutrition with supplemental arginine, RNA, and omega-3 fatty acids in patients after operation: Immunologic, metabolic, and clinical outcomes. *Surgery*. 1992;112(1):56–67.
10. Daly JM, Weintraub FN, Shou J, Rosato EF, Lucia M. Enteral nutrition during multimodality therapy in upper gastrointestinal cancer patients. *Ann Surg*. 1995;221(4):327–338.
11. Di Carlo V, Gianotti L, Balzano G, Zerbi A, Braga M. Complications of pancreatic surgery and the role of perioperative nutrition. *Dig Surg*. 1999;16(4):320–326.

(continues)

Table 5.5   *Studies of the Use of Nutrition Support Therapy in Surgical Cancer Patients, Continued*

12. Braga M, Gianotti L, Vignali A, Cestari A, Bisagni P, Di Carlo V. Artificial nutrition after major abdominal surgery: Impact of route of administration and composition of the diet. *Crit Care Med.* 1998;26(1):24–30.

13. Gianotti L, Braga M, Nespoli L, Radaelli G, Beneduce A, Di Carlo V. A randomized controlled trial of preoperative oral supplementation with a specialized diet in patients with gastrointestinal cancer. *Gastroenterology.* 2002;122(7):1763–1770.

14. DeWys WD, Begg C, Lavin PT, et al. Prognostic effect of weight loss prior to chemotherapy in cancer patients: Eastern Cooperative Oncology Group. *Am J Med.* 1980;69(4):491–497.

15. Farreras N, Artigas V, Cardona D, Rius X, Trias M, Gonzalez JA. Effect of early postoperative enteral immunonutrition on wound healing in patients undergoing surgery for gastric cancer. *Clin Nutr.* 2005;24(1):55–65.

16. Senkal M, Zumtobel V, Bauer KH, et al. Outcome and cost-effectiveness of perioperative enteral immunonutrition in patients undergoing elective upper gastrointestinal tract surgery: A prospective randomized study. *Arch Surg.* 1999;134(12):1309–1316.

17. Braga M, Gianotti L, Vignali A, Carlo VD. Preoperative oral arginine and Ω-3 fatty acid supplementation improves the immunometabolic host response and outcome after colorectal resection for cancer. *Surgery.* 2002;132(5):805–814.

18. de Luis DA, Izaola O, Cuellar L, Terroba MC, Aller R. Randomized clinical trial with an enteral arginine-enhanced formula in early postsurgical head and neck cancer patients. *Eur J Clin Nutr.* 2004;58(11):1505–1508.

19. Morlion BJ, Stehle P, Wachtler P, et al. Total parenteral nutrition with glutamine dipeptide after major abdominal surgery: A randomized, double-blind, controlled study. *Ann Surg.* 1998;227(2):302–308.

20. Gianotti L, Braga M, Vignali A, et al. Effect of route of delivery and formulation of postoperative nutritional support in patients undergoing major operations for malignant neoplasms. *Arch Surg.* 1997;132(11):1222–1229, discussion 1229–1230.

21. Sand J, Luostarinen M, Matikainen M. Enteral or parenteral feeding after total gastrectomy: Prospective randomised pilot study. *Eur J Surg.* 1997;163(10):761–766.

22. Shirabe K, Matsumata T, Shimada M, et al. A comparison of parenteral hyperalimentation and early enteral feeding regarding systemic immunity after major hepatic resection: The results of a randomized prospective study. *Hepatogastroenterology.* 1997;44(13):205–209.

23. Braga M, Gianotti L, Gentilini O, Parisi V, Salis C, Di Carlo V. Early postoperative enteral nutrition improves gut oxygenation and reduces costs compared with total parenteral nutrition. *Crit Care Med.* 2001;29(2):242–248.

24. Aiko S, Yoshizumi Y, Sugiura Y, et al. Beneficial effects of immediate enteral nutrition after esophageal cancer surgery. *Surg Today.* 2001;31(11):971–978.

25. Jiang XH, Li N, Li JS. Intestinal permeability in patients after surgical trauma and effect of enteral nutrition versus parenteral nutrition. *World J Gastroenterol.* 2003;9(8):1878–1880.

26. Hyltander A, Drott C, Unsgaard B, et al. The effect on body composition and exercise performance of home parenteral nutrition when given as adjunct to chemotherapy of testicular carcinoma. *Eur J Clin Invest.* 1991;21(4):413–420.

27. Aiko S, Yoshizumi Y, Matsuyama T, Sugiura Y, Maehara T. Influences of thoracic duct blockage on early enteral nutrition for patients who underwent esophageal cancer surgery. *Jpn J Thorac Cardiovasc Surg.* 2003;51(7):263–271.

28. Goonetilleke KS, Siriwardena AK. Systematic review of peri-operative nutritional supplementation in patients undergoing pancreaticoduodenectomy. *Jop.* 2006;7(1):5–13.

cancer patients. One prospective, randomized study of perioperative parenteral GLN in colorectal cancer patients indicated improved nitrogen balance with glutamine supplementation.[74] Most of the other available data focus on the use of GLN in the prevention of mucositis in bone marrow transplant patients.[75-89] At this time, there is not enough evidence to support the use of glutamine in surgical cancer patients, although this intervention may have other applications in cancer patients receiving chemotherapy.

The Ω-3 fatty acids, which are essential in the diet, favor production of prostaglandins in the 3-series (PGE_3) and leukotrienes in the 5-series. Studies of enteral Ω-3 fatty acid administration in pancreatic cancer patients indicate that Ω-3 fatty acid supplementation in the range of 2–3 g per day may help prevent weight loss.[90-92] Parenteral Ω-3 fatty acid supplementation in colorectal cancer patients increases leukotriene-5 levels and decreases TNF levels.[93] Some evidence indicates that surgical cancer patients who are losing weight may benefit from the use of a formula that contains Ω-3 fatty acids in doses of 2 g/day. However, clinical experience indicates poor compliance with oral nutritional supplements containing Ω-3 fatty acids owing to palatability issues.

Another amino acid, arginine (ARG), has been studied as an additive to enteral and parenteral preparations. ARG in combination with other immunonutrients has been associated with improvements in immune parameters such as leukotriene B_4, and decreases in the incidence of infection among patients undergoing elective upper and lower GI surgery for cancer.[94-98] Additionally, patients with colorectal cancer receiving perioperative parenteral ARG have been found to experience enhanced immune responsiveness when compared to controls.[94-96] ARG may be useful in some cancer patients undergoing surgery, although the advantages associated with the use of these formulas must outweigh the burden of their higher costs.

Nucleotides, administered in the form of nucleic acids, appear to stimulate nonspecific parameters of immune function, although the precise mechanism of action involved is not clearly understood.[98] Nucleotides are known to affect the growth of cells that experience rapid turnover, such as enterocytes. In animal models, supplementation with nucleotides improves jejunal adaptive growth after massive small bowel resection.[98] However, in one study of human patients with colorectal cancer, there was no effect on survival with nucleotide supplementation.[99] Similar to the situation with GLN, it does not appear that nucleotide supplementation provides any benefits for surgical oncology patients at this time.

Conversely, ingestion of formulas containing immunonutrients holds promise for improving nutrition in cancer patients. Studies investigating the use of a combination of arginine, RNA, and Ω-3 fatty acids perioperatively indicate improved immune parameters[100–107] and clinical outcomes with this type of supplementation.[3, 95, 96, 100–104] Because of the diversity of methods used in these studies, the relative effects of preoperative versus postoperative treatment have not yet been determined. For some of the nutrients, such as glutamine and arginine, more information is needed to determine the optimal dosing and administration. However, based on the results of studies utilizing a combination of arginine, RNA, and Ω-3 fatty acids with clinical endpoints, it appears that EN supplemented with these nutrients may be beneficial in malnourished patients who are undergoing major thoracic or abdominal procedures.[94, 104–107] Future studies exploring the benefits associated with consumption of these nutrients should focus on larger populations of cancer patients and elucidate the preferred timing of supplementation in relation to the surgical procedure. The rationale for utilizing these kinds of nutraceuticals is summarized in Table 5.6.

Palliative Specialized Nutrition Support

Despite published guidelines that state that the palliative use of NST is rarely appropriate,[108] this issue remains controversial.[6] The use of home PN in patients with a cancer diagnosis is becoming more frequent.[108, 109] In general, PN is indicated only in those patients with incurable cancer when they are receiving active anticancer therapy, are malnourished, and are unable to consume adequate oral or enteral nutrients for a significant period of time.[110] A small subset of terminally ill cancer patients (e.g., patients with ovarian cancer) not receiving cancer-directed therapy with dysfunctional GI tracts has been identified in whom long-term, home PN may provide palliative benefits[6] and improve quality of life; it may even lengthen survival.

It is important to remember that PN is complex, intrusive, and expensive. If patients are to benefit they (1) must be very strongly motivated and physically capable of participating in the their own care, (2) should have an estimated life expectancy of greater than 40 to 60 days, and (3) require strong social and financial support at home, including a dedicated in-home lay care provider. They must also fail trials of less invasive therapies, including aggressive medical management with antiemetics, narcotics, anticholinergics, and antidepressants.[111–115] Those patients with a life expectancy of less than 40 days are often well palliated with home intravenous fluid therapy. Most patients evaluated for palliative care with home PN do not meet these criteria.

Table 5.6   *Nutraceuticals: Therapeutic Rationale*

Substrate	Metabolic Activities	Clinical Use
Glutamine	• Most abundant amino acid in the human body, nonessential • Important substrate for rapidly proliferating cells such as lymphocytes, macrophages, enterocytes, fibroblasts, and renal epithelium • Nitrogen shuttle between tissues • Precursor for the synthesis of purines, pyrimidines, and amino acids	Potentially beneficial in stimulating postoperative return of gastrointestinal function and decrease in permeability[1,2]; may reverse postoperative immunodepression[3]
Arginine	• Nonessential amino acid, may become conditionally essential during periods of physiologic stress • Substrate in the urea cycle; roles in protein, creatinine, and polyamine synthesis • Affects nitrogen metabolism, wound healing, immune competence, and tumor metabolism	May improve immunologic indices postoperatively[4]; decreased incidence of postoperative fistula[5]
Nucleic acids	• Stimulatory effects on nonspecific parameters of immune function • Mechanism of action not understood	No clinical studies performed
Essential fatty acids	• Ω-3 polyunsaturated fatty acids (PUFAs) favor production of 3-series prostaglandins (PGE_3) and 5-series leukotrienes (immune-enhancing and anti-inflammatory) • Ω-3 PUFAs reduce production of 2-series prostaglandins (PGE_2) and 4-series leukotrienes (immunosuppressive and pro-inflammatory)	May improve postoperative inflammatory and immune response[6]; may decrease need for ventilator and length of stay in patients with major abdominal surgery[7]

PUFA, polyunsaturated fatty acids; PGE3, prostaglandin E3; PGE2, prostaglandin E_2; LOS, length of stay

Data Sources
1. De-Souza DA, Greene LJ. Intestinal permeability and systemic infections in critically ill patients: effect of glutamine. *Crit Care Med.* May 2005;33(5):1125–1135.
2. Morlion BJ, Stehle P, Wachtler P, et al. Total parenteral nutrition with glutamine dipeptide after major abdominal surgery: a randomized, double-blind, controlled study. *Ann Surg.* Feb 1998;227(2):302–308.
3. Yao GX, Xue XB, Jiang ZM, Yang NF, Wilmore DW. Effects of perioperative parenteral glutamine-dipeptide supplementation on plasma endotoxin level, plasma endotoxin inactivation capacity and clinical outcome. *Clin Nutr.* Aug 2005;24(4):510–515.

(continues)

Table 5.6   *Nutraceuticals: Therapeutic Rationale, Continued*

4. Song JX, Qing SH, Huang XC, Qi DL. Effect of parenteral nutrition with L-arginine supplementation on postoperative immune function in patients with colorectal cancer. *Di Yi Jun Yi Da Xue Xue Bao.* Jun 2002;22(6):545–547.
5. de Luis DA, Izaola O, Cuellar L, Terroba MC, Aller R. Randomized clinical trial with an enteral arginine-enhanced formula in early postsurgical head and neck cancer patients. *Eur J Clin Nutr.* Nov 2004;58(11):1505–1508.
6. Nakamura K, Kariyazono H, Komokata T, Hamada N, Sakata R, Yamada K. Influence of preoperative administration of omega-3 fatty acid-enriched supplement on inflammatory and immune responses in patients undergoing major surgery for cancer. *Nutrition.* Jun 2005;21(6):639–649.
7. Tsekos E, Reuter C, Stehle P, Boeden G. Perioperative administration of parenteral fish oil supplements in a routine clinical setting improves patient outcome after major abdominal surgery. *Clin Nutr.* Jun 2004;23(3):325–330.

Table Source:
Adapted with permission from: August DA, Huhmann MB. Nutritional Care of Cancer Patients. In: Norton J, Barie P, Bollinger R, et al., eds. *Surgery: Basic Science and Clinical Evidence.* 2nd ed. New York: Springer Publishing; 2006.

Nutrition Issues in Specific Gastrointestinal Malignancies

Esophageal Cancer

Esophageal cancer resections have significant nutritional consequences. In particular, patients with esophageal cancer often present with some degree of dysphagia and weight loss preoperatively.[116, 117] Approximately 79% to 100%[118–119] of these individuals are malnourished at presentation, and esophagectomy can worsen their malnutrition.

Reflux (because the lower esophageal sphincter is generally sacrificed with the resection), dysmotility of the remaining esophagus, gastric dysmotility secondary to resection of the vagus nerves with the esophagus, and dumping syndrome are common side effects of esophagectomy. Patients may complain of dysphagia postoperatively. This problem may be caused by multiple factors, including stricture, poor gastric emptying, or dysmotility. Stricture may occur after esophagectomy as a result of anastomotic ischemia, which is not uncommon when the stomach is mobilized as a conduit.[118, 120] Dilatation of the stricture can allow for normal oral intake, although it may require several dilatations to achieve "normal" swallowing. Disruptions of the vagal nerves can lead to altered sensations in the stomach, causing overeating and regurgitation.[118] Placement of a feeding jejunostomy tube during surgery allows for early enteral support. Postoperative diet modifications, including the consumption of small, frequent, energy-dense meals, can help in reducing regurgitation.

Dumping syndrome can also occur post esophagectomy. The rapid passage of hyperosmotic, undigested food into the small bowel with secondary hypersecretion of succus and extracellular fluid into the bowel lumen may cause hypotension, flushing, and diarrhea. This condition is a result of the rapid distention of the bowel. If left untreated, it can lead to weight loss, malnutrition, and increased mortality.[119] Postoperative diet changes, including limiting simple carbohydrates and liquids with meals, can assist in preventing the cramping, diarrhea, and flushing associated with dumping syndrome.

Gastric Cancer

Gastric resection can alter gastric reservoir function and vitamin B_{12} absorption. The capacity of the GI tract to "store" food following gastrectomy can vary greatly, which may lead to unintentional food regurgitation.[118, 121] Resection decreases stomach capacitance, with resultant compromise of reservoir function. Removal of either the pylorus or the lower esophageal sphincter (LES) may also be problematic. Post gastrectomy, the absence of the LES eliminates the barrier for the reflux of food and digestive juices. Reflux is observed in as many as 58% of patients who undergo esophagectomy[119] and 80% of patients who undergo a total gastrectomy.[120] If the procedure includes disruption of pyloric function or a gastrojejunostomy, bile reflux into the esophagus can occur. This complication is particularly difficult to manage because, unlike with acid, there are no drugs available to "neutralize" the irritant effects of bile on the esophageal squamous epithelium.

Dumping syndrome may also occur as a result of disruption of the pyloric sphincter and gastrojejunostomy. Restriction of simple carbohydrates and limiting liquids with meals can help to prevent dumping syndrome.

The acidic environment of the stomach assists in the release of vitamin B_{12} from food. Loss of intrinsic factor occurs with resection of the parietal cells in the proximal stomach and results in vitamin B_{12} malabsorption. Vitamin B_{12} deficiency can, in turn, lead to megaloblastic anemia and dementia.[121] Such a deficiency can develop as early as one year after total gastrectomy.[122] Patients in whom all of the proximal stomach is removed should be evaluated for the need for vitamin B_{12} replacement. Supplementation is available in enteral and parenteral formulations,[123] and routine prescription of 1000 mcg monthly intramuscular vitamin B_{12} is recommended for patients undergoing proximal or total gastrectomy to prophylactically prevent deficiency.[124]

Small Bowel Cancer

Small bowel resection, when carried out because of the presence of primary malignancy or malignancy in adjacent organs, can have significant effects on the ability to absorb both micronutrients and macronutrients. The small bowel plays a major role in nutrient absorption. Its anatomy, as well as the hormones that are released into the small intestine, affect the effectiveness of this absorption. Resection of any significant portion of the small bowel can result in decreased transit time, thereby producing malabsorption. Hormones released in response to the entry of food into the small intestine—for example, secretin, cholecystokinin, and enteropeptidase—affect pancreatic and gallbladder function as well as gastric emptying and feelings of satiety. The practitioner must evaluate these sources as potential etiologies in the cancer patient who has undergone a resection of the small intestine.

Micronutrient and macronutrient absorption is also altered based on the location and size of the resection. The duodenum is the primary site of absorption for calcium and magnesium. The jejunum is responsible for absorption of carbohydrate, protein, water-soluble vitamins, and iron. Jejunal resections can result in inappropriate secretion of digestive enzymes and accelerated gastric emptying. Lipid, fat-soluble vitamins, cholesterol, bile salts, and vitamin B_{12} are absorbed in the ileum. Patients with ileostomies must be educated about proper supplemental fluid and electrolyte intake because they have an increased risk for dehydration.[124, 125] Many of these individuals will have a need for increased sodium and water intake to balance increased losses in the stool. To counteract these losses, patients should be instructed to consume at least one liter more fluid daily than their stoma output.[125] Significant resection of the jejunum and ileum can also cause reduced intestinal absorption secondary to the loss of absorptive surface, or short bowel syndrome. Depending on the amount of intestine resected, fluid and electrolyte needs may not be met with oral feeding alone, such that enteral or parenteral nutrition intervention is required.[126]

The small bowel plays a significant role in bacterial homeostasis. An acidic environment in the small bowel lumen, which can occur after small bowel resection because of increased gastric acid secretion and decreased transit time, deactivates digestive enzymes and deconjugates bile acids, which in turn leads to further malabsorption. The malabsorbed food moves into the colon, where carbohydrate is fermented by bacteria into D-lactic acid. Build-up of D-lactic acid can cause metabolic acidosis characterized by increased serum D-lactate, an increased anion gap, and decreased serum bicarbonate.[127] This relatively rare neurologic syndrome occurs with short bowel syndrome or following jejuno-ileal bypass surgery. Symptoms include altered mental status, slurred speech, and ataxia, and typically present after the ingestion of high-carbohydrate feedings.[128] Carbohydrate restriction, antibiotics, and probiotics are generally recommended for the management or prevention of this adverse effect.[128, 129]

Bacterial growth in the small intestine is carefully regulated through several mechanisms, including the pH of stomach contents, intestinal peristalsis, and innate intestinal wall immune factors.[130] Massive bowel resection frequently leads to bacterial overgrowth, increasing the risk of bacterial translocation, and possibly sepsis. Bacterial overgrowth is diagnosed through culture or biopsy of the bowel or by a hydrogen breath test. Nutritional consequences of intestinal bacterial overgrowth include steatorrhea (fat malabsorption) as well as decreased intestinal micellar uptake of triglycerides, fatty acids, cholesterol, and lipophilic vitamins.[131]

Bacterial overgrowth is commonly treated with antibiotics and probiotics.[132] Probiotics are live microorganisms, such as lactobacillus or bifidobacterium, that may produce beneficial health effects in humans.[133–138]

Colon Cancer

The colon is responsible for fluid and electrolyte resorption. Resections of the terminal ileum and colon can, therefore, significantly affect the body's electrolyte and fluid balance. In response, the intestine may undergo structural and functional adaptation to increase fluid and nutrient absorption over a period of two years or more.[126]

The colon may contain as many as 10^{11} or 10^{12} bacterial cells/gram luminal contents.[6] Impaired intestinal peristalsis or anatomical abnormalities that alter luminal flow following surgery can cause bacterial overgrowth.[137] Dysfunctions of the gut barrier following colon resection have been hypothesized to lead to translocation of microorganisms, sepsis, shock, multisystem organ failure, and even death.[138] Bacterial overgrowth in the terminal ileum following ileocecal valve resection can adversely affect the specialized absorptive functions of the ileum. In particular, ileocolectomy has been associated with a significant increase in ileal and colonic bacterial counts.[139] As mentioned earlier, bacterial overgrowth can produce metabolic acidosis and malabsorption of both micronutrients and macronutrients.

Pancreatic Cancer

Digestion of starches, proteins, and lipids requires pancreatic enzymes. Pancreatic enzyme excretion can be impaired due to pancreatic duct obstruction, resection, or dysregulation. To compensate for this dysfunction, interventions may include oral administration of pancreatic enzymes, diet modification, and a physiologic shift of the site of digestion to the distal small intestine.[140] In general, derangements in postoperative pancreatic exocrine function are determined by type of resection, resection of adjacent organs, the underlying disease, and preoperative pancreatic function. The dysfunction often does not result in symptoms of obvious malabsorption such as diarrhea; instead, it may manifest as continued weight loss in spite of apparent adequate intake.

After major pancreatic surgery, enzyme replacement may be required. Pancreatic enzyme supplementation starts with 40,000–120,000 IU of lipase and is titrated according to patient response.[140] The addition of a proton-pump inhibitor assists in the prevention of early activation of enzymes by gastric acid.[140] Pancreaticocibal asynchrony occurs when pancreatic enzyme secretion is mistimed, resulting in malabsorption; it occurs in 16% to 43% of gastrectomy patients.[141] Oral pancreatic enzyme replacement in this setting is helpful in overcoming the malabsorption problem.

The type of pancreatic resection affects the extent of endocrine insufficiency. After a Whipple procedure (Figure 5.3), 20% to 40% of patients develop diabetes mellitus.[142] In some patients, hypoglycemia occurs as a result of postoperative insulin sensitivity in the presence of decreased glucagon secretion.[141, 142] Pylorus-preserving Whipple procedures seem to impair endocrine function more than a traditional Whipple procedure.[143] In some cases, such as in chronic pancreatitis, pancreatic head resection can improve endocrine secretion.[140] Functional islet cell, or neuroendocrine, tumors such as insulinomas, gastrinomas, glucagonomas, and VIPomas (vasoactive intestinal peptide-producing tumors), can cause a host of nutritional issues, ranging from hypoglycemia (insulinoma) to ulcers (gastrinoma).[144] Drugs such as octreotide can palliate the endocrine mediation effects of these tumors; however, the only curative option is surgery.[144, 145] Fortunately, complete resection alleviates these symptoms.

Cancers of the Liver and Gallbladder

The liver plays important roles in protein synthesis, glucose homeostasis, bilirubin excretion, and detoxication, among other functions.[146] Hepatic

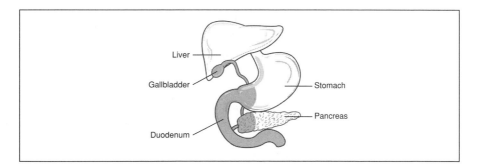

Figure 5.3 *Anatomy Removed in a Whipple Procedure*

Reprinted with permission from Cancer Research UK. Surgery to try to cure pancreatic cancer. Accessed at: http://www.cancerhelp.org.uk/help/default.asp?page=3124#whipple.

protein synthesis is altered in response to trauma and critical illness.[147] Whole-body protein synthesis is modified after surgery of moderate severity.[147] Production of positive acute-phase proteins (i.e., complement system, transport proteins, and antiproteases) increases with stress, whereas production of negative acute-phase proteins (i.e., albumin, prealbumin, and transferrin) decreases with stress.[147] Mediators of inflammation, including cytokines, seem to affect serum protein levels through two mechanisms: (1) alteration of normal synthesis and catabolism and (2) induction of capillary leak.[146]

The key functions carried out by the liver in nutrient metabolism include synthesis and degradation of glucose and glycogen, fatty acid metabolism, synthesis and degradation of serum proteins, detoxification of lipid-soluble toxins, and metabolism of bilirubin.[146] Poor nutritional status, which often manifests as fluid retention and low levels of serum proteins, is correlated to mortality in patients undergoing liver resections.[148] Preoperative liver disease may produce hypoalbuminemia, hyperglucagonemia, increased energy expenditure, depleted skeletal muscle mass, and anorexia prior to surgery.[149] In addition, patients may develop symptoms that limit food intake before and after liver surgery—for example, altered taste sensation, early satiety due to ascites, steatorrhea due to bile salt deficiency, anorexia, nausea, and vomiting.[150] Protein calorie malnutrition is evident in 20% of patients with compensated cirrhosis and in 60% of patients with liver insufficiency.[151]

Postoperative tolerance of liver resection and the liver's ability to regenerate and regain function after liver surgery vary greatly. The presence of malnutrition clearly affects the return of liver function and regeneration, and it has important implications for morbidity and mortality. Preoperative malnutrition is a predictor for first bleeding episode and survival, and is associated with both refractory ascites and postoperative complications.[152] Surgical techniques such as portal vein embolization can assist in preserving functional liver volume by inducing preoperative hepatic hypertrophy.[152] When the size of the liver is increased preoperatively, this organ may require less time to adapt to the resection, potentially limiting the previously mentioned complications. Despite this measure, however, patients still may need nutrition support postoperatively. Early EN after liver resection is associated with a lower rate of wound- and catheter-related complications and improved immune competence compared to PN.[153]

Perioperative Feeding Considerations

Maintenance of nutrition status perioperatively can be facilitated by careful preoperative planning and creation of a postoperative nutrition care plan.[154, 155]

Failure to consider nutrition and diet issues perioperatively can result in lost opportunities to maintain nutrition status and to avoid nutrition-related complications. The postoperative nutrition care plan should be determined and discussed with the patient prior to surgery.[154]

Historically, postoperative "bowel rest" has been recommended to promote anastomotic healing and prevent nausea and vomiting.[67] Early postoperative oral and enteral feedings are now recommended to encourage the return of gastrointestinal function by enhancing bowel hypertrophy and anastomotic healing.[155] Even in the absence of peristalsis, the small intestine regains the ability to absorb nutrients quickly after surgery.

It has become common practice to establish enteral feeding access during major gastrointestinal procedures.[156] Early enteral nutrition in malnourished surgical patients is associated with improved wound healing, maintenance of gut function, and improved gut immune function. It is also associated with decreased length of stay in intensive care.[156, 157] Furthermore, early resumption of oral/enteral feeding is only occasionally associated with undesirable side effects such as nausea, vomiting, colic, and anorexia.[65, 155, 158] In patients with established preoperative malnutrition, the benefits of enteral access outweigh the risks of enteral access-related complications.[6, 58, 159] For this reason, intraoperative placement of a gastrostomy or jejunostomy tube for enteral access should be strongly considered in patients who are malnourished preoperatively or in whom a prolonged period of poor oral intake is anticipated (7–14 days). Studies specifically assessing the use of NST for 7–14 days preoperatively[160] in moderately or severely malnourished patients indicate that this intervention provides a benefit in terms of both morbidity[1, 161, 162] and mortality.[1, 2, 57, 59, 162, 163]

In addition to planning for nutrition support access preoperatively, it is important to discuss the patient's transition to an oral diet. Upper gastrointestinal surgical resection may be associated with significant postoperative morbidity, including dumping syndrome, delayed gastric emptying, prolonged ileus, obstruction, gastroesophageal reflux, and post-gastrectomy syndrome (dumping, fat maldigestion, gastric stasis, and lactose intolerance).[2, 59, 162] These complications can lead to weight loss, malnutrition, and increased mortality.[164, 165]

Preoperative education by a registered dietitian (RD) to inform patients about both normal and abnormal postoperative events can assist patients in taking an active role in their recovery. As yet, few data have been published on the role of nutrition education in patients undergoing gastrointestinal cancer surgery. Several studies indicate that patients who receive preoperative education regarding expectations and pain management[121] experience less anxiety[166] and pain,[167, 168] and have improved outcomes[169, 170] and increased satisfaction.[171, 172] Preoperative nutrition education by an RD also has the potential to improve outcomes and facilitate a quicker return to oral diet (see Table 5.7).

Table 5.7   *Special Issues in Cancer Surgery Patients*

Category	Issue	Manifestation	Nutrition Intervention
Abnormal transit	Dumping syndrome	Early: Diarrhea, bloating, nausea, tachycardia immediately— 30 minutes after a meal Late: Hypoglycemic symptoms, dizziness 90–180 minutes after a meal	Small frequent meals Separation of solids and fluids at meals Reduction in simple carbohydrate and concentrated fat intake Increased soluble fiber intake[1]
	Reflux esophagitis	Regurgitation of food and digestive juices causing heartburn, nausea, or vomiting	Small frequent meals Use of antacids or sucralfate[2]
	Delayed gastric emptying/gastric stasis	Early satiety, postprandial fullness, heartburn, dysphagia, aspiration[2]	Small frequent meals Prokinetic agents[3]
	Pancreaticocibal asynchrony	Steatorrhea, frequent light greasy stools	Addition of pancreatic enzymes at meals and snacks
Malassimilation	Reduced intake, impaired absorption, disturbed metabolism, increased loss[1]	Micronutrient deficiencies	Enteral or parenteral replacement
Obstruction	Stricture, gastric outlet obstruction	Vomiting, constipation	Enteral or parenteral nutrition support depending upon extent Endoscopic balloon dilation or surgical stenting Promotility agent[2]
Pancreatic insufficiency	Pancreatic enzyme insufficiency	Steatorrhea, bloating	Pancreatic enzyme replacement[4]

Data Sources
1. Scholmerich J. Postgastrectomy syndromes—diagnosis and treatment. *Best Pract Res Clin Gastroenterol.* Oct 2004;18(5):917–933.
2. Lerut TE, van Lanschot JJ. Chronic symptoms after subtotal or partial oesophagectomy: diagnosis and treatment. *Best Pract Res Clin Gastroenterol.* Oct 2004;18(5):901–915.

(continues)

Table 5.7   *Special Issues in Cancer Surgery Patients, Continued*

3. Radigan A. Post-Gastrectomy: Managing the nutrition fall-out. *Practical Gastroenterology.* 2004 2004;28(6):63–75.
4. Kahl S, Malfertheiner P. Exocrine and endocrine pancreatic insufficiency after pancreatic surgery. *Best Pract Res Clin Gastroenterol.* Oct 2004;18(5):947–955.

Table Source: Reprinted with permission from Huhmann M, August D. General gastrointestinal and vascular surgery. In: Marian M., Russel M., Shikora S, eds., Clinical Nutrition for Surgical Patients. Sudbury, MA: Jones and Bartlett; 2007:99–128.

SUMMARY

Surgical oncology patients can develop complex nutritional issues. Preoperative nutrition assessment and planning can assist in decreasing the development or progression of malnutrition. Postoperative follow-up is also crucial for preventing deteriorations in nutritional status and addressing any procedure-related issues that may result in negative nutrition-related outcomes.

REFERENCES

1. Veterans Affairs Total Parenteral Nutrition Cooperative Study Group. Perioperative total parenteral nutrition in surgical patients. *N Engl J Med.* 1991;325(8):525–532.
2. Bozzetti F. Rationale and indications for preoperative feeding of malnourished surgical cancer patients. *Nutrition.* 2002;18(11–12):953–959.
3. Braga M, Gianotti L, Nespoli L, Radaelli G, Di Carlo V. Nutritional approach in malnourished surgical patients: A prospective randomized study. *Arch Surg.* 2002; 137(2):174–180.
4. Heyland DK, Novak F, Drover JW, Jain M, Su X, Suchner U. Should immunonutrition become routine in critically ill patients? A systematic review of the evidence. *JAMA.* 2001;286(8):944–953.
5. Heys SD, Ogston KN. Peri-operative nutritional support: Controversies and debates. *Int J Surg Investig.* 2000;2(2):107–115.
6. American Society for Enteral and Parenteral Nutrition. Guidelines for the use of parenteral and enteral nutrition in adult and pediatric patients. *JPEN J Parenter Enteral Nutr.* 2002;26(1)(suppl):1SA–138SA.
7. DeWys WD, Begg C, Lavin PT, et al. Prognostic effect of weight loss prior to chemotherapy in cancer patients: Eastern Cooperative Oncology Group. *Am J Med.* 1980;69(4):491–497.
8. Linn BS, Robinson DS, Klimas NG. Effects of age and nutritional status on surgical outcomes in head and neck cancer. *Ann Surg.* 1988;207(3):267–273.
9. Nguyen TV, Yueh B. Weight loss predicts mortality after recurrent oral cavity and oropharyngeal carcinomas. *Cancer.* 2002;95(3):553–562.

10. Haugstvedt TK, Viste A, Eide GE, Soreide O. Factors related to and consequences of weight loss in patients with stomach cancer: The Norwegian multicenter experience. Norwegian Stomach Cancer Trial. *Cancer.* 1991;67(3):722–729.

11. McCullum P, Poliseria C, eds. *The Clinical Guide to Oncology Nutrition.* Chicago, IL: American Dietetic Association; 2000.

12. Rivadeneira DE, Evoy D, Fahey TJ 3rd, Lieberman MD, Daly JM. Nutritional support of the cancer patient. *CA Cancer J Clin.* 1998;48(2):69–80.

13. Capra S, Ferguson M, Ried K. Cancer: Impact of nutrition intervention outcome—Nutrition issues for patients. *Nutrition.* 2001;17(9):769–772.

14. Parnes HL, Aisner J. Protein calorie malnutrition and cancer therapy. *Drug Saf.* 1992;7(6):404–416.

15. Bloch A, Charuhas P. Cancer and cancer therapy. In: Gottschlich M, ed. *The Science and Practice of Nutrition Support.* Dubuque, IA: Kendall Hunt; 2001:643–662.

16. Kern KA, Norton JA. Cancer cachexia. *JPEN J Parenter Enteral Nutr.* 1988;12(3):286–298.

17. Brennan MF. Total parenteral nutrition in the cancer patient. *N Engl J Med.* 1981;305(7):375–382.

18. Barber M. The pathophysiology and treatment of cancer cachexia. *Nutr Clin Prac.* 2002;17(4):203–209.

19. Tisdale MJ. Cachexia in cancer patients. *Nat Rev Cancer.* 2002;2(11):862–871.

20. MacDonald N, Easson AM, Mazurak VC, Dunn GP, Baracos VE. Understanding and managing cancer cachexia. *J Am Coll Surg.* 2003;197(1):143–161.

21. Tisdale MJ. Cancer cachexia: Metabolic alterations and clinical manifestations. *Nutrition.* 1997;13(1):1–7.

22. Tisdale MJ. Pathogenesis of cancer cachexia. *J Support Oncol.* 2003;1(3):159–168.

23. Lind D, Souba W, Copeland E. Weight loss and cachexia. In: Abeloff M, Armitage J, Lichter A, Niederhuber J, eds. *Clinical Oncology.* New York, NY: Churchill Livingstone; 1995:393–407.

24. Tisdale MJ. Tumor–host interactions. *J Cell Biochem.* 2004;93(5):871–877.

25. Dannhauser A, Van Zyl JM, Nel CJ. Preoperative nutritional status and prognostic nutritional index in patients with benign disease undergoing abdominal operations: Part I. *J Am Coll Nutr.* 1995;14(1):80–90.

26. Sungurtekin H, Sungurtekin U, Balci C, Zencir M, Erdem E. The influence of nutritional status on complications after major intraabdominal surgery. *J Am Coll Nutr.* 2004;23(3):227–232.

27. Hirsch S, de Obaldia N, Petermann M, et al. Nutritional status of surgical patients and the relationship of nutrition to postoperative outcome. *J Am Coll Nutr.* 1992;11(1):21–24.

28. Lacey K, Pritchett E. Nutrition Care Process and model: ADA adopts road map to quality care and outcomes management. *J Am Diet Assoc.* 2003;103(8):1061–1072.

29. Jensen GL. Inflammation as the key interface of the medical and nutrition universes: A provocative examination of the future of clinical nutrition and medicine. *JPEN J Parenter Enteral Nutr.* 2006;30(5):453–463.

30. Committee CoPCQM. Identifying patients at risk: ADA's definitions for nutrition screening and nutrition assessment. *J Am Diet Assoc.* 1994;94(8):838–839.

31. Sarhill N, Mahmoud F, Walsh D, et al. Evaluation of nutritional status in advanced metastatic cancer. *Support Care Cancer.* 2003;11(10):652–659.

32. Ottery FD. Definition of standardized nutritional assessment and interventional pathways in oncology. *Nutrition.* 1996;12(1)(suppl):S15–S19.

33. Detsky AS, McLaughlin JR, Baker JP, et al. What is subjective global assessment of nutritional status? *JPEN J Parenter Enteral Nutr.* 1987;11(1):8–13.

34. Luthringer S, Kulakowski K. Medical nutrition therapy protocols. In: McCallum P, Polisena C, eds. *The Clinical Guide to Oncology Nutrition.* Chicago, IL: American Dietetic Association; 2000:24–44.

35. Ottery F, Bender F, Kasenic S. The design and implementation of a model nutritional oncology clinic. *Oncology Issues: Integrating Nutrition into Your Cancer Program.* 2002;2–6.

36. Ferguson M. Patient-Generated Subjective Global Assessment. *Oncology (Huntingt).* 2003;17(2)(suppl)(2):13–14, discussion 14–16.

37. Guigoz Y, Vellas B, Garry PJ. Assessing the nutritional status of the elderly: The Mini Nutritional Assessment as part of the geriatric evaluation. *Nutr Rev.* 1996; 54(1 Pt 2):S59–S65.

38. Ferguson M, Capra S, Bauer J, Banks M. Development of a valid and reliable malnutrition screening tool for adult acute hospital patients. *Nutrition.* 1999;15(6):458–464.

39. Ferguson ML, Bauer J, Gallagher B, Capra S, Christie DR, Mason BR. Validation of a malnutrition screening tool for patients receiving radiotherapy. *Australas Radiol.* 1999;43(3):325–327.

40. Group MA. A consistent and reliable tool for malnutrition screening. *Nurs Times.* 2003;99(46):26–27.

41. Bauer J, Capra S. Comparison of a malnutrition screening tool with Subjective Global Assessment in hospitalised patients with cancer: Sensitivity and specificity. *Asia Pac J Clin Nutr.* 2003;12(3):257–260.

42. Association NCD. Skill-building success! *Link: NC Diet Assoc Newsletter.* 2004;3(1):5.

43. Services CfMaM. The assessment schedule for the RAI. In: Services CfMaM, ed. *Revised Long Term Care Resident Assessment Instrument User's Manual for the Minimum Data Set (MDS), Version 2.0.* Baltimore, MD: Centers for Medicare and Medicaid Services; 2002:1–40.

44. Hakel-Smith N, Lewis NM, Eskridge KM. Orientation to Nutrition Care Process standards improves nutrition care documentation by nutrition practitioners. *J Am Diet Assoc.* 2005;105(10):1582–1589.

45. American Dietetic Association. *International Dietetics and Nutrition Terminology (IDNT) Reference Manual: Standardized Language for the Nutrition Care Process.* Chicago, IL: Author; 2007.

46. NHS Center for Reviews and Dissemination. Nutrition support in patients with cancer. *Database Abstr Rev Effectiveness.* 2004;2.

47. Shike M, Russel DM, Detsky AS, et al. Changes in body composition in patients with small-cell lung cancer: The effect of total parenteral nutrition as an adjunct to chemotherapy. *Ann Intern Med.* 1984;101(3):303–309.

48. Hyltander A, Drott C, Unsgaard B, et al. The effect on body composition and exercise performance of home parenteral nutrition when given as adjunct to chemotherapy of testicular carcinoma. *Eur J Clin Invest.* 1991;21(4):413–420.

49. Popp MB, Wagner SC, Brito OJ. Host and tumor responses to increasing levels of intravenous nutritional support. *Surgery.* 1983;94(2):300–308.

50. Daly J, Thorn A. Neoplastic diseases. In: Kinney J, Jeejeebhoy K, Hill G, Owen O, eds. *Nutrition and Metabolism in Patient Care.* Philadelphia, PA: Saunders; 1988: 567–587.

51. Torosian MH. Stimulation of tumor growth by nutrition support. *JPEN J Parenter Enteral Nutr.* 1992;16(6)(suppl):72S–75S.

52. Pacelli F, Bossola M, Teodori L, et al. Parenteral nutrition does not stimulate tumor proliferation in malnourished gastric cancer patients. *JPEN J Parenter Enteral Nutr.* 2007;31(6):451–455.

53. Baron PL, Lawrence W Jr, Chan WM, White FK, Banks WL Jr. Effects of parenteral nutrition on cell cycle kinetics of head and neck cancer. *Arch Surg.* 1986;121(11):1282–1286.

54. Frank JL, Lawrence W Jr, Banks WL Jr, McKinnon JG, Chan WM, Collins JM. Modulation of cell cycle kinetics in human cancer with total parenteral nutrition. *Cancer.* 1992;69(7):1858–1864.

55. Heys SD, Park KG, McNurlan MA, et al. Stimulation of protein synthesis in human tumours by parenteral nutrition: Evidence for modulation of tumour growth. *Br J Surg.* 1991;78(4):483–487.

56. American Gastroenterological Association. Medical position statement: Parenteral nutrition. *Gastroenterology.* 2001;121(4):966–969.

57. Muller JM, Keller HW, Brenner U, Walter M, Holzmuller W. Indications and effects of preoperative parenteral nutrition. *World J Surg.* 1986;10(1):53–63.

58. August D, Huhmann M. Nutritional care of cancer patients. In: Norton JA, Barie PS, Bollinger RR, et al, eds. *Surgery: Basic Science and Clinical Evidence.* 2nd ed. New York, NY: Springer-Verlag; 2008:2123–2150.

59. Bozzetti F, Braga M, Gianotti L, Gavazzi C, Mariani L. Postoperative enteral versus parenteral nutrition in malnourished patients with gastrointestinal cancer: A randomised multicentre trial. *Lancet.* 2001;358(9292):1487–1492.

60. Koretz RL, Lipman TO, Klein S. AGA technical review on parenteral nutrition. *Gastroenterology.* 2001;121(4):970–1001.

61. Papapietro K, Diaz E, Csendes A, et al. Early enteral nutrition in cancer patients subjected to a total gastrectomy [in Spanish]. *Rev Med Chil.* 2002;130(10):1125–1130.

62. Braga M, Gianotti L, Gentilini O, Parisi V, Salis C, Di Carlo V. Early postoperative enteral nutrition improves gut oxygenation and reduces costs compared with total parenteral nutrition. *Crit Care Med.* 2001;29(2):242–248.

63. Aiko S, Yoshizumi Y, Sugiura Y, et al. Beneficial effects of immediate enteral nutrition after esophageal cancer surgery. *Surg Today.* 2001;31(11):971–978.

64. Huckleberry Y. Nutritional support and the surgical patient. *Am J Health Syst Pharm.* 2004;61(7):671–682, quiz 683–674.

65. Fearon KC, Luff R. The nutritional management of surgical patients: Enhanced recovery after surgery. *Proc Nutr Soc.* 2003;62(4):807–811.

66. Lipman TO. Grains or veins: Is enteral nutrition really better than parenteral nutrition? A look at the evidence. *JPEN J Parenter Enteral Nutr.* 1998;22(3): 167–182.

67. Braunschweig CL, Levy P, Sheean PM, Wang X. Enteral compared with parenteral nutrition: A meta-analysis. *Am J Clin Nutr.* 2001;74(4):534–542.

68. Beale RJ, Bryg DJ, Bihari DJ. Immunonutrition in the critically ill: A systematic review of clinical outcome. *Crit Care Med.* 1999;27(12):2799–2805.

69. Markman M. Prevention of paclitaxel-associated arthralgias and myalgias. *J Support Oncol.* 2003;1(4):233–234.

70. Savarese D, Boucher J, Corey B. Glutamine treatment of paclitaxel-induced myalgias and arthralgias. *J Clin Oncol.* 1998;16(12):3918–3919.

71. Savarese DM, Savy G, Vahdat L, Wischmeyer PE, Corey B. Prevention of chemotherapy and radiation toxicity with glutamine. *Cancer Treat Rev.* 2003;29(6): 501–513.

72. Stubblefield MD, Vahdat LT, Balmaceda CM, Troxel AB, Hesdorffer CS, Gooch CL. Glutamine as a neuroprotective agent in high-dose paclitaxel-induced peripheral neuropathy: A clinical and electrophysiologic study. *Clin Oncol (R Coll Radiol)*. 2005;17(4):271–276.

73. Vahdat L, Papadopoulos K, Lange D, et al. Reduction of paclitaxel-induced peripheral neuropathy with glutamine. *Clin Cancer Res*. 2001;7(5):1192–1197.

74. Morlion BJ, Stehle P, Wachtler P, et al. Total parenteral nutrition with glutamine dipeptide after major abdominal surgery: A randomized, double-blind, controlled study. *Ann Surg*. 1998;227(2):302–308.

75. Aquino VM, Harvey AR, Garvin JH, et al. A double-blind randomized placebo-controlled study of oral glutamine in the prevention of mucositis in children undergoing hematopoietic stem cell transplantation: A pediatric blood and marrow transplant consortium study. *Bone Marrow Transplant*. 2005;36(7):611–616.

76. Blijlevens NM, Donnelly JP, Naber AH, Schattenberg AV, DePauw BE. A randomised, double-blinded, placebo-controlled, pilot study of parenteral glutamine for allogeneic stem cell transplant patients. *Support Care Cancer*. 2005;13(10) 790–796.

77. Piccirillo N, De Matteis S, Sora F, et al. Glutamine parenteral supplementation in stem cell transplant. *Bone Marrow Transplant*. 2004;33(4):455, author reply 457.

78. Sykorova A, Horacek J, Zak P, Kmonicek M, Bukac J, Maly J. A randomized, double blind comparative study of prophylactic parenteral nutritional support with or without glutamine in autologous stem cell transplantation for hematological malignancies: Three years' follow-up. *Neoplasm*. 2005;52(6):476–482.

79. Ziegler TR, Young LS, Benfell K, et al. Clinical and metabolic efficacy of glutamine-supplemented parenteral nutrition after bone marrow transplantation: A randomized, double-blind, controlled study. *Ann Intern Med*. 1992;116(10):821–828.

80. Young LS, Bye R, Scheltinga M, Ziegler TR, Jacobs DO, Wilmore DW. Patients receiving glutamine-supplemented intravenous feedings report an improvement in mood. *JPEN J Parenter Enteral Nutr*. 1993;17(5):422–427.

81. Schloerb PR, Amare M. Total parenteral nutrition with glutamine in bone marrow transplantation and other clinical applications: A randomized, double-blind study. *JPEN J Parenter Enteral Nutr*. 1993;17(5):407–413.

82. Jebb SA, Marcus R, Elia M. A pilot study of oral glutamine supplementation in patients receiving bone marrow transplants. *Clin Nutr*. 1995;14(3):162–165.

83. Anderson PM, Ramsay NK, Shu XO, et al. Effect of low-dose oral glutamine on painful stomatitis during bone marrow transplantation. *Bone Marrow Transplant*. 1998;22(4):339–344.

84. Schloerb PR, Skikne BS. Oral and parenteral glutamine in bone marrow transplantation: A randomized, double-blind study. *JPEN J Parenter Enteral Nutr*. 1999; 23(3):117–122.

85. Coghlin Dickson TM, Wong RM, Offrin RS, et al. Effect of oral glutamine supplementation during bone marrow transplantation. *JPEN J Parenter Enteral Nutr*. 2000;24(2):61–66.

86. Pytlik R, Benes P, Patorkova M, et al. Standardized parenteral alanyl-glutamine dipeptide supplementation is not beneficial in autologous transplant patients: A randomized, double-blind, placebo controlled study. *Bone Marrow Transplant*. 2002;30(12):953–961.

87. Murray SM, Pindoria S. Nutrition support for bone marrow transplant patients. *Cochrane Database Syst Rev*. 2002;2:CD002920.

88. Piccirillo N, De Matteis S, Laurenti L, et al. Glutamine-enriched parenteral nutrition after autologous peripheral blood stem cell transplantation: Effects on immune reconstitution and mucositis. *Haematologica.* 2003;88(2):192–200.

89. Scheid C, Hermann K, Kremer G, et al. Randomized, double-blind, controlled study of glycyl-glutamine-dipeptide in the parenteral nutrition of patients with acute leukemia undergoing intensive chemotherapy. *Nutrition.* 2004;20(3): 249–254.

90. Jatoi A, Rowland K, Loprinzi CL, et al. An eicosapentaenoic acid supplement versus megestrol acetate versus both for patients with cancer-associated wasting: A North Central Cancer Treatment Group and National Cancer Institute of Canada collaborative effort. *J Clin Oncol.* 2004;22(12):2469–2476.

91. Fearon K, von Meyenfeldt MF, Moses A, et al. An energy and protein dense, high Ω-3 fatty acid oral supplement promotes weight gain in cancer cachexia. *Eur J Cancer.* 2001;37(suppl 6):S27–S28.

92. Moses AW, Slater C, Preston T, Barber MD, Fearon KC. Reduced total energy expenditure and physical activity in cachectic patients with pancreatic cancer can be modulated by an energy and protein dense oral supplement enriched with Ω-3 fatty acids. *Br J Cancer.* 2004;90(5):996–1002.

93. Wachtler P, Konig W, Senkal M, Kemen M, Koller M. Influence of a total parenteral nutrition enriched with omega-3 fatty acids on leukotriene synthesis of peripheral leukocytes and systemic cytokine levels in patients with major surgery. *J Trauma.* 1997;42(2):191–198.

94. Braga M, Gianotti L, Vignali A, Carlo VD. Preoperative oral arginine and Ω-3 fatty acid supplementation improves the immunometabolic host response and outcome after colorectal resection for cancer. *Surgery.* 2002;132(5):805–814.

95. Farreras N, Artigas V, Cardona D, Rius X, Trias M, Gonzalez JA. Effect of early postoperative enteral immunonutrition on wound healing in patients undergoing surgery for gastric cancer. *Clin Nutr.* 2005;24(1):55–65.

96. Senkal M, Zumtobel V, Bauer KH, et al. Outcome and cost-effectiveness of perioperative enteral immunonutrition in patients undergoing elective upper gastrointestinal tract surgery: A prospective randomized study. *Arch Surg.* 1999;134(12): 1309–1316.

97. Song JX, Qing SH, Huang XC, Qi DL. Effect of parenteral nutrition with L-arginine supplementation on postoperative immune function in patients with colorectal cancer. *Di Yi Jun Yi Da Xue Xue Bao.* 2002;22(6):545–547.

98. Heys SD, Gough DB, Khan L, Eremin O. Nutritional pharmacology and malignant disease: A therapeutic modality in patients with cancer. *Br J Surg.* May 1996; 83(5):608–619.

99. Evans ME, Tian J, Gu LH, Jones DP, Ziegler TR. Dietary supplementation with orotate and uracil increases adaptive growth of jejunal mucosa after massive small bowel resection in rats. *JPEN J Parenter Enteral Nutr.* 2005;29(5):315–320, discussion 320–311.

100. Daly JM, Lieberman MD, Goldfine J, et al. Enteral nutrition with supplemental arginine, RNA, and omega-3 fatty acids in patients after operation: Immunologic, metabolic, and clinical outcome. *Surgery.* 1992;112(1):56–67.

101. Daly JM, Weintraub FN, Shou J, Rosato EF, Lucia M. Enteral nutrition during multimodality therapy in upper gastrointestinal cancer patients. *Ann Surg.* 1995;221(4):327–338.

102. Di Carlo V, Gianotti L, Balzano G, Zerbi A, Braga M. Complications of pancreatic surgery and the role of perioperative nutrition. *Dig Surg.* 1999;16(4):320–326.

103. Braga M, Gianotti L, Vignali A, Cestari A, Bisagni P, Di Carlo V. Artificial nutrition after major abdominal surgery: Impact of route of administration and composition of the diet. *Crit Care Med.* 1998;26(1):24–30.

104. Gianotti L, Braga M, Nespoli L, Radaelli G, Beneduce A, Di Carlo V. A randomized controlled trial of preoperative oral supplementation with a specialized diet in patients with gastrointestinal cancer. *Gastroenterology.* 2002;122(7):1763–1770.

105. Tepaske R, Velthuis H, Oudemans-van Straaten HM, et al. Effect of preoperative oral immune-enhancing nutritional supplement on patients at high risk of infection after cardiac surgery: A randomised placebo-controlled trial. *Lancet.* 2001;358 (9283):696–701.

106. Bistrian BR. Practical recommendations for immune-enhancing diets. *J Nutr.* 2004;134(10)(suppl):2868S–2872S, discussion 2895S.

107. Lacour J, Laplanche A, Malafosse M, et al. Polyadenylic-polyuridylic acid as an adjuvant in resectable colorectal carcinoma: A 6½ year follow-up analysis of a multicentric double blind randomized trial. *Eur J Surg Oncol.* 1992;18(6):599–604.

108. Fainsinger RL, Gramlich LM. How often can we justify parenteral nutrition in terminally ill cancer patients? *J Palliat Care.* 1997;13(1):48–51.

109. Fan BG. Parenteral nutrition prolongs the survival of patients associated with malignant gastrointestinal obstruction. *JPEN J Parenter Enteral Nutr.* 2007;31(6):508–510.

110. Howard L. Home parenteral nutrition in patients with a cancer diagnosis. *JPEN J Parenter Enteral Nutr.* 1992;16(6)(suppl):93S–99S.

111. Bozzetti F. Home total parenteral nutrition in incurable cancer patients: A therapy, a basic humane care or something in between? *Clin Nutr.* 2003;22(2):109–111.

112. August DA, Thorn D, Fisher RL, Welchek CM. Home parenteral nutrition for patients with inoperable malignant bowel obstruction. *JPEN J Parenter Enteral Nutr.* 1991;15(3):323–327.

113. King LA, Carson LF, Konstantinides N, et al. Outcome assessment of home parenteral nutrition in patients with gynecologic malignancies: What have we learned in a decade of experience? *Gynecol Oncol.* 1993;51(3):377–382.

114. Cozzaglio L, Balzola F, Cosentino F, et al. Outcome of cancer patients receiving home parenteral nutrition: Italian Society of Parenteral and Enteral Nutrition (S.I.N.P.E.). *JPEN J Parenter Enteral Nutr.* 1997;21(6):339–342.

115. Baines M, Oliver DJ, Carter RL. Medical management of intestinal obstruction in patients with advanced malignant disease: A clinical and pathological study. *Lancet.* 1985;2(8462):990–993.

116. Larrea J, Vega S, Martinez T, Torrent JM, Vega V, Nunez V. The nutritional status and immunological situation of cancer patients [in Spanish]. *Nutr Hosp.* 1992; 7(3):178–184.

117. Hammerlid E, Wirblad B, Sandin C, et al. Malnutrition and food intake in relation to quality of life in head and neck cancer patients. *Head Neck.* 1998;20(6):540–548.

118. Lerut TE, van Lanschot JJ. Chronic symptoms after subtotal or partial oesophagectomy: Diagnosis and treatment. *Best Pract Res Clin Gastroenterol.* 2004;18(5): 901–915.

119. Scholmerich J. Postgastrectomy syndromes: Diagnosis and treatment. *Best Pract Res Clin Gastroenterol.* 2004;18(5):917–933.

120. Shibuya S, Fukudo S, Shineha R, et al. High incidence of reflux esophagitis observed by routine endoscopic examination after gastric pull-up esophagectomy. *World J Surg.* 2003;27(5):580–583.

121. Rey-Ferro M, Castano R, Orozco O, Serna A, Moreno A. Nutritional and immunologic evaluation of patients with gastric cancer before and after surgery. *Nutrition.* 1997;13(10):878–881.

122. Malouf M, Grimley EJ, Areosa SA. Folic acid with or without vitamin B_{12} for cognition and dementia. *Cochrane Database Syst Rev.* 2003;4:CD004514.

123. Adachi S, Kawamoto T, Otsuka M, Todoroki T, Fukao K. Enteral vitamin B_{12} supplements reverse postgastrectomy B_{12} deficiency. *Ann Surg.* 2000;232(2):199–201.

124. Oh R, Brown DL. Vitamin B_{12} deficiency. *Am Fam Physician.* 2003;67(5):979–986.

125. Phang PT, Hain JM, Perez-Ramirez JJ, Madoff RD, Gemlo BT. Techniques and complications of ileostomy takedown. *Am J Surg.* 1999;177(6):463–466.

126. Beyer P. Medical nutrition therapy for lower gastrointestinal tract disorders. In: Maham L, Escott-Stump S, eds. *Krause's Food, Nutrition, and Diet Therapy.* 11th ed. New York, NY: Elsevier; 2004:705–737.

127. Petersen C. D-Lactic acidosis. *Nutr Clin Pract.* 2005;20(6):634–645.

128. Azhar SS, Beach RE. D-Lactic acidosis in a diabetic patient with a short bowel. *J Am Board Fam Pract.* 2002;15(4):316–318.

129. Uchida H, Yamamoto H, Kisaki Y, Fujino J, Ishimaru Y, Ikeda H. D-Lactic acidosis in short-bowel syndrome managed with antibiotics and probiotics. *J Pediatr Surg.* 2004;39(4):634–636.

130. Neale G, Gompertz D, Schonsby H, Tabaqchali S, Booth CC. The metabolic and nutritional consequences of bacterial overgrowth in the small intestine. *Am J Clin Nutr.* 1972;25(12):1409–1417.

131. Bongaerts GP, Severijnen RS, Tangerman A, Verrips A, Tolboom JJ. Bile acid deconjugation by lactobacilli and its effects in patients with a short small bowel. *J Gastroenterol.* 2000;35(11):801–804.

132. Mogilner JG, Srugo I, Lurie M, et al. Effect of probiotics on intestinal regrowth and bacterial translocation after massive small bowel resection in a rat. *J Pediatr Surg.* 2007;42(8):1365–1371.

133. Quigley EM, Quera R. Small intestinal bacterial overgrowth: Roles of antibiotics, prebiotics, and probiotics. *Gastroenterology.* 2006;130(2)(suppl 1):S78–S90.

134. Seehofer D, Rayes N, Schiller R, et al. Probiotics partly reverse increased bacterial translocation after simultaneous liver resection and colonic anastomosis in rats. *J Surg Res.* 2004;117(2):262–271.

135. van Minnen LP, Timmerman HM, Lutgendorff F, et al. Modification of intestinal flora with multispecies probiotics reduces bacterial translocation and improves clinical course in a rat model of acute pancreatitis. *Surgery.* 2007;141(4):470–480.

136. Salminen S, von Wright A, Morelli L, et al. Demonstration of safety of probiotics: A review. *Int J Food Microbiol.* 1998;44(1–2):93–106.

137. Guarner F, Malagelada JR. Gut flora in health and disease. *Lancet.* 2003;361 (9356):512–519.

138. Husebye E. The pathogenesis of gastrointestinal bacterial overgrowth. *Chemotherapy.* 2005;51(suppl 1):1–22.

139. Neut C, Bulois P, Desreumaux P, et al. Changes in the bacterial flora of the neoterminal ileum after ileocolonic resection for Crohn's disease. *Am J Gastroenterol.* 2002;97(4):939–946.

140. Kahl S, Malfertheiner P. Exocrine and endocrine pancreatic insufficiency after pancreatic surgery. *Best Pract Res Clin Gastroenterol.* 2004;18(5):947–955.

141. Riediger H, Adam U, Fischer E, et al. Long-term outcome after resection for chronic pancreatitis in 224 patients. *J Gastrointest Surg.* 2007;11(8):949–959; discussion 959–960.

142. Slezak LA, Andersen DK. Pancreatic resection: Effects on glucose metabolism. *World J Surg.* 2001;25(4):452–460.
143. Buchler MW, Friess H, Muller MW, Wheatley AM, Beger HG. Randomized trial of duodenum-preserving pancreatic head resection versus pylorus-preserving Whipple in chronic pancreatitis. *Am J Surg.* 1995;169(1):65–69, discussion 69–70.
144. Pereira PL, Wiskirchen J. Morphological and functional investigations of neuroendocrine tumors of the pancreas. *Eur Radiol.* 2003;13(9):2133–2146.
145. Nikou GC, Toubanakis C, Nikolaou P, et al. VIPomas: An update in diagnosis and management in a series of 11 patients. *Hepatogastroenterology.* 2005;52(64): 1259–1265.
146. Fuhrman MP, Charney P, Mueller CM. Hepatic proteins and nutrition assessment. *J Am Diet Assoc.* 2004;104(8):1258–1264.
147. Barle H, Nyberg B, Essen P, et al. The synthesis rates of total liver protein and plasma albumin determined simultaneously in vivo in humans. *Hepatology.* 1997; 25(1):154–158.
148. Sanchez AJ, Aranda-Michel J. Nutrition for the liver transplant patient. *Liver Transpl.* 2006;12(9):1310–1316.
149. Schneider PD. Preoperative assessment of liver function. *Surg Clin North Am.* 2004;84(2):355–373.
150. Marchesini G, Marzocchi R, Noia M, Bianchi G. Branched-chain amino acid supplementation in patients with liver diseases. *J Nutr.* 2005;135(6)(suppl):1596S–1601S.
151. Kondrup J. Nutrition in end stage liver disease. *Best Pract Res Clin Gastroenterol.* 2006;20(3):547–560.
152. Schiff E, Sorrell M, Maddrey W, eds. *Schiff's Diseases of the Liver.* 10th ed. New York, NY: Lippincott Williams & Wilkins; 2006.
153. Richter B, Schmandra TC, Golling M, Bechstein WO. Nutritional support after open liver resection: A systematic review. *Dig Surg.* 2006;23(3):139–145.
154. Kudsk KA. Early enteral nutrition in surgical patients. *Nutrition.* 1998;14(6): 541–544.
155. Gabor S, Renner H, Matzi V, et al. Early enteral feeding compared with parenteral nutrition after oesophageal or oesophagogastric resection and reconstruction. *Br J Nutr.* 2005;93(4):509–513.
156. Date RS, Clements WD, Gilliland R. Feeding jejunostomy: Is there enough evidence to justify its routine use? *Dig Surg.* 2004;21(2):142–145.
157. Jensen GL, Sporay G, Whitmire S, Taraszewski R, Reed MJ. Intraoperative placement of the nasoenteric feeding tube: A practical alternative? *JPEN J Parenter Enteral Nutr.* 1995;19(3):244–247.
158. Andersen H, Lewis S, Thomas S. Early enteral nutrition within 24h of colorectal surgery versus later commencement of feeding for postoperative complications. *Cochrane Database of Systematic Reviews, Vol. 4*; 2005.
159. Klein S, Koretz RL. Nutrition support in patients with cancer: What do the data really show? *Nutr Clin Pract.* 1994;9(3):91–100.
160. Gerndt SJ, Orringer MB. Tube jejunostomy as an adjunct to esophagectomy. *Surgery.* 1994;115(2):164–169.
161. Bozzetti F, Gavazzi C, Miceli R, et al. Perioperative total parenteral nutrition in malnourished, gastrointestinal cancer patients: A randomized, clinical trial. *JPEN J Parenter Enteral Nutr.* 2000;24(1):7–14.
162. Wu GH, Liu ZH, Wu ZH, Wu ZG. Perioperative artificial nutrition in malnourished gastrointestinal cancer patients. *World J Gastroenterol.* 2006;12(15):2441–2444.

163. Meijerink WJ, von Meyenfeldt MF, Rouflart MM, Soeters PB. Efficacy of perioperative nutritional support. *Lancet*. 1992;340(8812):187–188.

164. Gupta D, Lammersfeld CA, Vashi PG, Burrows J, Lis CG, Grutsch JF. Prognostic significance of Subjective Global Assessment (SGA) in advanced colorectal cancer. *Eur J Clin Nutr*. 2005;59(1):35–40.

165. Radigan A. Post-gastrectomy: Managing the nutrition fall-out. *Pract Gastroenterol*. 2004;28(6):63–75.

166. Watt-Watson J, Stevens B, Katz J, Costello J, Reid GJ, David T. Impact of preoperative education on pain outcomes after coronary artery bypass graft surgery. *Pain*. 2004;109(1–2):73–85.

167. Danino AM, Chahraoui K, Frachebois L, et al. Effects of an informational CD-ROM on anxiety and knowledge before aesthetic surgery: A randomised trial. *Br J Plast Surg*. 2005;58(3):379–383.

168. Pager CK. Randomised controlled trial of preoperative information to improve satisfaction with cataract surgery. *Br J Ophthalmol*. 2005;89(1):10–13.

169. Sjoling M, Nordahl G, Olofsson N, Asplund K. The impact of preoperative information on state anxiety, postoperative pain and satisfaction with pain management. *Patient Educ Couns*. 2003;51(2):169–176.

170. Ratanalert S, Soontrapornchai P, Ovartlarnporn B. Preoperative education improves quality of patient care for endoscopic retrograde cholangiopancreatography. *Gastroenterol Nurs*. 2003;26(1):21–25.

171. Buzby GP, Mullen JL, Matthews DC, Hobbs CL, Rosato EF. Prognostic Nutritional Index in gastrointestinal surgery. *Am J Surg*. 1980;139(1):160–167.

172. Giraudet-Le Quintrec JS, Coste J, Vastel L, et al. Positive effect of patient education for hip surgery: A randomized trial. *Clin Orthop Relat Res*. 2003(414):112–120.

Chapter 6

Nutrition and Cancer Prevention

Nicole Stendell-Hollis, MS, RD

INTRODUCTION

Throughout history, changes and trends in food and beverage intake, physical activity habits, and body composition have accompanied the increases in industrialization and urbanization throughout the world. In general, diets have become more energy dense, while levels of physical activity have decreased as the population has become increasingly sedentary, resulting in increased rates of overweight and obesity worldwide. These changes correlate with shifts in cancer incidence throughout the world, with a doubling of global cancer rates projected to occur by 2030.[1]

Approximately one-third of the cancer deaths that occur yearly in the United States are estimated to be due to nutrition and physical activity factors, as well as weight status.[2] Cancer is caused by both internal factors (e.g., inherited mutations, hormones, immune conditions, and metabolic mutations) and external factors (e.g., tobacco, chemicals, radiation, and infectious organisms); these factors may work either collectively or in sequence to initiate or promote carcinogenesis. Although all cancers involve the malfunction of genes that control cell growth and division, only approximately 5% of cancers are attributed to hereditary factors. Hence, for those individuals who do not use tobacco, choices associated with diet, physical activity, and weight control are the most significant modifiable aspects of cancer risk.

Recent cancer prevention recommendations by organizations focused on chronic diseases, such as the American Cancer Society (ACS) and the World Cancer Research Fund/American Institute for Cancer Research (WCRF/AICR), focus on healthy diet choices, increased physical activity, and achievement and/or maintenance of a healthy weight. Specifically, the ACS's 2006 *Recommendations for Nutrition and Physical Activity for Cancer*

Prevention[3] emphasize the following ways to decrease one's risk for developing cancer:

- Maintain a healthy body weight throughout life.
- Adopt a physically active lifestyle.
- Consume a healthy diet with an emphasis on plant food sources.
- If you drink alcoholic beverages, limit consumption.

In concurrence with these recommendations, the WCRF/AICR's 2007 *Guidelines for Cancer Prevention* include the following points:[1]

- Be as lean as possible within the normal range of body weight.
- Be physically active as part of everyday life.
- Limit consumption of energy-dense foods and avoid sugary drinks.
- Eat mostly foods of plant origin.
- Limit intake of red meat and avoid processed meat.
- Limit alcoholic drinks.
- Limit consumption of salt and avoid moldy grains or legumes.
- Aim to meet nutritional needs through diet alone.
- Mothers should breastfeed if possible; children should be breastfed if possible.
- Cancer survivors: Follow the recommendations for cancer prevention.

Throughout this chapter, recommendations are made based on the evidence and defined as convincing, probable, or limited/suggestive. Table 6.1 provides definitions and criteria for these terms based on the review and strength of the evidence. This chapter summarizes the AICR's recent recommendations related to diet (Table 6.2), physical activity, and weight control for the prevention of cancer.[1]

Table 6.1   *Criteria for Judging the Evidence*

Convincing	Strong, high-quality evidence from numerous combinations of scientific studies, including epidemiological and experimental research, as well as proof of plausible biological mechanisms
Probable	Evidence is slightly less robust, but still generally justifies goals and recommendations
Limited/suggestive	Evidence is too limited to permit a probable judgment, but there is a suggestive direction of effect

Source: Adapted from World Cancer Research Fund/American Institute for Cancer Research. *Food, Nutrition, Physical Activity, and the Prevention of Cancer: A Global Perspective.* Washington, DC: Author; 2007.

Table 6.2 *Summary of the Role of Diet and Cancer Risk*

	Decreases Risk	*Increases Risk*
Meat, poultry, fish, and eggs	• Fish (limited) • Foods containing vitamin D (limited)	• Red meat (convincing) • Processed meat (convincing) • Cantonese-style salted fish (probable) • Foods containing iron (limited) • Smoked foods (limited) • Grilled (broiled) or barbequed (charbroiled) animal products (limited)
Plant foods	• Non-starchy vegetables (probable and limited) • Allium vegetables (probable) • Garlic (probable) • Fruits (probable and limited) • Foods containing folate and selenium (probable and limited) • Foods containing carotenoids and vitamin C (probable) • Carrots (limited) • Legumes (limited) • Foods containing pyridoxine, vitamin E, and quercetin (limited)	• Chili pepper (limited)
Grains, roots, tubers, and plantains	• Foods containing fiber (probable and limited)	• Aflatoxins (convincing)
Milk and dairy products	• Milk (probable and limited)	• Diets high in calcium (probable) • Milk, dairy products, and cheese (limited)
Fats and oils		• Total fat (limited) • Foods containing animal fats (limited) • Butter (limited)
Sugars and salt		• Salt (probable) • Salted and salty foods (probable) • Foods containing sugar (limited)
Water, fruit juices, soft drinks, and hot drinks		• Arsenic in drinking water (convincing, probable, and limited) • Maté (probable and limited) • High-temperature drinks (limited)

(continues)

Table 6.2   *Summary of the Role of Diet and Cancer Risk, Continued*

	Decreases Risk	Increases Risk
Alcohol		• Alcoholic drinks (convincing and probable)
Dietary supplements	• Calcium (probable) • Selenium (probable and limited) • Retinol and alpha-tocopherol (limited)	• Beta-carotene supplements (convincing) • Retinol and selenium supplements (limited)

Source: Adapted from World Cancer Research Fund/American Institute for Cancer Research. *Food, Nutrition, Physical Activity, and the Prevention of Cancer: A Global Perspective.* Washington, DC: Author; 2007.

The Role of Diet

Food and nutrients have the ability to modify cancer risk at a large number of sites by a variety of factors that influence cellular processes associated with carcinogenesis. DNA repair; cellular proliferation, differentiation, and apoptosis; hormonal regulation; inflammation and immunity; the cell cycle; and carcinogen metabolism have all been identified as processes that may be altered by diet, nutrients, or bioactive food compounds, thereby affecting cancer risk.[1]

Substantial changes have transpired in the patterns of foods and beverages available and consumed throughout the world. These trends have resulted in a reduction in some dietary deficiencies and improvements in overall nutrition, but also in unfavorable shifts in the composition of diets. The increased proportions of energy-dense foods now consumed by much of the world's population contain large amounts of fats, oils, and sugars—all of which contribute to an increased risk of some types of cancer. There are several plausible theories for this increase in cancer risk due to dietary choices, such as an excess intake of energy, increased exposure to red meat, insufficient intake of fruits and vegetables, and/or an imbalance of omega-3 and omega-6 fatty acids. All of these factors may further contribute to risk both alone and through an undesirable increase in body weight. These factors and others are discussed in more detail in this chapter.

Meat, Poultry, Fish, and Eggs

One notable change in dietary patterns is the increased accessibility of animal products, which traditionally have provided only a small percentage of the overall food availability. Meat consumption has tended to increase with economic development, with the ultimate result of worldwide meat consumption per person approximately doubling between 1961 and 2002. In general, animal products provide relatively high amounts of fat and energy, both of which contribute to the increased risk of some cancers.

Evidence from epidemiological studies illustrate a dose-response relationship between red meat consumption and colorectal cancer, and suggest red meat intake is a causative factor in esophageal, lung, pancreas, and endometrial cancers.[4] Several conceivable mechanisms for an underlying causative association between red meat intake and cancer have been proposed: the generation of potentially carcinogenic and mutagenic *N*-nitroso compounds by gastrointestinal bacteria[5]; the production of carcinogenic heterocyclic amines and polycyclic aromatic hydrocarbons due to cooking at high temperatures[6]; and possible excess iron exposure leading to excess generation of free radicals, oxidative stress, inflammation, and hypoxia.[7]

The term "processed meat" is defined inconsistently in the literature. For the purpose of this review, processed meat is defined as any meat that has been preserved by smoking, curing, salting, or addition of preservatives. Examples include ham, bacon, pastrami, salami, sausages, bratwursts, frankfurters, hotdogs, and sometimes minced meats. A considerable body of strong evidence from cohort studies indicates that processed meat is a contributory factor in colorectal cancer, and limited evidence suggests that processed meat is a contributory factor in esophageal, lung, stomach, and prostate cancers.[8] Several plausible mechanisms for explaining the carcinogenic capacity of these foods exist:

- Nitrates are commonly used as preservatives for meats, which may contribute to the production and exposure of *N*-nitroso compounds, thereby increasing the risk of cancer.
- Many processed meats contain high levels of salt and nitrites, which may negatively influence cancer risk.[9]
- Processed meats generally contain high amounts of fat and iron, which may increase the production of free radicals, thereby increasing cancer risk.
- Processed meats are likely to be cooked at high temperatures, increasing the production of heterocyclic amines and polycyclic aromatic hydrocarbons.

Probable evidence exists that Cantonese-style salted fish is associated with increased risk of nasopharyngeal cancer because of the high levels of the known carcinogens *N*-nitrosamines found in this product. Cantonese-style salted fish refers to the traditional method of preserving raw fish through drying and salting of fish, thereby contributing to fermentation and/or insect infestation of the fish and increasing the risk of cancer.

There is limited evidence that smoked, grilled (broiled), and barbequed (charbroiled) foods are causative factors in stomach cancer, as meats cooked at a high temperature, over an open flame, or charred or "well done" may lead to the development of heterocyclic amines or polycyclic aromatic hydrocarbons.

The evidence regarding poultry and eggs is too limited in amount, consistency, and/or quality to draw any conclusions. There are also limited data suggesting that eating fish and foods containing vitamin D may be protective against colorectal cancer owing to their involvement in inflammation, and cellular proliferation and differentiation, respectively.[10]

In conclusion, it is recommended to limit intake of red meat to no more than three (3–4 oz/serving) servings per week, and to avoid processed meats altogether.[1]

Plant Foods

Despite the numerous benefits of eating a plant-based diet, consumption of plant foods around the world varies and is generally lower than what is commonly recommended. Historically, diets have combined grains and legumes, thereby ensuring adequate protein consumption, while providing only small amounts of animal products. Nutrient-dense plant sources such as vegetables and fruits are rich sources of a variety of vitamins, minerals, phytochemicals, and fiber, but provide only a limited amount of energy. Nuts and seeds provide concentrated sources of micronutrients and essential fatty acids, and many herbs and spices have known beneficial pharmacological properties. Therefore, it is recommended to eat mostly foods of plant origin, with an average daily consumption of 21 oz of non-starchy vegetables and fruits and 25 g of unprocessed cereal grains and legumes.[1]

Non-starchy vegetables can be defined as green, leafy vegetables including broccoli, okra, eggplant, and bok choy, as well as roots and tubers such as carrots, artichokes, celery root, rutabaga, and turnips. A substantial amount of probable—although not convincing—evidence exists that non-starchy vegetables protect against mouth, pharynx, larynx, esophageal, and stomach cancers, and limited evidence suggests that non-starchy vegetables may protect against nasopharyngeal, lung, colorectal, ovarian, and endometrial cancers. Several hypotheses have been put forth to explain these protective effects. Non-starchy vegetables contain an abundance of potentially anticarcinogenic substances, including antioxidants such as carotenoids and vitamin C, dietary fiber, and numerous phytochemicals (glucosinolates, dithiolthiones, indoles, chlorophyll, flavonoids, allyl sulfides, and phytoestrogens). Bioactive food components (BAFC) may alter cancer risk through their antioxidant properties, modulation of detoxification enzymes, stimulation of the immune system, antiproliferative activities, and modulation of hormone concentrations and metabolism.[11] Non-starchy vegetables also contain substantial amounts of folate, which plays an important role in the synthesis and methylation of DNA, and which may prevent expression of the aberrant gene linked to several types of cancer.[12] Additionally, probable data exist that the allium vegetables (onions, garlic, leeks, chives, and shallots) lower the risk of stomach and colorectal cancers; limited evidence suggests carrots are protective against cervical cancer.

Cruciferous vegetables are increasingly receiving attention as potential anticarcinogenic agents because of their high concentrations of glucosinolates, which are metabolized to isothiocyanates (ITCs) and indoles in the digestion process. These metabolic products lessen the effects of polycyclic aromatic hydrocarbons and nitrosamines via the activation of glutathione-S-transferases (GSTs) and inhibition of cytochrome P450 isoenzymes. Additionally, ITCs have been shown to modify meat-derived urinary mutagens as well as mutations formed by tobacco carcinogens.[13] Despite this promising preliminary evidence, research has shown inconsistent results regarding cruciferous vegetables' potential to act as anticarcinogenic agents. Of course, it is difficult to pinpoint the specific anticarcinogenic effect of the various nutrients in foods in general, as most likely this effect arises through the additive and synergistic actions of the many nutrients present in whole fruits and vegetables.

Consistent, plausible evidence indicates that fruits probably protect against mouth, pharynx, larynx, esophageal, lung, and stomach cancers, with limited evidence for protection against nasopharyngeal, liver, and colorectal cancers.[14-16] Fruits are a rich source of vitamin C, phenols, and flavonoids, as well as other potentially bioactive phytochemicals; this nutritional content may explain fruits' shielding effect against certain types of cancer. Vitamin C is especially protective against cancer, as it readily traps free radicals and reactive oxygen species, thereby protecting against oxidative damage; it also regenerates other antioxidants such as vitamin E and inhibits the formation of carcinogens.[17] Some fruits contain high concentrations of the antioxidant-acting flavonoids, which have the ability to inhibit carcinogen-activating enzymes and DNA damage.[18] Finally, the antioxidant phytochemicals commonly found in fruits may diminish the free-radical damage generated by inflammation.

The evidence regarding specific carotenoids and other nutrients found within fruits and vegetables is summarized in Table 6.3, and the general mechanisms involved are discussed later in this section. Many of the protective effects of the carotenoids result from their antioxidant properties, which can prevent lipid oxidation and free-radical–induced oxidative stress.[17] Additionally, several of the carotenoids function as pro-vitamin A

Table 6.3   *Specific Nutrients and Evidence of a Protective Effect Against Select Cancer Risk*

	Probable Evidence	*Limited Evidence*
Carotenoids (pro-vitamin A, α-carotene, β-carotene, lycopene, and β-cryptoxanthin)	• Mouth • Pharynx • Larynx • Lung • Esophageal • Prostate	
Folate-containing foods		• Pancreas • Esophageal • Colorectal
Pyridoxine (vitamin B_6)-containing foods		• Esophageal
Vitamin C–containing foods	• Esophageal	
Vitamin E–containing foods		• Esophageal • Prostate
Selenium–containing foods	• Prostate	• Lung • Stomach • Colorectal
Quercetin–containing foods		• Lung

Source: Adapted from World Cancer Research Fund/American Institute for Cancer Research. *Food, Nutrition, Physical Activity, and the Prevention of Cancer: A Global Perspective.* Washington, DC: Author; 2007.

precursors, which, once converted to retinol, play a role in cellular differentiation, immuno-enhancement, and activation of carcinogenic-metabolizing enzymes.[17] Finally, lycopene—the most potent of the carotenoid antioxidants—demonstrates an antiproliferative effect, reduces plasma low-density lipoprotein cholesterol, improves immune function, and reduces inflammation.[19, 20]

The benefits of folate in relation to the prevention of cancer have previously been discussed. At the same time, it is important to note that in animal studies, high doses of folate have been shown to promote carcinogenesis. Thus dose is an important factor to consider when determining folate's effect on cancer prevention.

Pyridoxine (vitamin B_6) is involved in one-carbon metabolism and thus plays a role in the synthesis, repair, and methylation of DNA, as demonstrated in animal studies.[21] Vitamin E is another antioxidant that has been reported to enhance DNA repair and to prevent DNA damage, lipid peroxidation, and the activation of carcinogens such as nitrosamines.[17] Vitamin E has also been reported to enhance the immune system, which may play a role in the body's ability to shield against cancer.[17]

Selenoproteins, which are commonly found in foods containing selenium, have been shown to demonstrate anti-inflammatory and antioxidant properties primarily due to the activity of the glutathione peroxidases, which protect against oxidative damage, and the thioredoxin reductases, which regenerate oxidized ascorbic acid to its reduced antioxidant form.[22]

Lastly, the flavonoid quercetin has antioxidant properties as well as the ability to inhibit the expression of CYP1A1 (a cytochrome P450 enzyme that helps to metabolize toxins[23]), resulting in decreased formation of DNA adducts.[24] Elevated CYP1A1 activity has been correlated with an increased risk of lung cancer.[25]

While the evidence is inconsistent, limited data suggest that legumes and soy products may exhibit a protective effect against stomach and prostate cancers.[26] Ecological studies support a potential inverse dose-response relationship between soy intake and stomach and prostate cancer risk, perhaps due to soy's numerous BAFCs. Legumes and other soy foods are rich in BAFCs that exhibit anticarcinogenic effects, such as protease inhibitors, saponins, and phytoestrogens (genistein, daidzein),[27] all of which may modulate estrogen metabolism, demonstrate antioxidant properties, inhibit tumor angiogenesis, and influence apoptosis and cell growth.

The evidence for the protective effects of nuts and seeds is too limited in amount, consistency, and quality to draw any decisive conclusions. Limited evidence does suggest that chili pepper may increase the risk of stomach cancer. This increased risk is likely related to its pro-irritant effect, which may possibly increase the risk of inflammation in the stomach.[28]

Grains, Roots, Tubers, and Plantains

The starchy plant foods traditionally have served as the primary source of energy since societies and agriculture have evolved. Their whole, unprocessed forms represent a plentiful source of dietary fiber and other micronutrients. With the trends toward increased industrialization and urbanization, consumption of these whole foods has decreased, with more being consumed in the refined form of cereal grains. These processed foodstuffs are more energy dense and generally contain added fat, sugar, or salt, thereby lowering the overall nutrient value of the food. Roots and tubers, when eaten with their skins on, provide a rich source of fiber and micronutrients as well; however, most urbanized populations tend to eat them in a more processed form.

In general, the evidence that grains, roots, tubers, or plantains are able to modify cancer risk is not convincing. Probable data do suggest that foods containing fiber likely have a protective effect against colorectal cancer, with limited data suggesting that such fiber-containing foods may lower the risk of esophageal cancer. Rich sources of fiber include unprocessed grains, roots, tubers, and plantains, as well as fruits, vegetables, and legumes. Fiber's protective effect is thought to be due to its bulky, satiating effect and the fact that fiber-containing foods are also low in energy. Additionally, fiber dilutes fecal contents, increases stool weight, and decreases transit time, effectively removing potentially carcinogenic compounds within the intestinal tract, as well as fermentation by-products produced by the gut flora from various dietary carbohydrates.

Aflatoxins, which are naturally occurring mycotoxins produced by certain molds or fungi, are classified as human carcinogens.[29] Although most molds are destroyed by the cooking process, the toxins they produce may persist in the cooked foods. The main foods prone to contamination by aflatoxins are cereal grains and legumes, and this issue is considered to be the most problematic in countries with hot, humid climates and poor storage facilities. Aflatoxins become a worldwide problem when these contaminated foods are exported to other countries. Cohort and case-control studies have shown a convincing association between aflatoxin biomarkers and hepatocellular carcinoma, possibly due to its interaction with the *GST* genotype. Evidence shows that the positive *GSTM1/GSTT1* genotypes are protective against liver cancer from hepatitis infection combined with aflatoxin exposure, while the negative *GSTM1/GSTT1* genotypes increase risk.[30] Other conceivable mechanisms include the production of epoxide products of aflatoxin, which are commonly found in the liver and known to be genotoxic to the p53 gene, leading to the increased proliferation of abnormal cells and causing the progression of cancer.[31] Additionally, the synergistic effect of hepatitis infection and aflatoxin exposure may be explained by the increased production of the enzyme CYP1A2, which is responsible for the increased production of the genotoxic metabolites of aflatoxin. Likewise, the hepatitis virus may increase gene transversion, inhibit nucleotide repair, or act as a tumor promoter.[32] In any event, strong evidence supports the existence of a dose-response relationship between aflatoxin-contaminated foods and liver cancer.

In conclusion, it is recommended to consume unprocessed grains and/or legumes with every meal while limiting the intake of processed starchy foods.

Milk and Dairy Products

Until the late nineteenth century, cow's milk was primarily used as an artificial substitute for breast milk to feed infants, with adults consuming very little, if any, of this product. With the industrialization of cattle farming in the twentieth century, cow's milk became a staple food in the United States and other European countries, representing a major source of calcium as well as other vitamins, minerals, and protein.

Data from cohort studies suggest that milk is probably protective against colorectal cancer, with limited evidence suggesting it is protective against bladder cancer and a causative factor in prostate cancer. Interestingly, limited data suggest that cheese consumption may be a causative factor in colorectal cancer, despite milk and dairy products' protective effects against colorectal cancer. The ability of milk to decrease colorectal cancer risk likely results in part from its calcium content, which decreases cell proliferation and/or promotes cell differentiation; calcium also protects the gastrointestinal lining by binding to potentially damaging bile and fatty acids.[33]

Alternatively, calcium may actually increase prostate cancer risk by reducing circulating 1,25-dihydroxyvitamin D, which is thought to inhibit development of prostate cancer through its ability to regulate prostate growth and differentiation.[34] Other hypotheses seeking to explain the association between dairy products and prostate cancer point to the effects of the increased concentrations of insulin-like growth factors[35] or estrogens[36] found in these foods.

Finally, while no specific mechanism has been identified, cheese could plausibly cause colorectal cancer through an indirect mechanism related to its saturated fat content. Saturated fat may increase insulin production and expression in colorectal cells as well as stimulate the production of inflammatory mediators associated with carcinogenesis.[37]

Fats and Oils

Similar to meat and dairy consumption, fat and oil intake tends to increase with greater industrialization and urbanization. Specifically, commercially bred animals have a higher fat content than wild animals. On a global scale, production and consumption of animal fats and plant oils continues to increase. Contradicting previous reports, only limited evidence now suggests that diets high in fats and oils might be causative of some types of cancer.

Fats can be classified as either saturated or unsaturated, depending on their chemical structure. Liquid oils in general have higher concentrations of unsaturated fatty acids, whereas solid fats have higher concentrations of saturated fatty acids. The two essential polyunsaturated fatty acids, linoleic acid (Ω-6) and linolenic acid (Ω-3), are important lipid constituents whose amounts in the diet were once thought to be roughly equal. More recently, trends toward greater urbanization have caused vegetable oils, which are predominantly composed of Ω-6 fatty acids, to become more widely available. Thus the ratio of Ω-6 to Ω-3 fatty acids has gradually increased to between 10:1 and 20:1 in most high-income countries.[38] This imbalance in fatty acids is concerning because the Ω-3 fatty acids have a known immune-enhancing effect, whereas the Ω-6 fatty acids may have a suppressing effect on the immune system, thereby increasing cancer risk.[39]

Trans-fatty acids are unsaturated fatty acids that have been partially converted to saturated fatty acids by the hydrogenation process, resulting in chemically unsaturated fatty acids that behave like saturated fatty acids. This process alone has greatly increased the production and consumption of total fat and saturated fat throughout the world, thereby contributing to the steady increase in consumption of energy-dense foods and, indirectly, obesity.

Limited evidence suggests that consumption of total fat is a contributing factor in the progression of lung cancer, although no evidence for a plausible mechanism has been identified.[40] Of course, the primary modifiable cause of lung cancer remains the smoking of tobacco products.

Select, speculative data suggest that total fat intake is also causative of postmenopausal breast cancer, possibly due to the increased production of endogenous estrogen derived from dietary fat intake.[41] The recent results of the prospective low-fat dietary modification trial of the Women's Health Initiative (WHI), however, did not demonstrate a reduction in breast cancer risk among postmenopausal women consuming a low-fat (20–25% total energy intake) diet for more than 7 years,[42] perhaps due to poor adherence to the diet plan. Nevertheless, a small reduction in risk was observed among the subset of women entering the trial who had the highest dietary fat eating pattern at baseline. Further, an analysis of cancer incidence related to fat intake undertaken in 2007 from the WHI study showed that ovarian cancer risk is reduced in women who adhere to a low-fat eating pattern post menopause.[43] Additionally, low-fat diets are generally associated with higher fiber intake, which may assist in reducing total estrogen concentration in the body by decreasing intestinal reabsorption. Other likely mechanisms include a decrease in the sex hormone-binding globulin associated with increased body mass, leading to elevated concentrations of free estradiol,[44] or early menarche related to energy-dense diets, which is an established risk factor for breast cancer.[45]

Limited but consistent evidence suggests that consumption of animal fats is a contributing factor in colorectal cancer. However, in terms of cholesterol and *trans*-fatty acids, there is insufficient corroborative evidence specifically linking these lipids to cancer risk. The low-fat diet intervention studied in the WHI dietary modification trial participants, for example, showed no association between adoption of a low-fat diet post menopause and colorectal cancer risk.[43]

Sugars and Salts

Sugars and salts are most commonly consumed as ingredients in processed foods. Consumption of these foods is increasing globally. Specifically, intake of added sugars is rising with the trend toward increased ingestion of sugary beverages, such that sugars now account for a substantial quantity of total energy intake. The consumption of salt, though variable worldwide, has also generally risen with increasing availability. Excess sugar and salt intake has been associated with obesity and cardiovascular disease, respectively, in addition to certain cancers.[46, 47]

It is difficult to assess the overall effect of sugar as a modifier of cancer risk because of the inconsistencies in the classification of sugars. Sugars may, for example, be categorized as sucrose, maltose, lactose, glucose, fructose, refined sugars, high-fructose corn syrup, chemical sweeteners, or naturally occurring intrinsic sugars. Further, the United States Department of Agriculture (USDA) database for quantifying sugar in foods is relatively incomplete, making the use of this variable by epidemiological studies difficult at best. Additionally, sugar's contribution to body weight may influence cancer risk. While the data are hard to interpret, there is limited evidence that sugar intake is a contributory factor in the development of colorectal cancer.

Despite the World Health Organization's (WHO) recommendation of restricting salt consumption to less than 5 g per day, worldwide the consumption of salt has been estimated to vary from between 6 g and 18 g per day. A substantial body of probable evidence related to total salt intake, added table salt, and sodium intake supports salt's role as a mechanistic cause of stomach cancer, possibly related to damage to the stomach lining by excess salt intake.[48] Further, elevated salt intake has been shown to increase the formation of endogenous *N*-nitroso compounds,[49] demonstrate a synergistic effect with gastric carcinogenesis,[49] and contribute to gastric cancer in subjects with *Helicobacter pylori* infections who have also been exposed to a carcinogen.[50]

Beverages

When referring to beverages and cancer risk, this section focuses on water, fruit juices, soft drinks, and hot drinks; alcohol is considered separately later in the chapter.

Water quality and sufficiency is a worldwide public health issue, as water may be easily compromised by chemicals or microbiological contamination. Water is also an essential nutrient; without it, people die within a matter of days. Fruit juices are frequently diluted with water and contain added sugar, while soft drinks are made almost entirely from water, sugar, coloring, flavoring, and combinations of herbs and other ingredients to enhance taste. The primary hot drinks consumed worldwide are coffee and tea, both of which contain stimulants and other bioactive ingredients that are generally consumed with the addition of milk and sugar. A variety of herbal mixtures are also consumed, including maté, a South American tea-like beverage.

Overall, the evidence related to non-alcoholic drinks and cancer risk focuses on water supply contamination with arsenic or irritation to the oral cavity by the very-high-temperature consumption of maté or other hot beverages. Arsenic residues can result from agricultural, mining, and industrial processes, or from naturally occurring volcanic activity. Arsenic is a known human carcinogen.[51] WHO guidelines recommend that arsenic levels in drinking water not exceed 10 mcg/L, although in affected areas these levels may range from tens to thousands of micrograms per liter.[52] Other factors in the water supply that are known to increase cancer risk include contamination by *H. pylori* (associated with stomach cancer)[50] and infestation by schistosomes (parasitic worms found in the blood of humans and other mammals that are associated with bladder and liver cancer).[53]

Convincing data exist that arsenic in drinking water is causative of lung cancer, probable data demonstrate that arsenic in drinking water causes skin cancer, and limited data show that it causes kidney and bladder cancer. Several mechanisms have been proposed to explain how arsenic may be associated with increased cancer risk. Arsenic is known to cause changes in the methylation of oncogenes or tumor-suppressor genes; increase the generation of free radicals; and cause the depletion of reduced glutathione, leading to a chronic state of oxidative stress that can damage DNA and induce cell proliferation.[54]

Constant irritation to the epithelial surface by very hot beverages may increase cancer risk due to chronic inflammation. Evidence suggests that chemically irritating components within beverages may be a causative factor in cancer progression, although few data exist to confirm this relationship. It is generally believed that the increased risk derives from the extremely hot temperature or, more likely, from a combination of the high temperature and chemical irritants in the beverage.

The evidence is too limited in amount, consistency, and quality to draw any conclusions about the consumption of soft drinks and fruit juices and modulation of cancer risk. By contrast, tea—especially black and green tea—is known to contain various antioxidants and phenolic compounds that exhibit promising anticarcinogenic effects. However, the evidence has been inconsistent in suggesting regular tea consumption may be protective against certain types of cancer. Perhaps the inconsistencies in the data are related to the different cultures within which these teas are consumed. For example, the ways in which teas are prepared and drunk vary significantly between cultures in regard to how strong the tea is and whether it is consumed with or without milk and sugar; both of these factors may influence its anticarcinogenic potential.

Maté, which is prepared by steeping the dried leaves of yerba maté, is typically drunk scalding hot through a metal straw. This practice generates repetitive damage and inflammation to the mouth, pharynx, larynx, and esophagus, resulting in increased cancer risk. Although evidence on this issue is limited, it suggests that maté and other hot beverages may be a contributing factor in the progression of mouth, pharynx, larynx, and esophageal cancers.

Alcohol

Alcoholic drinks can be produced from the fermentation of many plants and some animal foods, with the alcohol content of the different beverages varying greatly. The main alcoholic drinks consumed include beers, ciders, wines, and liquors. These libations have been popular in most populations ever since alcohol's effects on mood were identified, although the level of intake varies widely depending on availability, price, culture or religion, and dependency. The active ingredient present in alcohol, ethanol, has been labeled a human carcinogen.[55]

Convincing evidence suggests that alcoholic drinks are causative of mouth, pharynx, larynx, and esophageal cancers, as well as breast cancer in women and colorectal cancer in men. Alcohol is a probable cause of liver cancer in men and women, and colorectal cancer in women. The reactive metabolites of alcohol, such as acetaldehyde, are likely to be carcinogenic.[56] Further, alcohol may modulate the production of prostaglandins, lipid peroxidation, and free radicals; enhance the penetration of carcinogens into cells through its solvency actions; and alter retinoid status effecting cellular growth, cellular differentiation, and apoptosis.[56]

Epidemiological studies suggest that in assessing alcohol's contribution to cancer risk, using breast cancer as an example, folate intake/status may be of particular importance. Women with low folate intake are especially vulnerable in terms of the cancer-promoting effects of alcohol intake.[57] Heavy alcohol consumers are also more likely to have nutrient deficiencies, which together with the previously mentioned factors may increase the risk of cancer development.

If alcoholic drinks are consumed, they should be limited to no more than two drinks per day for men and one drink per day for women. Sufficient folate intake should be promoted in those wishing to consume alcohol in any amount. Table 6.4 provides recommended portion sizes for various types of alcoholic beverages.

Table 6.4 *Recommended Serving Sizes for Alcoholic Beverages**

Beer: 12 ounces
Wine: 5 ounces
Distilled spirits: 1.5 ounces
Wine cooler: 10 ounces
*One drink is defined as having ½ ounce (approximately 14 g) of pure ethanol.

Dietary Supplements

In this section, dietary supplements such as vitamins, minerals, and phytochemicals are considered separately from whole foods and their subsequent effects on cancer risk. The manufacturing and marketing of dietary supplements has escalated ever since claims regarding their health-promoting benefits in the prevention of disease were postulated. The effect of these bioactive substances differs depending on the quantity consumed. Consequently, evidence from clinical studies is difficult to interpret because different combinations and concentrations are used in the various investigations. Moreover, while nutrients at lower doses may be protective against cancer risk, higher doses may actually be toxic or pathogenic, further complicating the interpretation of the evidence.

BAFCs are bioactive constituents of plant foods that are not considered to be essential, but whose consumption has been shown to have beneficial effects on health and in the prevention of diseases due to the substances' antioxidant, anticarcinogenic, anti-inflammatory, antimicrobial, and immunomodulatory effects.[11] Phytochemicals are classified as flavonoids, isoflavones, glucosinolates, terpenes, organosulfur compounds, saponins, capsaicinoids, or phytosterols; they are found in many vegetables, fruits, legumes, herbs, and teas.

Retinoids demonstrate antitumor actions, although their mechanisms of action are not well understood. Retinol is known to bind to cell receptors and promote cellular differentiation, alteration of membranes, and induction of immunological adjuvant effects,[58] suggesting that retinol supplements might be protective against squamous cell skin cancer. Conversely, limited data suggest that high-dose intake of retinol supplements is a causative agent for lung cancer in smokers. Convincing evidence also demonstrates a causative effect for high-dose beta-carotene supplements in lung cancer in smokers. Perhaps the protective association of carotenoid intake against cancer risk is lost or reversed at very high doses, or the protective effect of naturally occurring carotenoids is not due to the individual carotenoids but rather to the synergistic effect of all the carotenoids together, or in combination with other dietary constituents.

Alpha-tocopherol is thought to be the most biologically active of the eight different isomers that exist for vitamin E. This substance is known to inhibit cellular proliferation, directly activate certain enzymes, and demonstrate transcriptional control over several genes.[59] Alpha-tocopherol has also demonstrated the ability to inhibit the propagation of prostate tumors in animal models.[60] The research on this topic is sparse, but suggests that alpha-tocopherol supplementation might have a protective effect against prostate cancer.

1-25-dihydroxyvitamin D, a vitamin D metabolite, has antiproliferative, pro-differentiation, and apoptotic effects in some cells that are mediated by the vitamin D receptor. Additionally, a high level of sunlight exposure, which can convert 7-dehydrocholesterol into vitamin D_3 in the skin, has been correlated with lower breast cancer incidence and mortality in ecological studies.[61] These observations, together with experimental evidence, have inspired the hypothesis that high levels of vitamin D might reduce the risk of breast cancer. Notably, however, the effects of vitamin D are strongly correlated with its interactions with calcium, as both of these substances are growth-restraining and able to induce cell differentiation and apoptosis. Further complicating the interpretation of the data is the fact that the biologically active form of vitamin D is dependent on diet, supplements, and UV exposure to the skin. Inconsistent evidence from cohort and ecological studies implies that consumption of foods containing vitamin D and improvement in vitamin D status may be protective against colorectal and breast cancer, respectively.

Calcium plays an important role as a second messenger affecting numerous cellular functions throughout the body. Consistent evidence exist that calcium probably protects against colorectal cancer, possibly through its direct growth-restricting, differentiation, and apoptosis-inducing actions toward normal and tumor colorectal cells. Additionally, calcium may bind to bile and fatty acids, thereby decreasing injury to the intestinal lining. Evidence of varying quality has demonstrated a dose-response relationship between calcium intake and colorectal cancer; importantly, however, elevated levels of calcium intake have also been correlated with increased risk for prostate cancer.

An insufficient intake of selenium has been noted to cause a lack of selenoprotein expression; these proteins have numerous anti-inflammatory and antioxidant functions, as previously discussed. Selenoproteins appear to reach their maximal levels easily with normal dietary selenium intake and do not increase with supplementation. Nevertheless, it is postulated that supra-physiological concentrations might influence programmed cell death, DNA repair, carcinogen metabolism, the immune system, and antiangiogenic properties.[62] Strong, probable evidence suggests that selenium protects against prostate cancer; limited evidence indicates that it is protective against lung cancer. Conversely, some data suggest that selenium supplements may be causative of skin cancer.

A review completed by U.S. Preventive Services Task Force concluded that the evidence is either too limited or too inconsistent to make a recommendation in support of or against any type of supplement use for the prevention of cancer.[63] It is recommended that the general population achieve nutritional adequacy without the addition of dietary supplements. Supplements should be prescribed when dietary approaches are inadequate in achieving average daily intake goals.

Food Production, Preservation, Processing, and Preparation

The various methods of food preparation and preservation employed may also modify cancer risk. Nearly all foods and beverages are altered in some manner before they are consumed. Thus it is plausible that the various methods of processing and/or preservation might have protective, causative, or neutral effects on the risk of cancer.

The use of synthetic pesticides and herbicides has greatly increased since the middle of the twentieth century, with an estimated 2,500 tons of these chemicals being used worldwide in 2001. In many countries, the use of pesticides and herbicides is regulated to minimize the buildup of residues in foods and drinks. Although no epidemiological data exist that show current levels are carcinogenic, theoretical grounds for concern remain.

Another cause for concern is the use of veterinary drugs to treat and prevent infectious diseases and/or promote growth in industrial animal production. If any of these medications are found to be carcinogenic, they are removed from the market, of course. Nevertheless, the toxicity of such drugs remains constantly under review.

The use of genetic modification techniques for the production of foods for human and animal consumption is regulated in most, but not all, countries. Currently, the effect of gene modification on cancer risk is unknown because there are too few data available from which to draw any decisive conclusions.

The many methods for preserving foods include drying, fermenting, canning and bottling, pasteurizing, chemical preservation, and irradiation. The safety of such methods is continually reviewed, and to date no consistent associations between preservation and cancer risk have been identified.

Many processed foods contain additives that may be either synthetic or naturally occurring, such as bulking aids, colors, flavors, and solvents. Although these additives may serve useful functions, they may also be toxic, mutagenic, and/or carcinogenic. For that reason, these additives face constant scrutiny regarding their safety.

The naturally occurring aflatoxins, which are known carcinogens, are produced by certain molds or fungi in cereal grains and legumes. Although they are usually destroyed by the cooking process, the toxins they generate may remain if the grains or legumes are kept in hot, humid climates and poor storage facilities.

Lastly, preparation methods such as industrial cooking, steaming, boiling, stewing, baking, roasting, microwaving, frying, broiling, and barbequing may alter cancer risk, but currently the evidence is too limited in amount to draw any conclusions. It is recommended to avoid salted foods and moldy grains or legumes.

The Role of Physical Activity

Physical activity can be classified as occupational, household, transportation, or recreational, and can be further identified as vigorous, moderate, light, or sedentary, with a combination of frequency, intensity, and duration determining total physical activity levels. General levels of physical activity have declined in recent decades, with more machines performing the work that was previously done by hand, and transportation, which was once accomplished by walking or cycling, being carried out by automobiles. In most industrialized countries, people engage in some form of recreation, although in general they remain largely inactive, performing mostly sedentary activities.

Studies have found that physical inactivity is related to a higher overall cancer incidence and mortality.[64] Hypothesized mechanisms for the protective association of increased amounts of physical activity include the promotion of healthy levels of circulating hormones and the ability to consume more foods without accompanying weight gain. Additionally, the evidence indicates that the more people are physically active, the better their potential for lowering their cancer risk. No threshold level in regard to physical activity and cancer risk has been identified.

A number of mechanisms have been recognized as potential ways in which physical activity may protect against colorectal cancer, including reduction in insulin resistance, beneficial effects on body fat levels, beneficial effects on steroid hormones, and reduction of gastrointestinal transit time.[65] An abundant and convincing body of evidence demonstrates that higher levels of physical activity are associated with lower risk of colorectal cancer. Limited data suggest that physical activity is protective against premenopausal breast cancer and probably protective against postmenopausal breast cancer. The proposed protective mechanisms in these types of cancer are the beneficial effect on body fat levels, the reduction of circulating estrogen and androgens, and possible enhancement of the immune system.[65] Furthermore, studies consistently find that physical activity may lower the risk of endometrial cancer through mechanisms similar to those proposed for breast cancer.

The evidence regarding the protective effects of physical activity on lung and pancreatic cancers is limited but suggest that exercise may lower the risk of developing both types of cancer. No specific mechanisms for the reduction of lung cancer risk have been identified, and the association is complex, possibly reflecting reverse causation due to chronic lung disease. The mechanisms by which physical activity may lower pancreatic cancer risk include a reduction in insulin resistance and gastrointestinal transit time, with the latter factor having beneficial effects on the content and secretion of bile and affecting general pancreatic activity.

It is recommended that individuals be moderately physically active for at least 30 minutes or more every day and to limit their sedentary habits as much as possible.

The Role of Body Weight

The degree of body fatness, rates of growth and their outcome, and lactation all affect cancer risk throughout the lifespan. The rates of overweight and obesity doubled in many high-income countries between 1990 and 2005. Being overweight or obese increases the risk for a number of diseases, including dyslipidemia, hypertension and stroke, type II diabetes, coronary heart disease, and selected cancers, and shortens life expectancy.[66]

The distribution of body fat varies from person to person and is primarily determined by genetics. Body fat may accumulate subcutaneously or viscerally, as well as peripherally or abdominally. Estimates of body fat levels can be made by measuring waist-to-hip circumference or body mass index (BMI; see Table 6.5), with waist-to-hip circumference (or abdominal fatness) generally considered to be a better predictor of chronic diseases such as cardiovascular or metabolic disease. The WHO reference values for waist measurements are 37 inches for men and 31.5 inches for women, roughly correlating to a BMI of 25 kg/m². [1] Adult weight gain generally occurs as a result of accumulation of fat rather than lean tissue, and it

Table 6.5   *Body Mass Index Classification*

Classification BMI (kg/m²)
Underweight: BMI < 18.5
Normal weight: BMI = 18.5–24.9
Overweight: BMI = 25.0–29.9
Obese: BMI ≥ 30.0
Morbidly obese: BMI ≥ 40.0

may more accurately reflect body fatness than just an increase in body mass alone. The recommended median adult BMI is in the range of 21 to 23 kg/m². Ideally, the proportion of the population that is overweight or obese will not exceed the current level, or preferably be lower, in 10 years.

Body fatness has been acknowledged as a probable cause of esophageal, pancreatic, colorectal, postmenopausal breast (probable for premenopausal breast cancer), endometrial, and kidney cancers, and limited evidence indicates that it may cause liver and lung cancers. Evidence for a relationship between excess abdominal fat and increased cancer risk is convincing in regard to colorectal cancer, and excess abdominal fat is considered a probable cause of pancreatic, postmenopausal breast, and endometrial cancer. Lastly, adult weight gain has been identified as a probable cause of post-menopausal breast cancer.

There are several plausible mechanisms by which excess body and abdominal fat might modify cancer risk. First, elevated body fat levels increase the inflammatory response. Second, increased body fat levels increase the concentration of circulating estrogen. Third, excess body fat decreases insulin sensitivity.[67] Further, the elevated levels of insulin-like growth factor 1 (IGF-1), insulin, and leptin found in obese individuals can promote the growth of cancer cells.[68]

Growth during childhood is a predictor of age at sexual maturity as well as eventual attainment of adult height, and the rate of growth has metabolic and hormonal effects that can influence cancer risk throughout the lifespan. Based on the evidence, greater adult attained height appears unlikely to modify cancer risk directly, but it is a marker for genetic, environmental, hormonal, and nutritional factors affecting growth from preconception to the completion of linear growth. For every tissue or organ, unfavorable environmental influences—such as inadequate nutrients or energy obtained—during critical periods of development can restrict growth and impair future functioning, with the timing, severity, and duration determining the extent of the potentially negative impact.

Growth can be divided into three phases: fetal–infant, childhood, and puberty. Growth during the fetal–infant period is considered the most vulnerable to the availability of nutrients and energy. When nutrient intake is suboptimal, brain growth is protected relative to stature growth, which in turn is less affected than increases in body weight. Negative influences on growth during this period tend to affect a person's future adult height and body shape. For example, any nutrient deficiency during this critical period may result in a person's predisposition to excess body fatness because his or her energy intake exceeds the available nutrients' ability to lay down lean tissue mass; as a consequence, any excess of energy is stored as fat. In general, individuals characterized by a lower birth weight have a greater tendency to store fat, resulting in an increased risk of overweight and obesity. Speculative evidence has also led to the hypothesis that a greater birth weight is a probable cause of premenopausal breast cancer. The effects of lactation during the infant period on body weight and cancer risk will be considered separately.

Growth hormones, insulin-like growth factors, and sex hormone-binding proteins all affect height, growth, sexual maturity, fat storage, and other various processes that may be relevant to cancer development. For this reason, nutritional factors that alter height might also potentially influence cancer risk. Convincing evidence suggests that various factors influencing attainment of a greater adult height are causative agents for colorectal cancer and postmenopausal breast cancer. Of course, this risk is unlikely to be due to height alone, but instead probably reflects a combination of factors promoting linear growth in childhood. The data imply that a greater adult height is a probable cause of premenopausal breast, pancreatic, and ovary cancers, and limited data support the supposition that it is a cause of endometrial cancer.

Human milk is the natural, complete food for infants until six months of age, with no truly equivalent substitute. Not only does breast milk provide a complete source of nutrition, but it also provides immunologically active components. However, the hormones associated with amenorrhea and infertility are actually believed to be substances that modify cancer risk, probably due to the decreased lifetime exposure to menstrual cycles. Decreased exposure to certain hormones, such as androgen, can also influence cancer risk.[69] Abundant and consistent data demonstrate that lactation has a convincing protective effect against premenopausal and postmenopausal breast cancer, with limited evidence suggesting that it is protective against ovarian cancer. It is recommended that women exclusively breastfeed infants for the first six months of life and continue with complementary feeding thereafter.

Cancer Survivorship

The total number of cancer survivors worldwide continues to grow. In tandem, awareness of their unique needs has increased. In particular, lifestyle modifications' potential to prevent cancer recurrence and the need for improved quality of life both during and after cancer treatment have generated significant interest in recent decades. As yet, research into the effects of food, nutrition, physical activity, and body weight on cancer survivorship remains in the early stages. For that reason, recommendations regarding the prevention of future cancer events cannot not be made with certainty. Despite the lack of data on this issue, when possible and appropriate, the same recommendations made for primary cancer prevention should also be applied to cancer survivors to prevent future recurrence as well as to improve general quality of life. Specifically, it is recommended that all cancer survivors receive nutritional care from an appropriately trained professional and, if able, aim to follow the recommendations for diet, healthy weight, and physical activity.

SUMMARY

The role of diet, physical activity, and body composition in cancer prevention and recurrence is a subject of active research, as reflected by current cancer prevention recommendations by organizations focused on chronic diseases. The worldwide prevention of cancer remains a vital, and largely unsolved, challenge. Currently, the evidence suggests that appropriate modifications of food intake, physical activity levels, and body composition are effective ways of addressing this need. For that reason, clinicians should encourage their patients to consume an increased plant-based, low-fat, complex-carbohydrate-rich diet; to engage in increased physical activity; and to maintain a healthy body weight through small, attainable, lifelong behavior change. A summary of the recommendations is provided in Table 6.6.

Table 6.6 *Summary of the Recommendations for Nutrition, Physical Activity, and Body Composition for the Prevention of Cancer*

Meat, poultry, fish, and eggs	Limit intake of red meat to no more than three 3- to 4-oz servings per week, and avoid processed meats altogether.
Plant foods	Eat mostly foods of plant origin, with an average daily consumption of 21 oz of non-starchy vegetables and fruits and 25 g of unprocessed cereal grains and legumes.
Grains, roots, tubers, and plantains	Consume unprocessed grains and/or legumes with every meal, and limit the intake of starchy foods.
Alcohol	If alcoholic drinks are consumed, limit to no more than two drinks per day for men and one drink per day for women. Sufficient folate intake should be promoted in those wishing to consume alcohol in any amount.
Dietary supplements	The general population should strive to achieve nutritional adequacy without the addition of dietary supplements. Supplements should be prescribed when dietary approaches are inadequate in achieving average daily intake goals.
Food production, preservation, processing, and preparation	Avoid salted foods and moldy grains or legumes.
Physical activity	Be moderately physically active for at least 30 minutes or more every day, and limit sedentary habits as much as possible.
Body weight	Strive to maintain a median adult BMI between 21 and 23 kg/m².
Lactation	Exclusively breastfeed infants for the first six months of life, and continue with complementary feeding thereafter.
Survivorship	All cancer survivors should receive nutritional care from an appropriately trained professional and, if able, aim to follow the recommendations for diet, healthy weight, and physical activity.

Source: Adapted from World Cancer Research Fund/American Institute for Cancer Research. *Food, Nutrition, Physical Activity, and the Prevention of Cancer: A Global Perspective.* Washington, DC: Author; 2007.

REFERENCES

1. World Cancer Research Fund/American Institute for Cancer Research. *Food, Nutrition, Physical Activity, and the Prevention of Cancer: A Global Perspective.* Washington, DC: Author; 2007.
2. American Cancer Society. Cancer facts and figures—2007. http://www.cancer.org/downloads/stt/caff2007pwsecured.pdf. Accessed January 3, 2008.
3. American Cancer Society. ACS recommendations for nutrition and physical activity for cancer prevention. http://www.cancer.org/docroot/PED/content/PED_3_2X_Recommendations.asp?sitearea=PED. Accessed December 31, 2007.
4. Larsson SC, Wolk A. Meat consumption and risk of colorectal cancer: A meta-analysis of prospective studies. *Int J Cancer.* 2006;119:2657–2664.
5. American Institute for Cancer Research. Ingested nitrates and nitrites. http://monographs.iarc.fr/ENG/Meetings/94-nitratenitrite.pdf. Accessed December 31, 2007.
6. Hein D. Molecular genetics and function of NAT1 and NAT2: Role in aromatic amine metabolism and carcinogenesis. *Mutat Res.* 2002;506–507:65–77.
7. Huang X. Iron overload and its association with cancer risk in humans: Evidence for iron as a carcinogenic metal. *Mutat Res.* 2003;533:153–171.
8. Flood A, Velie EM, Sinha R, et al. Meat, fat, and their subtypes as risk factors for colorectal cancer in a prospective cohort of women. *Am J Epidemiol.* 2003;158:59–68.
9. De Stefani E, Oreggia F, Ronco A, et al. Salted meat consumption as a risk factor for cancer of the oral cavity and pharynx: A case control study from Uruguay. *Cancer Epid Biomarkers Prev.* 1994;3:381–385.
10. Kim YS, Milner JA. Dietary modulation of colon cancer risk. *J Nutr.* 2007;137:2576S–2579S.
11. Nishino H, Satomi Y, Tokuda H, et al. Cancer control by phytochemicals. *Curr Pharm Des.* 2007;13:3394–3399.
12. Mason JB, Choi SW. Folate carcinogenesis: Developing a unifying hypothesis. *Adv Enzyme Regul.* 2000;40:127–141.
13. Talalay P, Fahey JW. Phytochemicals from cruciferous plants protect against cancer by modulating carcinogen metabolism. *J Nutr.* 2001;131:3027S–3033S.
14. Notani PN, Jayant K. Role of diet in upper aerodigestive tract cancers. *Nutr Cancer.* 1987;10:103–113.
15. Jansen MC, Bueno-de-Mesquita HB, Feskens EJ, et al. Quantity and variety of fruit and vegetable consumption and cancer risk. *Nutr Cancer.* 2004;48:142–148.
16. Ngoan LT, Mizoue T, Fujino Y, et al. Dietary factors and stomach cancer mortality. *Br J Cancer.* 2002;87:37–42.
17. Byers T, Perry G. Dietary carotenes, vitamin C, and vitamin E as protective antioxidants in human cancers. *Annu Rev Nutr.* 1992;12:139–159.
18. Prasain JK, Barnes S. Metabolism and bioavailability of flavonoids in chemoprevention: Current analytical strategies and future prospectus. *Mol Pharm.* 2007;4:846–864.
19. Di Mascio P, Kaiser S, Sies H. Lycopene as the most efficient biological carotenoid singlet oxygen quencher. *Arch Biochem Biophys.* 1989;272:534–538.

20. Rafi M, Yadav P, Reyes M. Lycopene inhibits LPS-induced proinflammatory mediator inducible nitric oxide synthase in mouse macrophage cells. *J Food Sci.* 2007; 72:S69–S74.

21. Leklem J. Vitamin B-6. In: Shils M, Olson JA, Shike M, et al. *Nutrition in Health and Disease.* 9th ed. Baltimore, MD: Williams and Wilkins; 1999:413–422.

22. Geissler C, Powers H. *Human Nutrition.* 11th ed. London, England: Elsevier Churchill Livingstone; 2005.

23. Guengerich FP, Shimada T. Oxidation of toxic and carcinogenic chemicals by human cytochrome P-450 enzymes. *Chem Res Toxicol.* 1991;4:391–407.

24. Kang ZC, Tsai SJ, Lee H. Quercetin inhibits benzoa-pyrene-induced DNA adducts in human Hep G2 cells by altering cytochrome P-450 *1A1* gene expression. *Nutr Cancer.* 1999;35:175–179.

25. Wenzlaff AS, Cote ML, Bock CH, et al. CYP1A1 and CYP1B1 polymorphisms and risk of lung cancer among never smokers: A population-based study. *Carcinogenesis.* 2005;26:2207–2212.

26. Tokui N, Yoshimura T, Fujino Y, et al. Dietary habits and stomach cancer risk in the JACC Study. *J Epidemiol.* 2005;15:S98–S108.

27. Rao AV, Sung MK. Saponins as anticarcinogens. *J Nutr.* 1995;125:717S–724S.

28. López-Carrillo L, López-Cervantes M, Robles-Díaz G, et al. Capsaicin consumption, *Helicobacter pylori* positivity and gastric cancer in Mexico. *Int J Cancer.* 2003;106:277–282.

29. International Agency for Research on Cancer. Aflatoxins. *Monograph Evaluation Carcinogenic Risks to Humans.* 1993;56:245–395.

30. Kensler TW, Egner PA, Davidson NE, Roebuck BD, Pikul A, Groopman JD. Modulation of aflatoxin metabolism, aflatoxin-N7-guanine formation, and hepatic tumorigenesis in rats fed ethoxyquin: Role of induction of glutathione S-transferases. *Cancer Res.* 1986;46:3924–3931.

31. Bressac B, Kew M, Wands J, Ozturk M. Selective G to T mutations of p53 gene in hepatocellular carcinoma from southern Africa. *Nature.* 1991;350:429–431.

32. Groopman JD, Johnson D, Kensler TW. Aflatoxin and hepatitis B virus biomarkers: A paradigm for complex environmental exposures and cancer risk. *Cancer Biomark.* 2005;1:5–14.

33. Cho E, Smith-Warner SA, Spiegelman D, et al. Dairy foods, calcium, and colorectal cancer: A pooled analysis of 10 cohort studies *J Natl Cancer Inst.* 2004;96: 1015–1022.

34. Giovannucci E. Dietary influences of 1,25(OH)$_2$ vitamin D in relation to prostate cancer: A hypothesis. *Cancer Causes Control.* 1998;9:567–582.

35. Gunnell D, Oliver SE, Peters TJ, et al. Are diet–prostate cancer associations mediated by the IGF axis? A cross-sectional analysis of diet, IGF-I and IGFBP-3 in healthy middle-aged men. *Br J Cancer.* 2003;88:1682–1686.

36. Qin LQ, Wang PY, Kaneko T, Hoshi K, Sato A. Estrogen: One of the risk factors in milk for prostate cancer. *Med Hypotheses.* 2004;62:133–142.

37. Kampman E, Goldbohm RA, van den Brandt PA, et al. Fermented dairy products, calcium, and colorectal cancer in the Netherlands Cohort Study. *Cancer Res.* 1994;54:3186–3190.

38. Simopoulos A. The importance of the ratio of omega-6/omega-3 essential fatty acids. *Biomed Pharmacother.* 2002;56:365–379.

39. Gleeson M, Nieman DC, Pedersen BK. Exercise, nutrition, and immune function. *J Sports Sci.* 2004;22:115–125.

40. Knekt P, Seppanen R, Jarvinen R, et al. Dietary cholesterol, fatty acids, and the risk of lung cancer among men. *Nutr Cancer*. 1991;16:267–275.
41. Willett WC, Stampfer MJ, Colditz GA, et al. Dietary fat and the risk of breast cancer. *N Engl J Med*. 1987;316:22–28.
42. Prentice RL, Caan B, Chlebowski RT, et al. Low-fat dietary pattern and risk of invasive breast cancer: The Women's Health Initiative Randomized Controlled Dietary Modification Trial. *JAMA*. 2006;295:629–642.
43. Prentice RL, Thomson CA, Caan B, et al. Low-fat dietary pattern and cancer incidence in the Women's Health Initiative Dietary Modification Randomized Controlled Trial. *J Natl Cancer Inst*. 2007;99:1534–1543.
44. Heiss CJ, Sanborn CF, Nichols DL, et al. Associations of body fat distribution, circulating sex hormones, and bone density in postmenopausal women. *J Clin Endocrinol Metab*. 1995;80:1591–1596.
45. Kelsey JL, Gammon MD, John EM. Reproductive factors and breast cancer. *Epidemiol Rev*. 1993;15:36–47.
46. World Health Organization Technical Report Series, No. 797. *Diet, Nutrition and the Prevention of Chronic Diseases: Report of a Joint FAO/WHO Experts Consultation*. Geneva: World Health Organization; 2003.
47. Kono S, Hirohata T. Nutrition and stomach cancer. *Cancer Causes Control*. 1996;7: 41–55.
48. Bergin IL, Sheppard B, Fox JG. *Helicobacter pylori* infection and high dietary salt independently induce atopic gastritis and intestinal metaplasia in commercially available outbred Mongolian gerbils. *Dig Dis Sci*. 2003;48:475–485.
49. Takahashi M. Enhancing effect of a high salt diet on gastrointestinal carcinogenesis [in Japanese]. *Gan No Rinsho*. 1986;32:667–673.
50. Kusters JG, van Vliet AH, Kuipers EJ. Pathogenesis of *Helicobacter pylori* infection. *Clin Microbiol Rev*. 2006;19:449–490.
51. International Agency for Research on Cancer. Some drinking-water disinfectants and contaminants, including arsenic. *IARC Monogr Eval Carcinog Risks Hum*, 84. http://monographs.iarc.fr/ENG/Monographs/vol84/volume84.pdf. Accessed January 2, 2008.
52. World Health Organization. Arsenic in drinking water. Fact sheet no. 210. http://www.who.int/mediacentre/fastsheets/fs210/en/index.html. Accessed January 2, 2008.
53. Mayer DA, Fried B. The role of helminth infections in carcinogenesis. *Adv Parasitol*. 2007;65:239–296.
54. Kligerman AD, Tennant AH. Insights into the carcinogenic mode of action of arsenic. *Toxicol Appl Pharmacol*. 2007;222:281–288.
55. Garro AJ, Espina N, Farinati F, et al. The effects of chronic ethanol consumption on carcinogen metabolism and on O6-methylguanine transferase–mediated repair of alkylated DNA. *Alcohol Clin Exp Res*. 1986;10:73S–77S.
56. Seitz HK, Becker P. Alcohol metabolism and cancer risk. *Alcohol Res Health*. 2007;30:38–41, 44–47.
57. Linos E, Willett WC. Diet and breast cancer risk reduction. *J Natl Compr Canc Netw*. 2007;5:711–718.
58. Ross C. Advances in retinoid research: Mechanisms of Cancer Chemoprevention Symposium introduction. *J Nutr*. 2003;133:271S–272S.
59. Kline K, Yu W, Sanders BG. Vitamin E: Mechanisms of action as tumor cell growth inhibitors. *J Nutr*. 2001;131:161S–163S.

60. Basu A, Grossie B, Bennett M, et al. Alpha-tocopheryl succinate (alpha-TOS) modulates human prostate LNCaP xenograft growth and gene expression in BALB/c nude mice fed two levels of dietary soybean oil. *Eur J Nutr*. 2007;46:34–43.
61. Studzinski GP, Moore DC. Sunlight: Can it prevent as well as cause cancer? *Cancer Res*. 1995;55:4014–4022.
62. Ganther HE. Selenium metabolism, selenoproteins and mechanisms of cancer prevention: Complexities with thioredoxin reductase. *Carcinogenesis*. 1999;20:1657–1666.
63. U.S. Preventive Services Task Force. Routine vitamin supplementation to prevent cancer and cardiovascular disease. *Nutr Clin Care*. 2003;6:102–107.
64. Smith DG, Shipley MJ, Batty GD, Morris JN, Marmot M. Physical activity and cause-specific mortality in the Whitehall study. *Public Health*. 2000;114:308–315.
65. Friedenreich CM, Orenstein MR. Physical activity and cancer prevention: Etiologic evidence and biological mechanisms. *J Nutr*. 2002;132:3456S–3464S.
66. Burton BT, Foster WR, Hirsch J, VanItallie TB. Health implications of obesity: NIH consensus development conference. *Int J Obes Relat Metab Disord*. 1985;9:155–169.
67. McTiernan A. *Cancer prevention and management through exercise and weight control*. Boca Raton, FL: CRC Press; 2006.
68. Bostwick DG, Burke HB, Djakiew D, et al. Human prostate cancer risk factors. *Cancer*. 2004;101:2371–2490.
69. Lukanova A, Kaaks R. Endogenous hormones and ovarian cancer: Epidemiology and current hypotheses. *Cancer Epidemiol Biomarkers Prev*. 2005;14:98–107.

Chapter 7

Esophageal and Head and Neck Cancer

Elisabeth Isenring, PhD, AdvAPD*

INTRODUCTION

The term *head and neck cancer* (HNC) is used to describe a range of malignant tumors located in the head and neck area. Patients with *esophageal cancer* (EC) experience many of the same nutritional challenges as those with HNC and, therefore, will also be covered in this chapter. Disease-related malnutrition is common in patients with both EC and HNC[1, 2] and is associated with increased morbidity and mortality.[3, 4] HNC therapies include surgery, radiation therapy, chemotherapy, or a combination of these modalities. Treatments for EC and HNC are continually evolving and improving but may result in significant side effects for the patient. Strong evidence indicates that dietary counseling improves nutritional status and quality of life (QoL) in patients with EC or HNC.[5–7] Some evidence—albeit at a lower level, mainly from retrospective studies—also suggests that using tube feeding for patients who would otherwise be unable to manage sufficient dietary intake leads to earlier commencement of nutritional support[8] and less weight loss.[9, 10] A multidisciplinary approach is the preferred management method for patients with EC or HNC. Early referral and management by the dietitian and speech pathologist and effective management of symptoms by the medical team are vital for best nutritional and QoL outcomes.[11]

---

*AdvAPD = Advanced Accredited Practicing Dietitian of the Dietitians Association of Australia in recognition of expertise and leadership to the profession.

What Are HNC and EC?

HNC describes a range of malignant tumors located in the head and neck area, including the mouth, nose, throat, larynx, and sinuses. In the United States, the five main types of HNC include (1) oral and oropharyngeal cancer, (2) salivary gland cancer, (3) laryngeal and hypopharyngeal cancer, (4) nasopharyngeal cancer, and (5) nasal cavity and paranasal sinus cancer.[12] Most HNC tumors are squamous in nature, but more rarely patients may develop non-squamous tumors in the sinus and salivary glands.[13]

Cancer of the esophagus starts in the innermost layer of the esophageal wall and extends outward. Esophageal tumors are usually squamous cell carcinomas or adenocarcinomas.[14]

The most common presenting symptoms for patients with EC or HNC include a sore that does not heal, swallowing difficulties, and a lump on the neck.[12] Detecting HNC at an early stage increases the chance of a cure.[12] Five-year survival rates are good (approximately 90%) when HNC tumors are detected and treated early, but are much lower for advanced-stage tumors.[12]

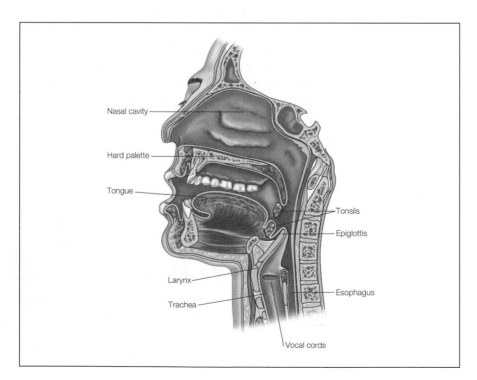

Figure 7.1 *Head and Neck Area*

Statistics and Risk Factors

In the United States, HNC accounts for 3–5% of all cancer cases.[15] An estimated 45,660 people were expected to be diagnosed with HNC, with 11,210 people predicted to die from HNC in 2007.[15] In 2007, an estimated 15,560 people in the United States were anticipated to be diagnosed with EC, with an estimated 13,940 deaths occurring from this disease in that year.[15]

Both EC and HNC tend to be more common in males. The most notable modifiable risk factors for developing HNC include the use of tobacco and/or marijuana and frequent, heavy consumption of alcohol.[16] For primary prevention of HNC, research suggests that consuming a diet characterized by high fruit and vegetable intake is important.[17] However, few studies have examined whether a diet meeting the recommended fruit and vegetable intake reduces the risk of cancer recurrence or improves survival.

A recent Australian study evaluating patients with adenocarcinomas of the esophagus ($n = 367$) compared with population-matched controls ($n = 1,580$) reported that obesity (body mass index [BMI] > 40 kg/m^2) increases the risk of esophageal adenocarcinoma (odds ratio [OR] 6.1; 95% confidence interval [CI] 2.7–13.6) independent of other factors, especially in males.[18] Persons with a BMI > 40 kg/m^2 and frequent gastroesophageal reflux symptoms had a significantly elevated EC risk (OR 16.5; 95% CI 8.9–30.6) compared to people with a BMI > 40 kg/m^2 but experiencing no reflux symptoms (OR 2.2; 95% CI 1.1–4.3) or having reflux but with a BMI < 40 kg/m^2 (OR 5.6; 95% CI 2.8–11.3).[18] These data suggest not only that obesity elevates the risk of EC, but also that obesity and gastroesophageal reflux symptoms may synergistically potentiate EC risk.

Consuming a balanced diet that meets fruit and vegetable dietary recommendations, avoiding or limiting alcohol consumption, and avoiding smoking appear to decrease the risk of developing HNC. These recommendations may also decrease the risk of developing EC, when combined with attaining and maintaining a healthy body weight and achieving effective management of gastroesophageal reflux symptoms.

Treatment

The management of EC and HNC has become increasingly complex with the trend toward combining treatment modalities and the introduction of new therapeutic technologies.[19] Advances in chemoradiation treatment and reconstructive surgery have made the treatment of EC and HNC dependent not only on tumor stage, primary subsite, and histology, but also on physician expertise and patient preference.[19] Several combinations of treatments are available for the management of EC and HNC, with advances continuing to occur. The treatment of choice for patients with EC or HNC should be determined by a multidisciplinary team and primarily depends on the size and location of the tumor, metastasis (if any) of the tumor, and the patient's overall health.[12] The continuum of cancer survivorship is associated with different nutritional needs and challenges, given that patients may be at any stage along the continuum: cancer treatment, recovery, living after recovery, or living with advanced cancer.[20]

Surgery

The aim of surgery is to remove the tumor with a margin of healthy tissue. If the cancer has spread, the neck lymph nodes may need to be removed as well. Surgery for major tissue removal (e.g., jaw, pharynx, or tongue) may require plastic surgery to replace missing tissue.[12]

The mode of treatment will affect nutritional outcomes. Surgical intervention, for example, can cause swallowing difficulties dependent on the degree and site of the resection. Resection of the floor of the mouth or base of the tongue places a patient at greater risk of requiring supplemental feeding.[21] A speech pathologist is likely to be required to provide ongoing review to help with speech and swallowing for patients having surgery on the base of the tongue. Side effects of surgery may include swelling, pain, and/or structural deformities, such as loss of teeth, making it difficult to chew or swallow and potentially limiting dietary intake (refer to Chapter 5).

Laser surgery may also be used to treat some forms of EC or HNC. Use of a laser (more formally, "light amplification by stimulated emission of radiation") entails manipulation of high-intensity light that can be directed to perform very precise surgical resection of surfaces or the lining of internal organs; this type of surgery is generally carried out through an endoscope. Laser surgery can be used alone but is often undertaken in combination with more traditional surgery, chemotherapy, or radiation therapy. Laser surgery is more precise than use of the traditional surgical scalpel, resulting in less bleeding and damage to healthy tissue. Laser surgery also carries a lower risk of infection. The main limitations of laser surgery are that the surgeon must undergo specialized training, the treatment is expensive, and the effects of laser surgery may not be permanent and may need to be repeated for the best treatment outcomes.[12]

Radiation Therapy

Radiation therapy acts by directing x-rays to cause damage to cell DNA so cells cannot replicate. Rapidly dividing cells (e.g., blood cells, hair cells, gut mucosa cells) are the most susceptible to radiation damage. Radiation therapy can also exacerbate tooth decay; for this reason, patients with HNC should see a dentist because damaged teeth may need to be removed prior to treatment. Potential side effects of radiation therapy include mucositis, odynophagia, thick saliva, xerostomia, trismus, pharyngeal fibrosis, and decreased appetite as a result of changes in the senses of smell and taste (see Chapter 4 for more detail).[22, 23] Radiation therapy to the thyroid gland in the neck area may lead to hypothyroidism, so patients should have their neck area checked regularly.[12]

Chemotherapy

Chemotherapy can be used alone or as either neoadjuvant (before) or adjuvant (after) therapy in combination with surgery or radiation therapy to treat patients with EC or HNC. For example, patients may receive both chemotherapy and radiation therapy prior to esophagectomy. Chemotherapy treatment is described in detail in Chapter 4.

Potential side effects of chemotherapy for HNC include nausea, vomiting, diarrhea, constipation, mucositis, trismus, dry mouth, and loss of appetite. Advances in the use of chemotherapy and radiation therapy together (concurrent chemoradiation) have led to improvements in survival and local/regional tumor control for patients with advanced HNC,[24] but often at the expense of significant toxicity to the patient. In particular, severe mucositis and weight loss have been expected toxicities of these new chemoradiation regimens.[25] Allen et al.[24] evaluated the acceleration of hyperfractionated chemoradiation for advanced HNC ($N = 46$) and found that this therapy was feasible but required enteral feeding tubes in most patients.

Long-term swallowing difficulties may be a problem following chemoradiation. As a consequence, ongoing liaison and review by the multidisciplinary team, including a dietitian and speech pathologist, may be required.

Immunotherapy

Immunotherapy—in particular, monoclonal antibody therapy—is a recent development for the treatment of metastatic squamous cell carcinoma of the head and neck region. The epidermal growth factor receptor (EGFR) monoclonal antibody inhibitor works by attaching itself to the surface of cancer cells, thereby preventing the EGFR from being activated. This approach stops the tumor cells from dividing and has the potential for preventing the cancer from growing. Currently, treatment with monoclonal antibody therapy can be very expensive and may be offered as part of a clinical trial. The most common side effect is a severe, acne-like rash, though some reports have indicated that monoclonal antibody therapy may also result in nausea and diarrhea.[12]

Nutritional Challenges Associated with HNC and EC

Cancer of the esophagus or head and neck can be particularly debilitating because it affects the critical functions of speech, swallowing, and breathing, as well as a patient's appearance and social functioning.[26] Patients with HNC have one of the highest malnutrition prevalence rates among all diagnostic groups, with 25–50% of these patients classified as nutritionally compromised prior to commencement of treatment.[2, 6, 27, 28] The treatment regimen itself can further compromise nutritional status. For example, HNC treatment advances such as combined chemoradiation compared with chemotherapy alone result in significant toxicity, which can increase the incidence of swallowing disorders and greatly elevate malnutrition risk.[19] Many patients are required to spend large amounts of time receiving medical treatment and waiting for appointments, which can disrupt routines and lead to missed meals. Anecdotal reports indicate that rural patients often need to travel long distances to receive treatment, and their alternate accommodation may not have suitable cooking facilities or the patient may not have the energy or skills to prepare suitable foods and fluids.

Malnutrition can have many negative consequences. Impaired nutritional status is associated with decreased QoL, physical function, and survival[28] and, therefore, with increased personal, social, and healthcare costs.[3, 4] These patients' inability to eat and drink adequately places a significant burden on both the healthcare system and the psychosocial well-being of the patient and his or her caregivers.[29] The functions of eating and drinking play a large role in social activity and participation, so it is not surprising that QoL in HNC is affected by these domains in particular.[26]

The results of studies investigating QoL in patients with HNC, however, are inconsistent. Despite demonstrating improved QoL, presumably associated with the nature of organ preservation treatments,[29] patient responses to treatment toxicity and the resultant impact on QoL remain to be fully investigated. Physicians are becoming increasingly aware that effective management of patients should include the assessment of a broader concept of outcomes such as QoL. Terrell[26] suggests that QoL may be a better predictor of survival than clinical outcomes alone.

Significant loss of body weight is not only suggestive of a poor prognosis and associated with decreased physical function and QoL, but can also affect treatment schedules. Weight loss during radiation therapy to the head and neck can diminish the safety and effectiveness of the treatment, as the patient may require repeat CT scans to keep critical structures to within accepted tolerance doses.[29] Significant amounts of weight loss can also affect the chemotherapy regimen, preventing the patient from receiving the optimal dosage.

Despite the association between malnutrition and poor outcomes, a malnutrition and survival cause–effect relationship has not yet been established.[30] This may be because of the nature of the cross-sectional or prospective study designs used to date, which can demonstrate associations but not necessarily causation, and because of the complex, multifactorial nature of disease-related malnutrition. It is often very challenging to conduct high-level clinical nutrition studies, for a variety of reasons: Such studies are difficult to complete in a blinded fashion, patients may not adhere to the nutritional recommendations, and it may not be ethically possible to conduct a randomized, controlled trial in malnourished patients.[31] Recent randomized controlled trials, however, have demonstrated that patients who experience less deterioration in nutritional status with nutrition intervention compared with usual care also have better physical function and QoL.[6, 7]

As previously discussed, nutrition-impact symptoms in patients with EC or HNC may be attributable to the tumor itself or may be side effects of the cancer treatment. In a study conducted in 205 patients with gastrointestinal cancer or HNC, the factors most significantly associated with nutritional status included tumor stage, tumor location, time since diagnosis, dietary intake, and previous treatment.[32] Nutrition-impact symptoms commonly experienced by patients with HNC include mucositis, xerostomia, trismus, pharyngeal fibrosis, and decreased appetite due to changes in the senses of smell and taste.[22, 23] Common nutrition-impact symptoms experienced by patients with EC include mucositis, esophageal pain, and dysphagia. More than 90% of patients with EC experience dysphagia, making it a very significant problem in this patient group.[33] Following treatment, swallowing function often deteriorates but then improves for as long as 12 months post-treatment. Swallowing function may then stabilize but often remains poorer compared to swallowing function prior to commencement of treatment.[34]

The loss of the ability to enjoy a meal can be distressing. Nguyen et al. showed that the severity of dysphagia in patients with swallowing difficulties after treatment for HNC is correlated with compromised QoL, depression, and anxiety.[35] Anecdotal evidence suggests that some patients with EC or HNC will require dietetic and speech pathology support for months after treatment has finished, and they may not ever return to managing a "normal" diet without supplementation.[29]

Nutritional Studies

Strong evidence exists that dietary counseling and supplements can increase dietary intake and prevent therapy-associated weight loss and interruptions to radiation therapy in patients with EC or HNC.[30] A study by Isenring et al. evaluated 60 oncology outpatients (51 males, 9 females; mean age 61.9 years ± 14.0 years) receiving radiation therapy to the head and neck or gastrointestinal area.[6] Intensive, individualized nutrition counseling by a dietitian, using a standardized protocol plus oral supplements as required, was compared to the standard practice of the center, which included general nutrition advice and nutrition handouts.[6] Outcomes were assessed upon commencement of radiation therapy and at 4, 8, and 12 weeks after starting treatment. The group receiving early and intensive nutrition intervention experienced less weight loss (−0.4 kg versus −4.7 kg; $P < 0.001$) over the 12-week study, which was associated with beneficial outcomes such as less deterioration in nutritional status, global QoL, and physical function.[6] Clinically, but not statistically, significant differences in fat-free mass were observed between the nutrition intervention and standard practice groups (0.5 kg versus −1.4 kg; $P = 0.195$).[6] Compared with the standard practice group, patients receiving nutrition intervention had a higher energy intake (28–31 kcal/kg/day versus 25–29 kcal/kg/day; $P = 0.022$) and protein intake (1.1–1.3 g/kg/day versus 1.0–1.1 g/kg/day; $P = 0.001$).[6] The investigators suggest one of the main reasons the patients receiving nutrition intervention were successful in maintaining body weight was the intensity and frequency of the nutrition counseling, which also included follow-up for approximately 6 weeks after completing radiation therapy.

A study conducted by Ravasco et al.[7] in Portugal randomized 75 patients with HNC receiving preoperative chemoradiation to receive either (1) dietary counseling alone, (2) oral supplements, or (3) an ad libitum diet. On completion of radiation treatment, significant increases were noted in dietary intake (compared to baseline) in patients receiving dietary counseling (521 kcal/day, $P = 0.002$; 26 g of protein/day, $P = 0.006$) and supplements (322 kcal/day, $P = 0.05$; 35 g of protein/day, $P = 0.001$), while the dietary intake of the ad libitum group decreased (−400 kcal/day, $P < 0.01$; −15 g of protein/day, $P < 0.01$). Three months following the commencement of radiation therapy, improved QoL was associated with improved nutritional intake and nutritional status.[7] Nutrition-impact symptoms such as anorexia, nausea, and xerostomia improved the most in the dietary counseling group (90% improved) compared with patients receiving supplements (67% improved) and those on the ad libitum diet (51% improved).[7] It appears that the individualized nature of the nutrition counseling helped patients manage nutrition-impact symptoms and led to better tailoring of the diet so as to increase intake. This study confirms the importance of early nutritional assessment and appropriate dietary counseling to meet patient needs and to improve nutritional status and QoL.

Dawson et al.[36] demonstrated that a dietary supervision program, which included regular and ongoing reviews by the dietitian approximately every 2 weeks, was effective in reducing weight loss (6.6% versus 9.8%; $P < 0.05$) in 43 patients with squamous cell carcinoma of the oral cavity treated by surgery and radiation therapy compared with 26 historical controls. This result occurred despite the fact that patients receiving the intervention had more advanced disease. These study results highlight the importance of assessing the nutritional status of patients on presentation and then both during and following cancer treatment.

Dietary counseling studies conducted in patients with HNC demonstrate that the decline in nutritional status all too often reported is not inevitable. The randomized controlled trials conducted by Isenring[6] and Ravasco[7] showed that dietary counseling with or without supplements can lead to improved dietary intake, nutritional status, and QoL outcomes. Few dietary counseling studies have been conducted specifically in patients with EC, although the study by Isenring et al.[6] did include some patients with this type of cancer. Further research is required to prove definitively whether dietary counseling will lead to beneficial outcomes in a more homogenous group of patients with EC. Despite the limited amount of research in this area, it is recommended that patients at risk for malnutrition—which would include the majority of EC and HNC patients—receive regular and individualized nutrition intervention.[30]

Goals of Nutritional Management

Ongoing nutrition-impact symptoms due to the tumor, its treatment, and/or the treatment's side effects can lead to unintentional weight loss and disease-related malnutrition. Maintaining body weight or minimizing weight loss for patients at nutritional risk is a major goal of the nutritional management of patients with EC and HNC. It has been known for many years that weight loss is a predictor of poor outcome in EC and HNC.[37] The goals of nutritional management during treatment should include preventing or minimizing nutritional deficiencies; preserving muscle tissue; minimizing nutrition-impact symptoms such as decreased appetite, nausea, or bowel function changes; and maximizing QoL.[20, 30] Treatment side effects such as early satiety, fatigue, and anorexia are possible to ameliorate with the appropriate dietary intake.[38]

There is limited evidence regarding the optimal time for initiation of nutrition support. The European Society of Parenteral and Enteral Nutrition (ESPEN) has developed a consensus statement that recommends nutrition therapy should commence if undernutrition already exists, if it is anticipated that the patient will be unable to eat for 7 or more days, or if the patient has had an inadequate energy intake (less than 60% estimated energy expenditure) for 10 or more days.[30] Professional practice suggests it is easier to prevent or slow the malnutrition trajectory than to reverse chronic malnutrition. In weight-losing patients with inadequate dietary intake, nutrition support (dietary counseling with or without supplements) should be provided to improve or maintain nutritional status and QoL.[30]

Nutritional depletion in EC and HNC patients is a well-known phenomenon, and several researchers have recommended initiating nutritional management of these patients on presentation.[5, 6, 37] All patients with EC or HNC should be regarded as being "at risk" for nutritional deficiency irrespective of their tumor stage.[6, 37] Unfortunately, because of the under-recognition of the consequences of malnutrition, and because of the limited resources available for nutrition diagnosis and treatment, referral of high-nutritional-risk patients is not always done consistently in practice.

Ideally, all EC and HNC patients should be referred to nutrition services for a complete nutrition assessment prior to commencing treatment. This nutrition assessment should be conducted using a valid and reliable nutrition assessment tool for use in patients with cancer, such as the scored Patient Generated-Subjective Global Assessment (PG-SGA).[39, 40] The PG-SGA is useful to assess nutritional status, guide nutrition intervention, and monitor outcomes in patients with cancer. Appropriate nutritional management (Table 7.1) and physical activity recommendations before, during, and

Table 7.1   *Key Points for Nutritional Management of Patients with Esophageal and Head and Neck Cancer*

• Implement routine nutrition screening.
• Refer high-risk patients for nutrition and swallowing assessment.
• Consider whether patient may require a gastrostomy/jejunostomy. (Discuss this possibility with the multidisciplinary team, patient, and caregiver).
• Monitor weight regularly (ideally weekly during radiation therapy, at every chemotherapy session, or at every outpatient appointment).
• Aim for weight maintenance (or at the very least minimize weight loss) during treatment.
• Manage nutrition-related symptoms as a multidisciplinary team.
• Nutritional management may include texture modification, high-energy and high-protein dietary modifications, supplements, and/or tube feeding if patient has an inadequate dietary intake.

after treatment should be implemented to ensure best patient care and optimal outcomes.[20, 41]

Dietary Recommendations During Treatment

Because a patient's dietary intake may be compromised due to either the tumor or the chosen therapy, a consultation with a registered dietitian for individualized nutrition strategies is recommended.[20] To increase dietary intake, alterations in food and fluid temperature, changes in food texture and consistency, and increased frequency of meals and snacks may be necessary. Frequent high-carbohydrate meals may be beneficial for patients who experience nausea. Patients with swallowing difficulties should use a thickening agent under the direction of a speech pathologist. Patients may want to utilize ready-made thickened fluids and puddings available commercially.

Earlier pilot studies suggested zinc sulfate lozenges might be considered beneficial for patient with an altered sense of taste. A recent, large ($N = 169$) double-blind, placebo-controlled trial conducted in HNC patients undergoing radiation therapy did not demonstrate decreased incidence of taste alterations or changes in the interval to taste recovery,[42] suggesting that zinc sulfate was not beneficial in preventing taste changes.

During mucositis and inflammation, acidic and very hot foods and sometimes even frozen foods may not be well tolerated. Other patients, however, report that cool or frozen foods help soothe the sore mouth, so this may be a personal preference. Sugar-free chewing gums and sweets, along with alcohol-free mouth rinses, can help with a dry mouth. Artificial saliva sprays and oral lubricants may be useful, though their benefit appears to be based on personal preference. Mouth care is important, however, so many centers recommend that patients use a made-at-home salt water and/or bicarbonate of soda mouth rinse. For a dry mouth, carrying around a water bottle and sipping frequently as well as keeping a glass of water by the bedside can be beneficial.

Because of their lifestyle prior to diagnosis, some EC and HNC patients will have had an inadequate diet for some time. In addition to protein and energy malnutrition, patients with EC or HNC may be at risk for vitamin and mineral deficiencies. As part of the nutritional management of these patients, it is important to replenish not only protein and energy intakes, but also vitamin and mineral intakes. Dietary intakes of vitamins and minerals should not be greater than the recommended dietary intakes (RDI), as excess amounts of these nutrients may interfere with treatment.[20] It is important that patients notify their medical team of any medications and vitamin, mineral, or herbal supplements they may be taking.

Alcohol is an irritant, even in the small amounts found in mouth washes. Given this property, it is reasonable to recommend that alcohol intake be avoided or limited in patients with or at risk of mucositis and those receiving radiation therapy to the head and neck area.[20]

Tube Feeding

When nutrition-impact symptoms cannot be adequately managed to allow for oral intake sufficient to meet dietary requirements, enteral feedings are highly effective. ESPEN enteral feeding guidelines are based on a consensus that tube feeding can be used if an obstructing EC or HNC interferes with swallowing[30] and, therefore, limits dietary intake. Currently, there are no universally accepted standards for determining which patients should receive tube feeding.[29] The literature, however, identifies particular patient characteristics that are associated with significant weight loss and the placement of feeding tubes (Table 7.2).

Mangar et al.[43] performed a retrospective review of 160 patients receiving radiation therapy to the head and neck area and found that 50 patients required enteral feedings. In their study, factors predictive of requiring enteral feedings include pre-treatment weight loss, low serum albumin and protein, stage 3–4 disease, performance status of 2–3, and smoking greater than 20 cigarettes per day.

Table 7.2   *Characteristics of Patients with Esophageal and Head and Neck Cancer Associated with Greater Likelihood of Severe Weight Loss or Need for Alternative Feeding Methods*

Diagnosis	Pharyngeal/hypopharyngeal primary tumors Base-of-tongue tumors Nasopharyngeal tumors T4 tumors Moderately or poorly differentiated cancer
Treatment	Excision of base of tongue or pharynx Mandibulectomy Reconstruction with a pectoralis major flap Chemoradiation Postoperative radiotherapy
Weight loss	Pretreatment weight loss > 7% BMI Preoperative weight loss > 10 lb (5 kg)

Source: Reprinted by permission of Cancer Forum. http://www.cancer.org.au/File/Policy Publications/CancerForumNov06.pdf

Enteral feedings are effective in increasing energy, protein, and micronutrient intake and maintaining body weight compared with dietary intake alone.[44] Bozzetti et al.[45] demonstrated that nasogastric feedings prevented deterioration in nutritional status in dysphagic, malnourished patients with EC receiving chemoradiation compared with those on a standard oral diet.

In a small, retrospective study involving 151 patients, 15 of whom required enteral feedings, Beer et al.[28] found that patients receiving an early percutaneous enteral gastrostomy (PEG) within 2 weeks of commencing radiation therapy maintained nutritional status and had less treatment interruptions than those patients in whom placement of a PEG was delayed between 2 weeks and 3 months after commencing radiation therapy. Prophylactic gastrostomy insertion results in earlier commencement of nutrition support and less weight loss compared with receiving tube feeding later during treatment.[5, 8, 46] Patients with prophylactic gastrostomy tubes also have fewer hospital admissions for dehydration or malnutrition[47, 48] and maintain QoL during treatment compared with patients who rely on dietary intake alone.[49] Some studies have found that patients prefer PEGs compared to nasogastric feeding tubes because PEGs are associated with greater mobility, better cosmetic appearance, and better QoL.[2] However, nasogastric and PEG feedings have been found to be equally effective in preserving body weight in patients with HNC undergoing radiation therapy[2]; hence the method of feeding (nasogastric or gastrostomy/jejunostomy) should reflect the anticipated length of feeding required.[5]

When considering a prophylactic gastrostomy/jejunostomy, discussions should involve the patient, caregiver, and multidisciplinary team as well as the speech pathologist, who can help with swallowing rehabilitation. The goal is to avoid long-term dependence on enteral feedings. Nutritional guidelines, including those dealing with follow-up and use of enteral feeding, are more likely to be followed if a dietitian is a part of the multidisciplinary team.[45] Odelli et al.[50] demonstrated that in EC patients receiving chemoradiation, early and regular nutrition assessment and intervention ($n = 24$), including tube feeding for patients assessed as being at severe nutrition risk, and a multidisciplinary approach, compared with no nutrition plan ($n = 24$), resulted in less weight loss (-4.2 kg $\pm$ 6.4 kg versus -8.9 kg ±5.9 kg; $P = 0.03$) and higher radiation therapy completion rates (92% versus 50%; $P = 0.001$).

The evidence is inconsistent regarding the role of nutrition intervention in tumor response or survival.[51] A secondary analysis of a large, prospective evaluation of patients ($N = 1,073$) with locally advanced HNC who were undergoing definitive radiation therapy concluded that those patients who received nutrition support before starting treatment had poorer overall survival and locoregional control at five years.[52] Although this study is relatively large, it did have several limitations. The main limitation is that it was a secondary analysis of a trial designed to investigate different radiation fractionation schedules; it was not designed as a nutrition trial. Hence, the nutritional data collected were very broad—namely, whether patients received nutritional support (supplements or enteral feeding) before, during, or after treatment and patients' weight loss at these time points. No thorough nutrition assessment was undertaken, and no data on the adherence to the nutrition intervention were collected. Due to its post hoc nature, this study does not describe causality. It does, however, suggest that future research in this area should measure locoregional control and mortality outcomes as well as more patient-centered outcomes such as QoL.

Cancer Cachexia

The loss of body weight resulting from cachexia differs significantly from the weight loss due to starvation.[31] Cancer cachexia is characterized by weight loss and cytokine-induced metabolic derangements such as insulin resistance, increased lipolysis, and increased protein turnover, and is associated with decreased appetite, weight loss, and metabolic alterations.[30] Although there is no definitive method for diagnosing cancer cachexia, clinical signs of anorexia, muscle wasting, and unintentional weight loss of 5% or more of body weight in 6 months not due to mechanical obstruction, treatment, or side effects are suggestive of cancer cachexia.[31] Weight loss due to obstruction, treatment, and/or side effects, that is expected to cease once treatment is ceased, should not be described as cachexia,[31] but rather as due to inadequate dietary intake.

Some patients with EC or HNC may not be formally classified as cachectic, but some of their nutrition-impact symptoms (e.g., dysphagia), may not resolve once treatment ceases and will require ongoing dietary and speech pathology review. Therefore, the primary nutritional goal of addressing inadequate oral intake in these patients is to increase dietary intake to a level sufficient to meet their requirements.

Weight loss due to cachexia may not be reversible because the abnormal host metabolism may limit the success of any nutritional interventions.[53] Indeed, cancer cachexia is challenging to treat. In addition to providing adequate energy and protein intake, other agents for limiting cachexia have been investigated, including fish oil (eicosapentaenoic acid) and other pharmacotherapies (refer to Chapter 15). Further research into the effectiveness of these agents is required. Several guidelines for the nutritional management of cancer cachexia have been developed.[30, 31] Likewise, specific guidelines for the nutritional management of radiation therapy patients[5, 30] and medical oncology patients have been developed.[30]

Preoperative Nutrition

Early preoperative nutritional assessment assists in the identification of mal-nourished patients who are at risk of refeeding syndrome due to extended periods with minimal dietary intake or abuse of alcohol. Refeeding syndrome can be a serious complication of too-rapid feeding in malnourished patients and can precipitate a number of metabolic and pathological complications that can lead to a range of clinical complications, including death.[54] In patients assessed as being at risk of refeeding syndrome, it is important to control carbohydrate intake and consider providing B vitamins prior to initi-ating nutrition support. Protocols have been developed to anticipate, pre-vent, and treat refeeding syndrome.[54]

For patients identified as being malnourished during the preoperative nutrition assessment, it is important to commence appropriate nutrition sup-port early. The implementation of 7 to 10 days of preoperative nutrition in patients with HNC can improve QoL and decrease postoperative infectious complications by 10% compared with patients who lost 12–20% of their ideal body weight and who are at increased risk of postoperative sepsis.[55]

Immunonutrition

While standard high-energy and -protein feeds (1 kcal/mL) were used in the enteral feeding studies discussed earlier, immunonutrition is being used more widely in surgical patients. Immunonutrition formulas include specific nutrients that have modulating effects on immune and inflammatory responses.

Despite advances in surgical techniques, major surgery is still associated with a high rate of postoperative morbidity. Surgery can lead to aberrational functioning of the immune system, including increased production of pro-inflammatory cytokines and reduced production of humoral factors, which may play a role in the genesis of postoperative complications.[56] A recent meta-analysis of 17 randomized controlled trials conducted in patients undergoing upper and lower gastrointestinal surgery (one study involved patients with HNC) demonstrated that the use of a specific immunonutri-tional product (IMPACT) preoperatively, perioperatively, and postoperatively resulted in a significant reduction in the overall incidence of infectious com-plications and a reduced length of hospital stay.[57] Subgroup analysis revealed that preoperative intervention resulted in fewer abdominal abscesses, wound infections, urinary tract infections, episodes of sepsis, and anastomotic leaks (46% less prevalent). Perioperative application resulted in fewer cases of pneumonia, urinary tract infections, and episodes of sepsis. Postoperative application was associated with a significant reduction in the incidence of abdominal abscesses but no improvement in the incidence of other postoperative complications, suggesting that this approach has a lower efficacy. The researchers concluded that immunonutrition conferred significant clinical benefits in patients undergoing major elective gastrointestinal surgery. While a considerable body of evidence suggests that immunonutrition is likely to reduce postoperative complications in patients undergoing gastrointestinal or neck surgery,[57] the evidence is less convincing for HNC. Further studies are required to investigate the impact of preoperative versus perioperative immunonutrition in EC and HNC patients.

Mucositis can be a serious and compromising side effect of some anti-cancer therapies.[58] Specialized nutrition supplements containing glutamine have been developed to help prevent or manage mucositis symptoms. As yet, evidence does not definitively show that glutamine is beneficial in preventing or minimizing the development of mucositis.[30] Well-designed, randomized, double-blinded, placebo-controlled trials are required to demonstrate the benefits of specialized glutamine-containing products for mucositis and nutritional status compared with traditional supplements in patients with EC and HNC.

Physical Activity

Some evidence suggests that physical activity, including resistance exercise, can improve physical function[59, 60] and QoL[60] in HNC survivors. A study conducted in 59 patients with HNC (mean age = 58 ± 12.8 years; time since diagnosis = 18.6 ± 51.9 months) demonstrated that the strongest independent correlates of physical activity were enjoyment of the physical activity and frequency of symptoms.[61] It appears that the best strategies for encouraging exercise in HNC patients are to focus on appreciating the enjoyment element of the exercise and to manage symptoms and treatment-related barriers.

Nutrition After Treatment

Currently, there is no evidence to suggest that any specific micronutrients are beneficial in decreasing the risk of cancer recurrence following treatment for EC or HNC. A randomized, placebo-controlled, double-blinded clinical trial investigating the effect of a beta-carotene supplement (50 mg) compared with placebo in 264 HNC patients reported no advantages in cancer recurrence or survival rates.[62] The World Cancer Research Fund report recommends that protective nutrients be obtained from food rather than from dietary supplements.[41]

The general recommendations for cancer survivors after cancer treatment are to follow general nutrition and exercise guidelines, maintain a healthy weight, and adopt a healthy lifestyle.[20] Cancer survivors should also follow the recommendations for cancer prevention.[41] Some patients may experience long-term swallowing problems and difficulty with eating resulting in weight loss, so long-term follow-up and management of these individuals' nutritional status is important. Treatment for HNC may also lead to problems with swallowing and dry mouth, and patients may require a modified-texture diet for a year or more. Pursuing swallowing rehabilitation, preventing gastrostomy/jejunostomy dependency, and managing late side effects that might affect nutritional status should also be considered.[5]

SUMMARY

As advances in the multimodal management of EC and HNC continue, it is vital that nutrition management strategies keep pace if healthcare providers are to optimize patient outcomes (Table 7.3). A multidisciplinary team approach, effective symptom management, and early and ongoing access to a dietitian, a speech pathologist, and the medical team are important in improving patient-centered outcomes, including QoL. Strong evidence demonstrates the benefits of individualized dietary counseling in patients with HNC. Lower levels of evidence, mainly from retrospective studies, suggest that enteral feedings result in less weight loss compared with dietary

Table 7.3 *Nutritional Support Strategies for Patients with Esophageal or Head and Neck Cancer*

• Longer-term follow-up
• Mortality data
• Health economic analyses
• Benefits of dietary counseling in patients with EC
• Well-designed prospective studies to identify which patients with EC or HNC would benefit from prophylactic tube feeding
• Preoperative versus perioperative immunonutrition during surgical resection
• Long-term effects of combined treatment, including chemoradiation, on swallowing and nutritional outcomes

intake alone in patients who are not able to meet their dietary requirements orally. The existing paradigm is that malnutrition in patients undergoing treatment for EC or HNC is inevitable. Early, individualized, and intensive nutrition intervention, however, has been shown to prevent or minimize nutritional deficits in patients with EC and HNC. Thus effective, multidisciplinary treatment and early and ongoing nutrition intervention by the registered dietitian is vital to optimize QoL and clinical outcomes in patients with EC or HNC.

REFERENCES

1. Shike M. Nutrition therapy for the cancer patient. *Hematol Oncol Clin North Am.* 1996;10:221–234.
2. Lees J. Incidence of weight loss in head and neck cancer patients on commencing radiotherapy treatment at a regional oncology centre. *Eur J Cancer Care (Engl).* 1999;8:133–136.
3. Nitenberg G, Raynard B. Nutritional support of the cancer patient: Issues and Dilemmas. *Crit Rev Oncol Hematol.* 2000;34:137–168.
4. van Bokhorst-de van der Schueren MAE, van Leeuwen PAM, Sauerwein HP, Kuik DJ, Snow GB, Quak JJ. Assessment of malnutrition parameters in HNC and their relation to postoperative complications. *Head Neck.* 1997;19:419–425.
5. Isenring EA, Hill J, Davidson W, et al. Evidence-based practice guidelines for nutritional management of patients receiving radiation therapy. *Nutrition and Dietetics.* 2008;65(suppl 1):1–20.
6. Isenring E, Capra S, Bauer J. Nutrition intervention is beneficial in oncology outpatients receiving radiotherapy to the gastrointestinal, head or neck area. *Br J Cancer.* 2004;9:447–452.
7. Ravasco P, Monteiro-Grillo I, Marques Vidal P, Ermelinda Camilo M. Impact of nutrition on outcome: A prospective randomized controlled trial in patients with head and neck cancer undergoing radiotherapy. *Head Neck.* 2005;27:659–668.
8. Scolapio J, Spangler P, Romano MM, et al. Prophylactic placement of gastrostomy feeding tubes before radiotherapy in patients with head and neck cancer. *J Clin Gastroenterol.* 2001;33:215–217.
9. Tyldesley S, Sheehan F, Munk P, et al. The use of radiologically placed gastrostomy tubes in head and neck cancer patients receiving radiotherapy. *Int J Radiat Oncol Biol Phys.* 1996;36:1205–1209.
10. Beaver ME, Matheny KE, Roberts DB, Myers JN. Predictors of weight loss during radiation therapy. *Otolaryngol Head Neck Surg.* 2001;125:645–648.
11. Riddle B, Davidson W, Elliot R, Balsillie F, Porceddu S. Collaborative management of acute side effects for head and neck cancer patients receiving radiotherapy. *Asia Pac J Clin Oncol.* 2005;(suppl 1):A18.
12. People Living With Cancer. Head and neck cancer. www.plwc.org. Accessed September 11, 2007.
13. Licitra L, Locati LD, Bossi P, Cantu G. Head and neck tumors other than squamous cell carcinoma. *Curr Opin Oncol.* 2004;16:236–241.
14. Blot WJ. Alcohol and cancer. *Cancer Res* 1992;52(suppl):2119S–2123S.

15. American Cancer Society. Cancer facts and figures 2007. http://www.cancer.org/docroot/STT/content/STT_1x_Cancer_Facts_Figures_2007.asp. Accessed September 11, 2007.

16. Jaber MA, Porter SA, Gilthorpe MS, Bedi R, Scully C. Risk factors for oral epithelial dysplasia: The role of smoke and alcohol. *Oral Oncol.* 1999;35:151–156.

17. Marshall JR, Boyle P. Nutrition and oral cancer. *Cancer Causes Control.* 1996; 7:101–111.

18. Whiteman DC, Sadeghi S, Pandeya N, et al. Combined effects of obesity, acid reflux and smoking on the risk of adenocarcinomas of the esophagus. *Gut.* October 11, 2007 [e-print].

19. Forastiere A, Trotti A, Pfister D, Grandis J. Head and neck cancer: Recent advances and new standards of care. *J Clin Oncol.* 2006;24:2603–2605.

20. Doyle C, Kushi LH, Byers T, et al. Nutrition, Physical Activity and Cancer Survivorship Advisory Committee. Nutrition and physical activity during and after cancer treatment: An American Cancer Society guide for informed choices. *CA Cancer J Clin.* 2006;56:323–353.

21. Schweinfurth JM, Boger GN, Feustel PJ. Preoperative risk assessment for gastrostomy tube placement in head and neck cancer patients. *Head Neck.* 2001;23:376–382.

22. Delaney GP, Fisher RJ, Smee RI, Hook C, Barton MB. Split-course accelerated therapy in head and neck cancer: An analysis of toxicity. *Int J Radiat Oncol Biol Phys.* 1995;32:763–768.

23. Rademaker AW, Vonesh EF, Logemann JA, et al. Eating ability in head and neck cancer patients after treatment with chemoradiation: A 12-month follow-up accounting for dropout. *Head Neck.* 2003;25:1034–1041.

24. Allen AM, Elshaikh M, Worden FP, et al. Acceleration of hyperfractionated chemoradiation regimen for advanced head and neck cancer. *Head Neck.* 2007; 29:137–142.

25. Ang KK, Harris J, Garden AS, et al. Concomitant boost radiation plus concurrent cisplatin for advanced head and neck carcinomas: Radiation therapy oncology group phase II trial 99-14. *J Clin Oncol.* 2005;23:3008–3015.

26. Terrell JE. Quality of life assessment in head and neck cancer patients. *Hematol Oncol Clin North Am.* 1999;13:849–865.

27. Mekhail TM, Adelstein DJ, Rybicki LA, Larto MA, Saxton JP, Lavertu P. Enteral nutrition during the treatment of head and neck carcinoma: Is a percutaneous endoscopic gastrostomy tube preferable to a nasogastric tube? *Cancer.* 2001;91: 1785–1790.

28. Beer KT, Krausse KB, Zuercher T, Stanga Z. Early percutaneous endoscopic gastrostomy insertion maintains nutritional state in patients with aerodigestive tract cancer. *Nutrition and Cancer.* 2005;52:29–34.

29. Davidson W, Isenring E, Brown T, Riddle B. Nutritional management of patients with head and neck cancer: Integrating research into practice. *Cancer Forum.* 2006;30:183–187.

30. Arends J, Bodoky G, Bozzetti F, et al. ESPEN guidelines of enteral nutrition: Nonsurgical oncology. *Clin Nutr.* 2006;25:245–259.

31. Bauer J, Ash S, Davidson W, et al. Evidence based practice guidelines for the nutritional management of cancer cachexia. *Nutr Dietetics.* 2006;63(suppl 2): S5–S32.

32. Ravasco P, Monteiro-Grillo I, Marques Vidal PM, Camilo ME. Nutritional deterioration in cancer: The role of disease and diet. *Clin Oncol.* 2003;15:443–450.

33. Sial SH, Catalano MF. Gastrointestinal tract cancer in the elderly. *Gastroenterol Clin North Am* 2001;30:565–590.

34. Mittal BB, Paulouski BR, Haraf DJ, et al. Swallowing dysfunction: Preventative and rehabilitation strategies in patients with head and neck cancers treated with surgery, radiotherapy, and chemotherapy: A critical review. *Int J Radiat Oncol Biol Phys.* 2003;57:1219–1230.

35. Nguyen NP, Sallah S, Karlsson U, Antoine JE. Combined chemotherapy and radiation therapy for head and neck malignancies: Quality of life issues. *Cancer.* 2002; 94:1131–1141.

36. Dawson ER, Morley SE, Robertson G, Souter DS. Increasing dietary supervision can decrease weight loss in oral cancer patients. *Nutr Cancer.* 2001;41:70–74.

37. Brookes GB. Nutritional status: A prognostic indicator in head and neck cancer. *Otolaryngol Head Neck Surg.* 1985;93:69–74.

38. Capra S, Bauer J, Davidson W, Ash S. Nutritional therapy for cancer-induced weight loss. *Nutr Clin Prac.* 2002;17:210–213.

39. Bauer J, Capra S, Ferguson M. Use of the scored Patient-Generated Subjective Global Assessment as a nutrition assessment tool in patients with cancer. *Eur J Clin Nutr.* 2002;56:779–785.

40. Ottery FD. Patient-Generated Subjective Global Assessment. In: McCallum P, Polisena C, eds. *The Clinical Guide to Oncology Nutrition.* Chicago, IL: American Dietetic Association; 2000:11–23.

41. World Cancer Research Fund and American Institute for Cancer Research. Food, nutrition, physical activity and the prevention of cancer: A global perspective. http://www.dietandcancerreport.org/downloads/summary/english.pdf. Accessed November 5, 2007.

42. Halyard MY, Jatoi A, Sloan JA, et al. Does zinc sulphate prevent therapy-induced taste alterations in head and neck cancer patients? Results of phase III double-blind, placebo-controlled trial from the North Central Cancer Treatment Group (N01C4). *Int J Radiation Oncology Biol Phys.* 2007;67:1318–1322.

43. Mangar S, Slevin N, Mais K, Sykes A. Evaluating predictive factors for determining enteral nutrition in patients receiving radical radiotherapy for head and neck cancer: A retrospective review. *Radiation Ther Oncol.* 2006;78:152–158.

44. Hearne BE, Dunaj JM, Daly JM, et al. Enteral nutrition support in head and neck cancer: Tube vs. oral feeding during radiation therapy. *J Am Dietetic Assoc.* 1985; 85:669–674.

45. Bozzetti F, Cozzagilo L, Gavazzi C, et al. Nutritional support in patients with cancer of the esophagus: Impact on nutritional status, patient compliance to therapy and survival. *Tumori.* 1998;84:681–686.

46. Wood K. Audit of nutritional guidelines for head and neck cancer patients undergoing radiotherapy. *J Hum Nutr Dietet.* 2005;18:343–351.

47. Lee JH, Machtay M, Unger LD, et al. Prophylactic gastrostomy tubes in patients undergoing intensive irradiation for cancer of the head and neck. *Arch Otolaryngol Head Neck Surg.* 1998;124:871–875.

48. Piquet M, Ozsahin M, Larpin I, et al. Early nutrition intervention in oropharyngeal cancer patients undergoing radiotherapy. *Support Care Cancer.* 2002;10: 502–504.

49. Fietkau R. Principles of feeding cancer patients via enteral or parenteral nutrition during radiotherapy. *Strahlenther Onkol.* 1998;174(suppl III):47–51.

50. Odelli C, Burgess D, Bateman L, et al. Nutrition support improves patient outcomes, treatment tolerance and admission characteristics in oesophageal cancer. *Clin Oncol*. 2005;17:639–645.
51. Elia M, van Bokhorst-de van der Schueren MAE, Garvey J, et al. Enteral (oral or tube administration) nutritional support and eicosapentaenoic acid in patients with cancer: A systematic review. *Int J Oncol*. 2006;28:5–23.
52. Rabinovitch R, Grant B, Berkey B, et al. Impact of nutrition support on treatment outcome in patients with locally advanced head and neck squamous cell cancer treated with definitive radiotherapy: A secondary analysis of RTOG trial 90-03. *Head Neck*. 2006;28:287–296.
53. De Blaauw I, Deutz NEP, von Meyenfeldt MF. Metabolic changes in cancer cachexia: First of two parts. *Clin Nutr*. 1997;16:169–176.
54. Stanga Z, Brunner A, Leuenberger M, et al. Nutrition in clinical practice: The refeeding syndrome: Illustrative cases and guidelines for prevention and treatment. *Eur J Clin Nutr*. August 15, 2007 [e-print].
55. Bertrand PC, Piquet MA, Bordier I, Monnier P, Roulet M. Preoperative nutritional support at home in head and neck cancer patients: From nutritional benefits to the prevention of alcohol withdrawal syndrome. *Curr Opin Clin Nutr Metab Care*. 2002;5:435–440.
56. Faist E, Wichmann M, Kim C. Immunosuppression and immunomodulation in surgery and trauma. *Curr Opt Crit Care*. 1997;3:293–297.
57. Waitzberg DL, Saito H, Plank LD, et al. Postsurgical infections are reduced with specialized nutrition support. *World J Surg*. 2006;30:1592–1604.
58. Sonis ST, Elting LS, Keefe D, et al. Perspectives on cancer-therapy induced mucosal injury. *Cancer*. 2004;100(suppl 9):1995–2025.
59. McNeely ML, Armijo OS, Magee DJ. A systematic review of the effectiveness of physical therapy interventions for temporomandibular disorders. *Phys Ther*. 2006;86:710–725.
60. Rogers LQ, Courneya KS, Robbins KT, et al. Physical activity and quality of life in head and neck cancer survivors. *Support Care Cancer*. 2006;14:1012–1019.
61. Rogers LQ, Courneya KS, Robbins KT, et al. Physical activity correlates and barriers in head and neck cancer patients. *Support Care Cancer*. 2008;16:19–27.
62. Mayne ST, Cartmel B, Baum M, et al. Randomized trial of supplemental beta-carotene to prevent second head and neck cancer. *Cancer Res*. 2001;61:1457–1463.

Chapter 8

Breast Cancer

Deborah Straub, MS, RD

INTRODUCTION

Much interest exists about the role nutrition plays in the etiology, treatment, and recurrence of breast cancer. To date, hundreds of studies have been published on nutrition's influence on the etiology of breast cancer, but much of this research is limited in scope and inconclusive. Nutrition care during breast cancer treatment should address not only the usual side effects associated with cancer treatment, but also the consequences of early menopause caused by treatment and the drug therapies that lower endogenous estrogen production. Many women treated for breast cancer use complementary and alternative medicine (CAM) to manage menopausal symptoms, and it is imperative that they obtain further knowledge about the risk versus benefit of supplementation. Data dealing with nutrition's potential to prevent recurrence of breast cancer are very limited, although a few clinical trials in this area have been completed or are in progress.

Breast Cancer Incidence

Breast cancer is the most common cancer in women. In 2008, it is estimated that 184,460 new cases of invasive breast cancer will be diagnosed.[1] During the period of 2001–2004, breast cancer incidence decreased by 3.5% per year. Breast cancer rates had been continuously increasing for more than two decades. This recent decrease may be due to the decline in the use of hormone replacement therapy (HRT) following publication of the results of the Women's Health Initiative (WHI) in 2002, which linked HRT use with increased risk of breast cancer and heart disease. It may also reflect a slight decrease in mammography utilization.

An estimated 67,770 new cases of ductal carcinoma in situ (DCIS) are expected to be identified in 2008. Incidence rates of this noninvasive form of breast cancer have leveled off since the late 1990s, which may also reflect the decrease in mammography utilization.

Breast cancer is second only to lung cancer as the most common cause of cancer death in women. An estimated 40,930 breast cancer deaths are expected in 2008. Death from breast cancer has steadily declined since 1990—a trend attributable to a combination of early detection and advancements in treatment. Five-year survival rates for all races are 98% for localized cancer, 84% for regional cancer, and 27% for distant female breast cancer.

Breast Anatomy and Estrogen Metabolism

The anatomy of the breast consists of primarily fat, connective tissue, epithelial cells, and glandular tissue arranged into lobules and ducts. The lobules are the milk-producing glands of the breast. Ducts connect the lobules to the nipple. Epithelial cells line the lobules and the ducts. A variety of hormones—including estrogen, progesterone, insulin and growth factors—contribute to breast tissue development during puberty, pregnancy, and lactation. After menopause, the glandular tissue atrophies as estrogen and progesterone levels decline.

The female hormone estrogen is found in three forms: estradiol, estrone, and estriol. The most potent of these is estradiol. Estrogens circulate in the blood bound to sex-hormone-binding globulin (SHBG). Only unbound estrogens can enter target tissue cells and induce biological activity. Prior to menopause, estrogens are synthesized from cholesterol in the ovaries in response to pituitary hormones. The amount of estrogen produced after menopause, however, is significantly less than the amount produced prior to menopause. After menopause, estrogen is produced primarily by the aromatization of adrenal androstenedione to estrone in the peripheral tissues. Estrogens are also produced by the aromatization of androgens in fat cells. In postmenopausal women, the ovaries continue to make small amounts of testosterone, which is converted to estradiol.

The metabolism of estrogen takes place predominantly in the liver through Phase I (hydroxylation) and Phase II (methylation, glucuronidation, and sulfation) pathways. Estrogen is excreted in the urine and feces.

Estrogens have a wide range of actions, such that they affect almost all systems of the body in a tissue-specific manner. Estrogens bind with high affinity to estrogen receptors (ER) in target cells. When estrogen is bound to the receptor, it initiates transcription of the estrogen-responsive target gene. Two forms of estrogen receptors are distinguished—alpha and beta—that differ in terms of their tissue distribution, binding affinity, and biological function. Different target cells may respond differently to estrogen depending on the ratio of receptor subtypes. The actions of the selective estrogen modulators (SERMs) known as tamoxifen and raloxifene are examples of this phenomenon: These drugs act as estrogen in some tissue (bone) and block its action in other tissues (breast).

Cellular Classification of Breast Cancer

Breast cancers are primarily carcinomas of the epithelial cells. Breast cancer is classified based on whether the cancer arose from the epithelial cells of the ducts or the lobules and whether the cells infiltrated through the duct or the lobule into the fatty tissue of the breast. Invasive (or infiltrating) ductal carcinoma (IDC; see Figure 8.1) is the most common type of invasive breast cancer, accounting for 80% of invasive breast cancers. Invasive (infiltrating) lobular carcinoma (ILC; see Figure 8.2) represents 10% of invasive breast

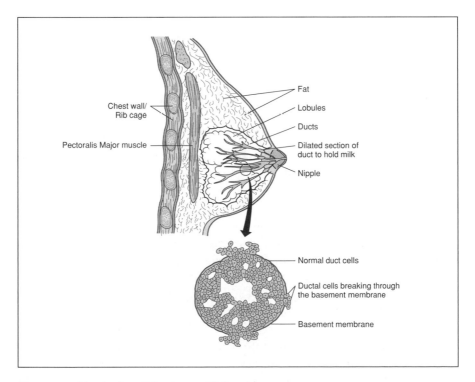

Figure 8.1   *Invasive Ductal Carcinoma (IDC)*

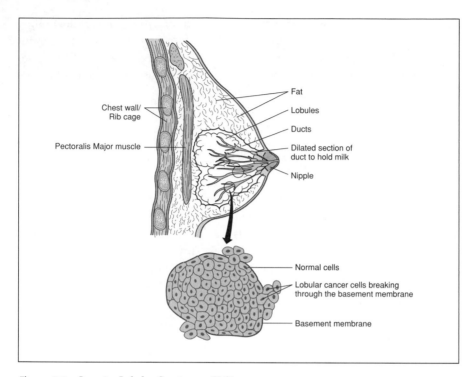

Figure 8.2   *Invasive Lobular Carcinoma (ILC)*

cancers. Noninvasive breast cancers include DCIS (Figures 8.3, page 191, and 8.4, page 192) and lobular carcinoma in situ (LCIS). LCIS is not a true cancer, but it does increase a woman's risk of developing invasive breast cancer in the ispsilateral or in the contralateral breast. Inflammatory breast cancer is a rare but aggressive type of breast cancer; it accounts for 1–5% of all breast cancer cases. Its symptoms may include redness, swelling, and warmth without a distinct tumor. Other less common ductal breast cancers include medullary, mucinous, papillary, and tubular carcinomas. Paget's disease of the nipple is rare and is responsible for only 1% of all breast cancers.

Breast cancer subtypes with distinct gene expression profiles have been identified through the use of microarray analysis.[2] The two major subtypes of the estrogen receptor-positive (ER-positive) tumors are luminal A and luminal B. Luminal A tumors tend to have a higher expression of ER-related genes and a lower expression of proliferative genes than do luminal B tumors. The major subtypes of the ER-negative tumors are those involving the human epidermal growth factor 2 (HER-2) and the basal-like subtype. Most ER-negative tumors tend to be HER-2 positive. The basal-like

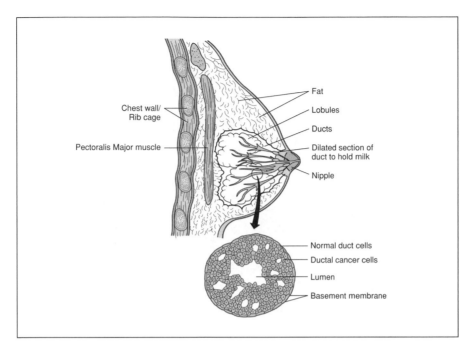

Figure 8.3 *Ductal Carcinoma in Situ (DCIS)*

subtype tends to have a low expression of ER, progesterone receptor (PR), and HER-2. In general, HER-2-positive and basal-like subtypes are more aggressive than the luminal A tumors. The luminal A subtype appears to be associated with the best prognosis.

Breast Cancer Risk

As noted earlier, breast cancers are primarily carcinomas of the epithelial cells. Estrogen modulates the structure and growth of epithelial cells. Thus estrogen exposure is a well-established risk factor for breast cancer.[3] Cumulative, excessive estrogen exposure over the course of a lifetime contributes to breast cancer risk and may be a cause of this disease. Early menarche, late menopause, not having children, or having children after age 30 all increase a woman's breast cancer risk.[4] Such prolonged estrogen exposure can cause direct genotoxic effects by increasing breast cell proliferation and random genetic errors affecting cellular differentiation and gene expression. The mechanisms of carcinogenesis include the metabolism of estrogen to

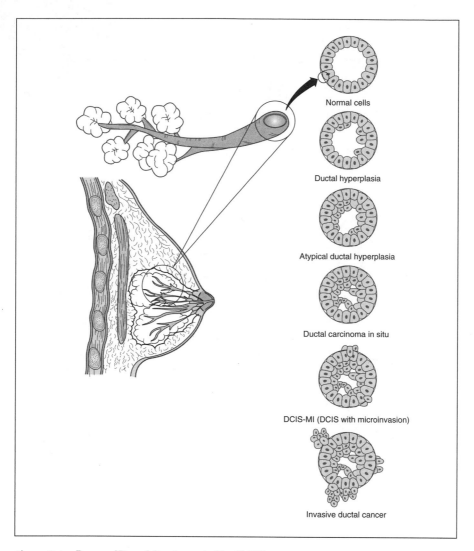

Figure 8.4   *Range of Ductal Carcinoma in Situ (DCIS)*

mutagenic, genotoxic metabolites and the stimulation of tissue growth. These processes cause initiation, promotion, and progression of breast cancer.

Risk prediction models can be helpful in assessing a woman's risk for breast cancer. The Breast Cancer Risk Assessment Tool (available at http://www.cancer.gov/bcrisktool) is a computer assessment tool developed by the National Cancer Institute and the National Surgical Adjuvant Breast and Bowel Project (NSABP).[5] It estimates breast cancer risk over the woman's next five years and over a lifetime and is based on the Gail model. The risk factors included in this tool include age, age at menarche, age at first live birth, breast cancer among first-degree relatives, and breast biopsies. The Breast Cancer Risk Assessment Tool was developed and validated for primarily non-Hispanic white women in the United States who are age 35 or older. More research is needed to refine and validate this model for other racial and ethnic groups.

Other risk factors for breast cancer have been identified but have not yet been incorporated into the Breast Cancer Risk Assessment Tool, as independent validation studies are lacking for these risk factors. In a large prospective study involving 1 million women who underwent screening mammography, researchers identified statistically significant risk factors for both premenopausal and postmenopausal women.[6] In premenopausal women, risk of breast cancer diagnosis was significantly associated with age, breast density, number of first-degree relatives with breast cancer, and a prior breast procedure. A prior breast procedure was associated with an approximately 50% increase in risk even without knowledge of the type or result of the prior breast procedure. Breast density was strongly associated with increased risk among women with extremely dense breasts, with this characteristic conferring almost a fourfold greater risk than having breasts composed primarily of fat. In postmenopausal women, risk increased with age, breast density, family history of breast cancer, a prior breast procedure even without knowledge of the type of prior procedure or the outcome, hormonal therapy, age at natural menopause, and a prior false-positive mammogram. Other factors associated with increased risk in postmenopausal women included higher body mass index (BMI), late age at the birth of the first child or being nulliparous, and the use of hormone replacement therapy. The study did not distinguish among the various types of hormone therapy.

In another study, radiation exposure to the chest for treatment during childhood or young adulthood cancers was found to significantly increase the risk of breast cancer in adulthood.[7] The risk was highest if the radiation was given during adolescence.

Genetic Breast Cancer

Genetic breast cancer, in which one dominant cancer gene is passed on to future generations, accounts for only 5–10% of all breast cancer cases. Most breast cancer cases are sporadic, meaning that there is no family history; indeed, 70–80% of women who get breast cancer do not have a family history of this disease.

A number of genetic mutations have been identified that increase the risk of breast cancer. Notably, mutations in the tumor suppression genes *BRCA1* and *BRAC2* confer up to a 50–80% lifetime chance of developing breast cancer. *BRCA* mutations are most often found in Jewish women of Ashkenazi (Eastern European) origin, but can appear in any racial or ethnic group.

Screening

The goal of screening is to detect breast cancer when it is more likely to be at an early stage, have a better prognosis, and be more successfully treated. Screen-detected breast cancers with or without clinical breast exams are associated with reduced morbidity and mortality. The American Cancer Society has established screening guidelines for breast cancer.[8] Mammography screening is the primary tool for early detection and is recommended annually for women starting at age 40. Women who are at high risk of developing breast cancer (greater than 20% lifetime risk) should have an annual breast magnetic resonance imaging (MRI) scan in addition to an annual mammogram.[9]

Diagnosis

A diagnostic mammogram is performed when a suspicious finding is identified on a screening mammogram. A breast ultrasound (US) and a breast MRI may be performed to obtain additional information. If imaging studies show suspicious findings, a biopsy will be performed.

The National Comprehensive Cancer Network (NCCN) has established diagnostic workup and treatment guidelines for breast cancer.[10] The workup for invasive cancer includes a history and physical examination, complete blood count, platelets, liver function tests, chest imaging, diagnostic bilateral mammogram, US as necessary, optional breast MRI, and a pathology review, including the determination of tumor estrogen/progesterone receptor status (ER/PR), human epidermal growth factor receptor 2 (HER-2/neu) status, and surgical margins. A bone scan, abdominal computed tomography (CT) scan, or positron emission tomography (PET) scan may also be performed depending on the stage of the cancer and the laboratory findings.

Treatment

The treatment of local disease may consist of surgery, radiation therapy (RT), or both. The management of systemic disease, if present, may involve cytoxic chemotherapy, endocrine therapy, biologic therapies, or combinations of these modalities. Treatment is determined by numerous factors, including disease stage, tumor histology, clinical and pathologic characteristics of the tumor, axillary node status, tumor hormone receptor status, level of HER-2/neu expression, presence or absence of detectable metastatic disease, comorbid conditions, the patient's age, and menopausal status. Molecular profiling of breast cancers using array technology has confirmed that breast cancer is a heterogeneous group of diseases that are marked by differences in prognosis and response to therapy.[11] Molecular predictive models are beginning to influence treatment strategies.

Staging

The American Joint Committee on Cancer's (AJCC) TNM system is used to stage breast cancer. Five stages of breast cancer are distinguished based on the tumor (T) size and spread to the chest wall or skin; the degree of lymph node involvement (N) (Figures 8.5 and 8.6); and metastasis to distant organs (M).

- Stage 0 includes DCIS and LCIS. DCIS is the earliest form of breast cancer, in which the cancer cells are still within the duct and have not invaded the surrounding fatty breast tissue. DCIS is usually treated with lumpectomy, RT, and tamoxifen citrate. LCIS is not considered true breast cancer by most oncologists, but is a marker for increased future risk and is treated with tamoxifen.

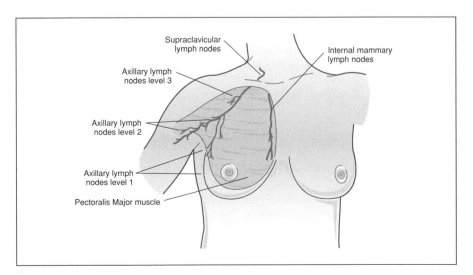

Figure 8.5 *Axillary Lymph Nodes*

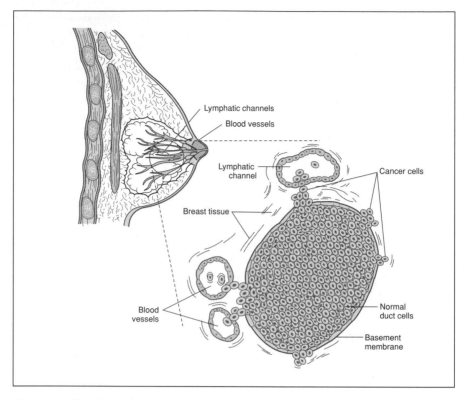

Figure 8.6 *Vascular and Lymphatic Invasions*

- Stages I–IV are classified by increasing tumor size, number of positive lymph nodes, and metastases to distant locations. The most common sites for metastatic breast cancer are the bone, liver, brain, or lung.

Local Treatment

Surgery

Breast-conserving lumpectomy and mastectomy are the two types of surgery used to locally remove breast cancer. With lumpectomy, the tumor and healthy tissue surrounding the tumor are removed; the surgical procedure is then usually followed by RT. With mastectomy, the entire breast, including the nipple, is removed. Women may elect to have reconstruction surgery at the same time as mastectomy, after mastectomy, or not at all. Survival rates for breast-conserving surgery plus RT are equal to those for mastectomy in case of Stage I and Stage II breast cancers.

Sentinel node biopsy is the preferred method of determining lymph node involvement. If the sentinel node is positive, an axillary dissection is performed. Complications of surgery vary with the type of surgery performed and the number of lymph nodes removed. Side effects are less common and less severe with sentinel node dissection, but are more common and more severe with full axillary lymph node dissection. Side effects of lymph node dissection include nerve damage, limitation of arm and shoulder movement, and lymphedema of the arm.

Radiation Therapy

Most women treated with breast-conserving surgery require follow-up treatment with RT. RT may also be indicated after mastectomy if the patient has extensive lymph node involvement. External-beam whole-breast radiation therapy with a boost to the tumor bed is the most common form of radiation employed. Brachytherapy or interstitial radiation involving the placement of radioactive seeds may be an option in some cases.

Side effects of radiation to the breast include swelling and heaviness in the breast, sunburn-like skin changes, hair loss in the treated area, and fatigue. Most symptoms occur during the second or third week of treatment and resolve within 2–4 weeks after RT completion. Changes in breast tissue and skin generally resolve in 6–12 months. Long-term risks associated with RT to the breast include rib fractures and secondary cancers caused by the radiation. Women treated with RT to the left breast are more likely than women treated with RT to the right breast to develop cardiac disease, including myocardial infarction and chest pain.[12]

Systemic Therapy

Chemotherapy

The decision to initiate adjuvant polychemotherapy involves balancing the risk of recurrence from local therapy alone, the degree of benefit from chemotherapy (CT), the toxicity of the therapy, and existing comorbidities. Neoadjuvant CT may be given to reduce the size of the tumor prior to surgery. Chemotherapy is also used to treat metastatic breast cancer.

Multi-gene testing of the tumor to predict responsiveness to chemotherapy and prognosis is currently available. However, the NCCN believes that none of the available tests has been adequately studied to recommend its use in clinical practice.

The severity of side effects of chemotherapy depend on the specific agent used, the dose, the length of treatment, existing comorbidities, and individual tolerance.

Adjuvant Endocrine Therapy

Adjuvant endocrine therapy is instituted for breast cancers that are estrogen or progesterone receptor-positive (ER-positive, PR-positive). The two SERMs used for treatment of breast cancer, tamoxifen and raloxifene (Evista®), compete with estrogen for receptor sites in target tissues such as the breast.

Tamoxifen is used for adjuvant treatment for premenopausal breast cancer. It is also used to reduce the risk of breast cancer in women with LCIS and DCIS.[13] This drug exerts estrogen-like activity on the skeletal and cardiovascular systems, reducing bone loss and improving lipid levels. Side effects of tamoxifen include hot flashes, night sweats, and vaginal dryness. Serious adverse effects include an increased risk of cataracts, endometrial cancer, and pulmonary embolism.

The U.S. Food and Drug Administration approved raloxifene for reducing the risk of invasive breast cancer in postmenopausal women with osteoporosis and in postmenopausal women at high risk for invasive breast cancer.[14] Raloxifen has not been approved for use in decreasing breast cancer risk in women with DCIS.

Aromatase inhibitors (AIs) are used to decrease estrogen levels in postmenopausal women through aromatase inhibition. Members of this drug class include anastrozole (Arimidex®), letrozole (Femara®), and exemestane (Aromasin®), all of which are used only in postmenopausal women. Nutrition-related side effects of AIs include loss of bone mineral density (BMD). Some agents may also have a negative effect on patients' lipid profiles.[15] For example, letrozole has been associated with increased total serum cholesterol, low-density cholesterol, apolipoprotein B, and serum-lipid risk ratios related to cardiovascular disease. An updated safety analysis of the Breast Cancer International Group (BIG) 1-98 study found that cardiovascular adverse events were relatively rare with letrozole, however.[16] A large ongoing phase III trial comparing anastrozole with letrozole will provide head-to-head safety evaluations of the two drugs. Because most women presenting with early-stage breast cancer can expect long-term survival, the assessment of cardiovascular adverse effects of AIs is important.

Targeted Therapy

Trastuzumab (Herceptin®) is used to treat HER-2/neu-positive tumors, which tend to be more aggressive. Overexpression of the HER-2/neu protein increases the rate of cell growth and division. Trastuzumab is a recombinant DNA-derived monoclonal antibody that selectively binds to HER-2, thereby inhibiting the proliferation of tumor cells that overexpress HER-2.

Ovarian Ablation

In an effort to decrease estrogen levels, premenopausal women may elect to have an oophorectomy. Side effects of this treatment include early menopause, which may be associated with hot flashes, night sweats, and bone loss.

Prognosis

The most significant prognostic factors predicting future recurrence or death from breast cancer include patient age, stage, comorbidity, tumor size, tumor grade, number of involved axillary lymph nodes, and possibly HER-2/neu level of expression. Algorithms are available that estimate rates of recurrence. A validated computer-based model, Adjuvant! Online, estimates 10-year disease-free and overall survival and is available at www.adjuvantonline.com.

Nutrition and Lifestyle Factors in the Etiology of Breast Cancer

All cancers start as a single cell that has lost control of its normal growth and replication processes. Carcinogenesis is a multistage process consisting of three phases: initiation, promotion, and progression. Initiation occurs when the cell has been exposed to an agent that results in the first genetic mutation, but by itself initiation is not sufficient for a cancer to develop. Instead, the initiated cell must be activated by a promoting agent that causes cellular proliferation—that is, the process called promotion. Initiated and promoted cells eventually form a tumor mass during the process of progression. At the end of the carcinogenesis process, the cell will have some or all of the characteristics of a cancer cell: growth signal autonomy, insensitivity to anti-growth signals, limitless replicative potential, evasion of apoptosis, sustained angiogenesis, tissue invasion, and metastasis. Factors related to food, nutrition, and physical activity can influence the various cellular processes involved in carcinogenesis.

In 2007, a joint panel of the World Cancer Research Fund (WCRF) and American Institute for Cancer Research published its findings on the role of food, nutrition, and physical activity in cancer prevention (Figure 8.7).[17] In their report, the panel members judged the weight of the evidence for the role of nutrition and lifestyle factors in the etiology of breast cancer. Premenopausal and postmenopausal breast cancers were considered separately

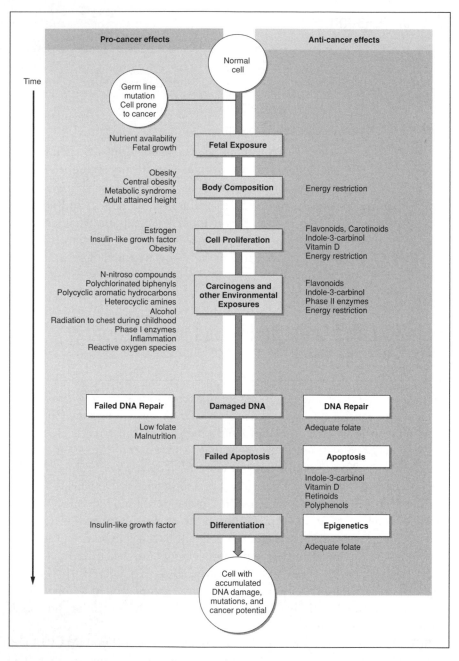

Figure 8.7 *The Influences of Food, Nutrition, Obesity and Physical Activity on the Cellular Processes Linked to Breast Cancer*

in the report. Premenopausal cancers are thought to be mainly genetically driven, with the environment and nutrition playing smaller roles in their genesis. In the genetically associated cancers, a healthy diet may result in the delayed onset of the disease. Diet modulation is most likely to influence postmenopausal disease, which is more prolonged in onset. The panel's findings related to breast cancer risk are summarized next.

POSTMENOPAUSAL BREAST CANCER

- *Convincing evidence:* The consumption of alcoholic drinks, body fatness, and adult attained height increase risk; lactation decreases risk.
- *Probable evidence:* Physical activity decreases risk; abdominal fatness and adult weight gain increase risk.
- *Limited suggestive evidence:* Total fat intake increases risk.

PREMENOPAUSAL BREAST CANCER

- *Convincing evidence:* Lactation decreases risk; consumption of alcoholic beverages increases risk.
- *Probable evidence:* Body fatness decreases risk; adult-attained height and greater birth weight increase risk.
- *Limited suggestive evidence:* Physical activity decreases risk.

The panel found limited evidence and could not draw a conclusion about other food and nutritional factors, including, but not limited to, soy, fiber, vegetables and fruits, tea, isoflavones, meat, folate, calcium, vitamin D, dietary patterns, culturally defined diets, and environmental chemicals. The lack of strong evidence for a relationship between diet and breast cancer may be real or it may reflect challenges related to study designs, including measurement errors in self-reporting intake by study participants, the focus on diet during adult life versus early life and puberty, follow-up periods that are too short to identify dietary factors, subgroups of women who are more susceptible to the influence of diet, or potential harmful effects of pesticides that negate the benefits of vegetable and fruit consumption.[18] Few studies have focused on the role of diet during gestation, or before or during puberty, and the risk of breast cancer. The influence of diet on breast cancer risk may be most important during mammary gland development.

Lactation

There is convincing evidence that breastfeeding decreases the risk of breast cancer in both premenopausal and postmenopausal women, according to the WCRF panel. Most studies show a decreased risk with increased duration of breastfeeding. Specifically, pooled analysis from 47 epidemiological studies showed a decreased risk of 4.3% for each 12 months of breastfeeding.[19]

Protection may be conferred by the lower exposure to estrogen during the amenorrhea associated with breastfeeding, increased differentiation of breast cells, exfoliation of breast tissue during lactation, and massive epithelial apoptosis at the end of lactation, which may eliminate cells with potential DNA damage. Little is known about dietary exposures during pregnancy or lactation on future breast cancer risk in the mother or the infant.

In rodents, in utero exposure to a diet high in polyunsaturated fatty acids (n-6) or genistein increases ER-α receptors, causing an increase in unopposed cell proliferation and increased mammary tumorigenesis.[20] In rodents, a diet high in genistein or n-6 fatty acids alters normal mammary gland development, which in turn may increase future breast cancer risk. It is unknown how these and other dietary exposures might modulate estrogen, estrogen receptor sites, or breast development during pregnancy or lactation, and what effects these changes might have on future breast cancer risk in women and their offspring.

Weight, Adult-Attained Height, and Postmenopausal Breast Cancer

As mentioned earlier, the WCRF panel determined that adult weight gain is a probable risk factor for postmenopausal breast cancer. The increased risk of breast cancer in this scenario may be due to higher estrogen levels: Circulating levels of estrogen are twice as high in overweight women. The higher estrogen levels are caused by the endogenous production of estrogen by the aromatization of adrenal androgens in the adipose tissue. Overweight women also have lower levels of SHBG as compared to normal weight women, and consequently have more bioavailable estrogen. Being overweight is also associated with increased levels of insulin and insulin-like growth factor 1 (IGF-1), which produces a hormonal environment that favors carcinogenesis and depresses apoptosis. Inflammation is also associated with overweight, especially abdominal adiposity. Chronic inflammation may be involved in the initiation and the progression of cancer by damaging DNA, increasing proliferation, inhibiting apoptosis, and increasing angiogenesis.

Epidemiologic data from the Nurses' Health Study found a direct association between weight gain since age 18 and postmenopausal breast cancer risk, especially in women who had never used postmenopausal replacement therapy (PMT).[21] In this prospective cohort, 49,514 women aged 30 to 55 years who were free of cancer were followed for as long as 26 years. Weight gain of 25 kg or more since age 18 was associated with an increased risk of breast cancer relative risk (RR) equal to 1.45, compared to women who maintained their weight. In women who never took PMT, the RR was 1.98. The data suggest that 15% of breast cancers could be attributed to weight gain of 2 kg or more since age 18 years and that 4.4% could be attributed to weight gain of 2.0 kg or more since menopause. Women who lost 10 kg or more since menopause and kept it off and never used PMT reduced their risk of breast cancer (RR = 0.45) compared to women who maintained their weight. The weaker association of weight gain in women who used PMT may be due to the high levels of circulating exogenous estrogens in these women, unrelated to their weight and adiposity.

The WCRF panel also found convincing evidence that postmenopausal breast cancer risk increases with adult-attained height. Tallness itself is probably not the cause of breast cancer. Rather, height acts as a surrogate for childhood nutritional factors affecting hormonal and metabolic systems that are related to cancer risk, including alterations in levels of growth hormone, insulin-like growth factors, sex hormone binding proteins, and the age of sexual maturation.

Body Fatness, Greater Weight at Birth, Greater Attained Height, and Premenopausal Risk

In premenopausal women, greater body fatness probably decreases the risk of breast cancer, according to the WCRF panel. The mechanism by which body fatness protects against breast cancer in premenopausal women is still speculative at this time. Proposed mechanisms include irregular menstrual cycles and ovulatory infertility in adulthood, with subsequent alteration in hormone levels.

Premenopausal breast cancer risk increases with greater weight at birth and greater adult-attained height. The mechanisms are speculative. The factors leading to greater birth weight and attained height may affect the long-term programming of hormonal systems. It is not likely that tallness itself is a risk factor, but rather the factors that promote growth during gestation and in childhood.

Alcohol

Convincing evidence exists that regular alcohol consumption increases the risk of breast cancer in both premenopausal and postmenopausal women in a dose-responsive manner. Pooled analysis of six prospective studies found a linear increase in breast cancer risk of 9% for each additional 10 g/day of alcohol consumed. The specific type of alcohol did not strongly influence risk.[22] Another pooled analysis from 53 epidemiological studies found a similar linear increase in breast cancer risk of 7% for each 10 g of alcohol consumed per day.[23] The risk was the same for ever-smokers and never-smokers. The authors estimated that 4% of breast cancers in developed countries could be attributed to alcohol consumption if the observed relationship is causal.

In one study, alcohol consumption was associated with ER-positive breast cancer in postmenopausal women but not with ER-negative breast cancer.[24] A number of hormonal and nonhormonal mechanisms have been proposed to explain the positive association between alcohol and breast cancer. Alcohol may affect a number of hormone-dependent pathways by inducing the production of endogenous estrogens, decreasing the metabolic clearance of estradiol, stimulating the proliferation of ER-positive cells, and increasing ER-alpha activity through inactivation of the *BRAC1* gene. Hormone-independent pathways include the induction of carcinogenesis and DNA damage by acetaldehyde (the reactive metabolite of ethanol), lipid peroxidation, and the production of reactive oxygen species.

Adequate folate status may partially mitigate the increased breast cancer risk associated with moderate alcohol consumption.[25] Folate adequacy should be ensured in women who consume alcohol.

Dietary Fat

The relationship between dietary fat intake and breast cancer risk has been controversial, with mostly observational studies showing inconsistent results. The WCRF panel determined that there is limited evidence suggesting total dietary fat intake increases the risk of postmenopausal breast cancer, but not premenopausal breast cancer. The panel also decided that there is insufficient evidence to draw conclusions about the risk of breast cancer and the various types of fatty acids.

The National Institutes of Health/AARP's (NIH-AARP) Diet and Health Study—a prospective study involving 188,736 postmenopausal women—did find a modest increase in the risk of breast cancer in women who were not using menopausal hormone therapy and who had higher total dietary fat intake.[26] Women who consumed 40% of their total calories in the form of fat (90 g/day, highest quintile) had an 11% higher incidence of invasive breast cancer than women who consumed 20% of calories as fat (24.2g/day, lowest quintile).

In the Women's Health Initiative (WHI)—a randomized, controlled, primary prevention trial involving 48,835 postmenopausal women, ages 50 to 70—reducing the total fat consumed to 20% of total calories did not result in a statistically significant reduction in invasive breast cancer over an 8.1-year follow-up period.[27] However, those women in the intervention group who consumed the highest percentage of energy in the form of fat at baseline (≥36.8% of calories from fat, ≥76 g/day) did see a significant reduction in their risk of invasive breast cancer risk (hazard ratio = 78) when compared to the comparison group. It may be that a subgroup of women with very-high-fat diets would benefit the most from switching to a low-fat dietary pattern.

If a causal relationship between breast cancer risk and dietary fat does exist, it may reflect any of several mechanisms that affect the initiation and growth of breast cancer. These include increased endogenous production of estrogen with higher-fat diets, an increase in bioavailable estrogen with higher-fat diets, modulation of the immune system, and regulation of gene function.

Red Meat, Processed Meat, and Heterocyclic Amines

Studies of meat consumption, red meat consumption, heterocyclic amines, and breast cancer risk have produced conflicting results. The WCRF has determined that there is limited evidence to support the relationship between these dietary factors and cancer risk, but a definitive conclusion cannot be reached. Nevertheless, it seems prudent to advise women to decrease red meat and processed meat consumption, as some evidence supports a link between intake of these foods and breast cancer.

In a prospective study involving 90,659 premenopausal women (Nurses' Health Study II), red meat intake was strongly associated with an elevated risk of ER-positive, PR-positive breast cancer, but not ER-negative, PR-negative breast cancer.[28] Compared with the practice of eating three or fewer servings of red meat per week, RR increased with increased consumption as follows: 1.14 for more than 3–5 servings per week, 1.42 for more than 5 servings per week to 1 or fewer servings per day, and 1.97 for more than 1.5 servings per day.

In the UK Women's Cohort Study, which enrolled 35,371 participants, women with the highest total meat consumption (poultry, red meat, and processed meat) had the highest risk of both premenopausal and post-menopausal breast cancer.[29] High total meat consumption (>103 g/day) compared with no meat consumption was associated with a premenopausal cancer hazard ratio (HR) of 1.20, high processed meat consumption (>20 g/day) compared with no meat consumption was associated with a HR of 1.45, and high red meat consumption (>57 g/day) compared with no meat consumption was associated with a HR of 1.32. The effect was larger in postmenopausal women for all types of meat, including red and processed meat. High total meat consumption (57 g/day) compared with no meat consumption was associated with a HR of 1.63, high processed meat consumption (>20 g/day) compared with no meat consumption was associated with a HR of 1.64, and high red meat consumption (>57 g/day) compared with no meat consumption was associated with a HR of 1.56.

Several mechanisms have been proposed to explain the positive association between meat consumption and breast cancer. In particular, heterocyclic amines, which are produced when meats are charbroiled, fried, or cooked until well done, have been implicated in increasing cancer risk. Heterocyclic amines are estrogenic and stimulate ER and PR gene expression in vitro. Processed meats contain nitroso compounds, which are known carcinogens and may also be involved in breast cancer etiology.

It has been suggested that individuals who have inherited polymorphisms in *N*-acetyltransferase 1 and 2 (*NAT1*, *NAT2*) genes and in glutathione *S*-transferase M1 and T1 genes (*GSTM1*, *GSTT1*), and who consume meat (especially charbroiled meat) are at increased risk for breast cancer. *NAT1* and *NAT2* are involved in phase II acetylation of heterocyclic amines.

GSTM1 and GSTT1 confer protection against oxidative stress by reducing hydrogen peroxide levels and by regenerating vitamins C and E. A study in the Netherlands found that the GSTM1 null genotype (i.e., absence of the gene on the chromosome) increases breast cancer risk irrespective of meat consumption.[30] A statistically significant relationship was not found for breast cancer risk and polymorphisms in NAT1, NAT2, GSTM1, or GSTT1, and levels of meat consumption were not identified in this study.

Women should be advised to decrease their red meat consumption to three or fewer times per week and to avoid processed meats. Well-done and char-broiled meats should be avoided; roasting, stewing, and slow cooker (Crock-Pot) techniques are the preferred methods of meat preparation.

Vegetarian Diets

A vegetarian diet does not appear to protect against breast cancer. A meta-analysis of five mortality studies comparing vegetarians with health-conscious meat-eaters did not find a statistically significant difference in mortality from breast cancer in the two groups.[31] Rates of breast cancer remain high among Adventist populations despite their healthy lifestyle, which includes following a lacto-ovo vegetarian diet.[32]

Macrobiotic Diets

The macrobiotic diet is a popular complementary approach to the treatment of cancer. The dietary pattern promoted by macrobiotics is vegetarian and emphasizes minimally processed foods. The Great Life pyramid was introduced by Michio Kushi, a proponent of macrobiotics[33]; it specifies the recommended macrobiotic diet. The diet consists of 40–60% by weight whole cereal grains, including brown rice, barley, millet, oats, wheat, corn, rye, buckwheat, and other whole grains; 20–30% by weight vegetables; 5–10% by weight beans and bean products, including tofu, tempeh, and natto; and daily consumption of sea vegetables. Fish, nuts, seeds, and fruit are recommended to be consumed on a weekly basis. Dairy, eggs, poultry, and red meat are to be consumed no more that once a month, if at all.

There are no direct studies examining the effects of the macrobiotic diet in cancer prevention and survival. This diet does eliminate red meat, which is associated with increased breast cancer risk. Because the macrobiotic diet does not provide adequate vitamin B_{12}, vitamin D, and calcium, these nutrients should be taken in supplement form by any persons following the diet. Women who elect to follow this diet should be educated on how to meet protein and calorie requirements. A macrobiotic diet may be difficult to adhere to during chemotherapy if the patient develops significant appetite and taste changes, or nausea and vomiting.

Vegetables, Fruit, and Fiber

The WCRF has determined that a conclusion cannot be drawn regarding the effect of dietary fiber or consumption of a diet high in vegetables and fruit on breast cancer risk. Epidemiological studies in this area have yielded inconsistent results. However, interest exists in specific bioactive compounds found in vegetables and fruit that may confer protection against cancer. According to the WCRF, there is limited, inconclusive evidence that cruciferous vegetables, flavonoids, green tea, and phytoestrogens may play a role in decreasing breast cancer risk.

Cruciferous Vegetables

The cruciferous vegetables of the Brassica genus include broccoli, Brussels sprouts, cabbage, collards, cauliflower, kale, kohlrabi, mustard greens, bok choy, Chinese cabbage, turnips, and rutabagas. Cruciferous vegetables are rich in glucosinolates, a group of sulfur-containing compounds. The hydrolysis of glucosinolates by the plant enzyme myrosinase results in biologically active compounds that include indoles. More than 100 glucosinolates with unique hydrolysis products have been identified in plants. These water-soluble compounds may leach into cooking water; microwaving at high power and steaming and boiling vegetables can also inactivate myrosinase.

Evidence that cruciferous vegetables decrease the risk of breast cancer in population-based studies is limited and inconsistent.[34] In addition, genetic polymorphisms may influence the activity of glutathione *S*-transferases (GST) and mediate the effects of cruciferous vegetable intake on cancer risk.[35]

Indole-3-carbinol (I3C) is a constituent of cruciferous vegetables that may offer chemopreventive benefits by shifting the metabolism of 17β-estradiol from 16-α-hydroxyestrone (16αOHE$_1$) to 2-hydroxyestrone (2OHE$_1$). The 16αOHE$_1$ metabolite is thought to be genotoxic and tumorigenic, compared to the 2OHE$_1$ metabolite. In postmenopausal women, increasing the consumption of cruciferous vegetables significantly increases the urinary ratio of 2OHE$_1$ to 16αOHE$_1$.[36] However, the relationship between urinary 2OHE$_1$ to 16αOHE$_1$ and breast cancer risk is unclear. Other proposed anticarcinogenic properties of cruciferous vegetables include their ability to induce apoptosis and inhibit angiogenesis.

The NIH is studying IC3 supplements in preventing breast cancer in nonsmoking women who are at high risk for breast cancer.[37] The long-term effects of IC3 supplementation in humans are not known, and women should be advised not to use these supplements until more is known about their potential risks versus their benefits. More generally, women should be encouraged to increase their consumption of cruciferous vegetables.

Flavonoids

Flavonoids are a group of more than 5,000 polyphenolic compounds that occur naturally in plant foods. Laboratory studies have shown that flavonoids act as anticarcinogens by inhibiting aromatase activity, tumor cell proliferation, and the formation of reactive oxygen species.

Epidemiological studies suggest that foods high in specific flavonoids are associated with a decreased risk of breast cancer. In a retrospective, population-based, case-controlled study of 1,434 women with breast cancer and 1,440 controls, the consumption of specific flavonoids was associated with a decrease in postmenopausal breast cancer risk.[38] Odds ratios (OR) for breast cancer risk were reduced in women with consumption of flavonoids in the highest quintile versus those with consumption in the lowest quintile. The effect was strongest for flavonols (found in onions, cherries, broccoli, tomatoes, tea, red wine, and berries), for which the OR was 0.54; the corresponding ORs were 0.61 for flavones (found in parsley, thyme, and cereal), 0.74 for flavan-3-ols (found in apples, tea, chocolate, red wine, and berries), and 0.69 for lignans (found in flaxseeds, legumes, and whole grains). The data did not support an inverse association between isoflavones (found in soy), anthocyanidins (found in blueberries and raspberries), or flavanones (found in citrus) and breast cancer risk.

The catechins in tea have also been studied for their potential anticarcinogenic properties. Tea is a popular beverage worldwide, and it has been brewed from the *Camellia sinensis* plant for more than 5,000 years. The method used in its processing results in black, green, oolong, or white tea. Black tea is produced by allowing the picked tea leaves to dry indoors, ferment, and oxidize. Green tea is produced by steaming the tea leaves, which inactivates enzymes and preserves the catechin content. Oolong tea is a partially fermented tea. White tea is the least processed of teas and consequently has even greater antioxidant activity than green tea. White tea is harvested before the leaves are fully opened and when the buds are still covered by fine white hair; the leaves are then picked and air-dried. White tea is widely available in the United States but is more expensive than other types of tea.

Studies of the health properties of tea have generally focused on green tea. Both green and white teas are rich in the flavonols known collectively as catechins. Catechins found in tea include epigallocatechin gallate (EGCG), epigallocatechin (EGC), epicatechin gallate (ECG), and epicatechin (EC). Green tea has been proposed to have anticarcinogenic properties as a result of the activity of EGCG. ECCG may protect against cancer by promoting selective apoptosis, suppressing angiogenesis, preventing oxidative damage to DNA, and enhancing the detoxification of carcinogens, including heterocyclic amines.[39]

Population studies suggest that green tea consumption does not decrease the risk of breast cancer. Most of these studies have been conducted in Asia; to date, few large-scale epidemiological studies or randomized controlled intervention trials have been carried out in Western populations. Ultimately, the protective effect of green tea may depend on the genotype of an individual. In a population-based, case-controlled study of Asian American women in Los Angeles, a significant inverse relationship was found to exist between tea consumption, breast cancer rate, and polymorphisms in the catechol-O-methyltransferase (*COMT*) gene.[40] Women with at least one low-activity *COMT* allele who drank tea had a significantly reduced risk of breast cancer (adjusted OR = 0.48) compared with non-tea drinkers. This benefit was observed in drinkers of both green and black teas. Breast cancer risk did not differ between tea and non-tea drinkers who were homozygous for the high-activity *COMT* allele. The *COMT* gene is involved in the methylation of catechins, and the researchers theorize that tea catechins consumed by women with the low-activity *COMT* allele were *O*-methylated and excreted less rapidly, thus conferring a greater cancer-protection benefit.

Phytoestrogens

Phytoestrogens are plant compounds that can bind to ERs. These substances act as SERMs, as they have both estrogenic and anti-estrogenic effects, depending on the expression of the ER subtype in the target cell and the amount of endogenous estrogen present. In premenopausal women, phytoestrogens appear to exert antiestrogenic effects; in postmenopausal women, they may exert estrogenic effects and minimize menopausal symptoms. These compounds may influence estrogen metabolism through several mechanisms: (1) by promoting C-2 hydroxylation over 16α hydroxylation; (2) by increasing SHBG levels, thereby reducing free estrogens; (3) by inhibiting aromatase activity; and (4) by binding to ERs.

The major types of phytoestrogens are isoflavones and lignans, which are discussed next.

Isoflavones

Isoflavones are found in soy, legumes, alfalfa, clover, licorice root, and kudzu root. Two isoflavones, genistein and daidzein, are found in soy, for example. The effects of genistein are well documented. The molecular structure of this compound is similar to that of estradiol-17β. Genistein binds to both ERα and ERβ, but it has a weaker transcriptional potency and, consequently, weaker estrogenic properties.

There has been much interest in—and controversy about—the role of soy in breast cancer risk. To date, the data on the beneficial or adverse effects of isoflavones and soy have been contradictory and inconclusive.[41] It is theorized that isoflavone intake during childhood and adolescence may decrease breast cancer risk by affecting cellular differentiation. Conversely, isoflavones given to women at the time of menopause may stimulate the proliferation of breast cells and, in theory, increase breast cancer risk.

More research is needed before recommending soy to women with ER-positive breast cancer, and supplementation with isoflavone preparations should be avoided. Preliminary evidence also suggests that genistein and daidzein can interfere with the efficacy of the drug tamoxifen.[42] Given this concern, women on tamoxifen should avoid consuming a diet high in soy or isoflavone supplements.

Lignans

Lignans are compounds found in fiber-rich foods including flaxseed, whole grains, legumes, and vegetables. Flaxseeds are the richest source of lignans (enterodiol and enterolactone) in the diet.

Lignans have been shown to modify estrogen metabolism, stimulate SHBG production in the liver, inhibit aromatase activity in adipose cells, and decrease cellular proliferation in breast cells. In a small, randomized, double-blind, placebo-controlled study of postmenopausal women, supplementation with 25 g of ground flaxseed/day (in the form of a muffin) resulted in increased excretion of the less biologically active estrogen metabolite 2-OHE1; the excretion of 16α-hydroxyestrone did not increase.[43]

In another study, 31 women with newly diagnosed breast cancer were randomized to daily intake of a muffin containing 25 g flaxseed or a control (placebo) muffin.[44] Their tumor tissue was analyzed for tumor cell proliferation and apoptosis both at the time of diagnosis and at the time of definitive surgery. In the intervention group, significantly reduced cell proliferation and increased apoptosis were observed compared to the control group at the time of definitive surgery.

Although these results are certainly interesting, more research is needed before flaxseed might be recommended to women who have breast cancer. In theory, flaxseed could interfere with the antiestrogenic effects of tamoxifen as a result of its phytoestrogen properties.

Allium Vegetables

The allium family of vegetables, which includes garlic, onions, and shallots, may have anticarcinogenic properties. Allium vegetables have high concentrations of organosulfur compounds, which may selectively inhibit or induce certain P-450 enzymes; they are also high in antioxidant activity due to their flavonoid content. To date, few data on their role in breast cancer risk have been collected. A recent Italian case-controlled study failed to find a protective role for garlic and onion consumption and breast cancer risk.[45]

Folate

Folate, in the polyglutamate form, occurs naturally in dark-green leafy vegetables, legumes, and fruits. Synthetic folic acid is available in supplements and fortified foods. Several mechanisms have been proposed for the role of folate inadequacy and carcinogenesis. Folate and vitamin B_{12} are coenzymes needed to regenerate methionine from homocysteine. Methionine in the form of S-adenosylmethione is the principal methyl donor for DNA methylation. Folate inadequacy, in theory, may lead to hypomethylation and, therefore, to gene mutation or altered gene expression. Inadequacy of folate may increase cancer risk by the misincorporation of uracil for thymine during DNA synthesis and by impaired DNA repair. Both of these processes can cause DNA strand breaks and chromosome damage.

Epidemiologic evidence supporting an inverse relationship between folate intake and breast cancer risk is inconclusive. In fact, some studies suggest that high folate intake may increase breast cancer risk. In the prospective, the randomized Prostate, Lung, Colorectal and Ovarian Cancer Screening Trial (PLCO), high folate intake due to supplementation was associated with an increased risk of breast cancer in postmenopausal women.[25] Women who consumed more than 400 mcg/day of supplemental folic acid had a 19% greater risk of postmenopausal breast cancer than women who did not take supplemental folic acid. Women in the highest quintile of total folate intake from food and supplements (> 853 mcg/day) had a 32% greater risk than women in the lowest quintile (≤ 335.5 mcg/day). Folate from food was not associated with increased risk.

As yet, researchers have not identified the mechanisms underlying the reported relationship between increased risk of breast cancer and high folate intake. A very high folate intake might potentially promote the growth of an existing cancer or cause epigenetic changes in gene-regulatory mechanisms, leading to gene silencing and cancer development. Ultimately, both deficiency and excess of folate may contribute to breast cancer carcinogenesis.

The combination of folate deficiency and alcohol use also appears to be positively associated with breast cancer risk. In the PLCO Trial women in the highest quintile in terms of alcohol consumption (> 7.62 g/day or approximately 0.5 serving/day) had a 37% greater risk than women in the lowest quintile of alcohol consumption (< 0.01 g/day).[25] The risk associated with alcohol consumption was highest in women with low total folate intake (< 335.5 mcg/day). Women in the lowest quintile of folate intake who consumed 0.5 drink per day had twice the risk of developing postmenopausal breast cancer compared to women in the lowest quintile of folate intake who consumed less than 0.01 g of alcohol per day.

Given this apparent linkage, folate adequacy should be ensured in women who consume alcohol. At the same time, more research is needed to elucidate fully the relationship between folic acid and breast cancer carcinogenesis.

Vitamin D and Calcium

Vitamin D is found in fatty fish such as salmon, sardines, mackerel, and tuna. Wild salmon is higher in vitamin D than farm-raised salmon. Vitamin D is also found in fortified foods such as milk, orange juice, and breakfast cereals. Multivitamins and some calcium supplements also contain vitamin D.

Two forms of supplemental vitamin D are available: vitamin D_3 (also known as cholecalciferol) and vitamin D_2 (also known as ergocalciferol). Cholecalciferol is manufactured through the ultraviolet irradiation of 7-dehydrocholesterol from lanolin; it is the preferred form of supplementation because it has more biological activity. Ergocalciferol is manufactured through the ultraviolet irradiation of ergosterol from yeast, and is less biologically active than cholecalciferol. Humans can produce vitamin D when the skin is exposed to ultraviolet radiation from the sun or from tanning booths.

An estimated 1 billion people worldwide are vitamin D insufficient or deficient. Obese individuals are particularly at risk for vitamin D deficiency. Because vitamin D from the diet or from sunlight is efficiently deposited in the body fat stores, it is not bioavailable. This process leads to low serum levels in obese persons.

The active form of vitamin D, 1,25-dihydroxyvitamin D, directly or indirectly controls more than 200 genes, including genes involved in the regulation of cellular proliferation, differentiation, apoptosis, and angiogenesis. Breast tissue expresses 25-hydroxyvitamin D-1α hydroxylase and produces 1,25-dihydroxyvitamin D locally to control genes that prevent cancer by regulating cellular proliferation and differentiation. It has been theorized that if a cell becomes malignant, 1,25-dihydroxyvitamin D can induce apoptosis and prevent angiogenesis, thereby decreasing the ability of the malignant cell to survive.

Prospective and retrospective studies suggest that serum levels of 25-hydoxyvitamin D less than 20 ng/mL are associated with a 30–50% increased risk of breast, colon, and prostate cancer and a greater risk of mortality.[46] The few intervention studies that have focused on calcium and/or vitamin D have shown a reduction in breast cancer in women who take these supplements. In a four-year, population-based, double-blind, randomized, placebo-controlled trial involving 1,179 women, risk of all cancers—including breast cancer—was reduced in the intervention group receiving 1,400–1,500 mg of calcium and 1,100 IU of vitamin D_3 per day and in the group receiving 1,400–1,500 mg of supplemental calcium per day.[47]

The optimal intake of vitamin D for cancer protection purposes is not known. The recommended daily intake of vitamin D developed by the Institute of Medicine is thought by most experts to be inadequate.[46] Most experts agree that without adequate sun exposure, children and adults require approximately 800–1,000 IU of vitamin D per day. Supplementation should be in the form of cholecalciferol. Assessment of vitamin D status using serum 25(OH) levels can be helpful in determining individual needs. Optimal vitamin D levels have not been established. Holick has defined vitamin D deficiency measured by 25(OH) vitamin D as less than 20 ng/mL, insufficiency as 21–29 ng/mL, sufficiency as more than 30 ng/mL, and toxicity as more than 150 ng/mL.[46] Other sources have proposed an optimal range of 40–65 ng/mL.[48]

Environmental Pollutants

A total of 216 chemicals have been identified in at least one animal study as increasing the incidence of mammary tumors.[49] These substances include industrial chemicals, chlorinated solvents, products of combustion, pesticides, dyes, radiation, drinking water disinfectant by-products, pharmaceuticals and hormones, natural products, and research chemicals. Of these chemicals, 73 are present in consumer products or as contaminants in food, 35 are air pollutants, 25 are associated with occupational exposure, and 29 are produced in the United States in large amounts. Laboratory research indicates that many environmental toxins cause mammary gland tumors in animals by mimicking estrogen or by increasing the susceptibility of the mammary gland to carcinogenesis.

The epidemiologic evidence that environmental pollutants play a role in human breast cancer risk is limited, although support for the relationship is building.[50] Meaningful evidence indicates that polycyclic aromatic hydrocarbons (PAHs) and polychlorinated biphenyls (PCBs) increase the risk of breast cancer in women with certain genetic polymorphisms including *GSTM1*. PAHs include products of combustion from air pollution, tobacco smoke, and cooked food and are prevalent in our environment. PCBs were used in the production of electrical equipment in the past, but were banned in the 1970s. The primary source of PCB exposure is through consumption of fish from rivers contaminated with the industrial pollutant. PCBs are found in high concentrations in breast milk, and they accumulate in fat. Although breast milk contains PCBs, the American Academy of Pediatrics remains a staunch advocate of breastfeeding infants because of the health, nutritional, immunological, developmental, psychological, social, economic, and environmental benefits associated with this practice.[51]

Additional epidemiologic research is needed on breast cancer risk and other chemicals that act as endocrine disruptors, including chlorinated solvents, diesel exhaust, dibutyl phthalate, ethylene oxide, perfluorooctanoic acid, and bisphenol A.

Nutrition Care During and After Cancer Treatment

Nutrition Assessment

Evaluation of nutritional status is important during and following treatment. Traditional nutrition assessment includes medical history, diet and weight history, laboratory data, and anthropometric measurements. The Mini Nutritional Assessment (MNA) and the Scored Patient-Generated Subjective Global Assessment (PG-SGA) are two tools that have been studied in the cancer population. Of these tools, the PG-SGA has been validated for use in cancer patients but is time-consuming and must be administered by a trained individual.[52] The MNA is a simple tool that can be managed by a nontrained person but is validated only for use in the elderly population.

In a study comparing the two tools in cancer patients, the MNA was found to have high sensitivity but low specificity: It adequately identified patients in need of nutrition intervention but also categorized patients as requiring nutrition intervention when it was not needed.[53] The PG-SGA appears to be more applicable in cancer patients than the MNA, but if staffing and resources are limited, its use may not be realistic. A modification of the MNA could be developed to increase its specificity in the cancer setting.

In clinical practice, many individuals with breast cancer who are treated on an outpatient basis may not require the use of any of these tools. Metastatic breast cancer is more likely to trigger the need for nutrition intervention. Lifestyle and nutrition issues related to survivorship, such as weight gain, exercise, vegetable and fruit intake, and prevention and treatment of the metabolic syndrome—all of which may influence the risk of recurrence—are common nutritional concerns in this population. For this reason, a system for identifying patients and providing education is important. Patients should be asked about the use of CAM, as there is potential for drug–supplement interactions. In one study, two-thirds of women who received traditional treatment for breast cancer also used one or more CAM therapies that they believed could prevent cancer recurrence and/or improve their quality of life.[54]

Nutritional Implications of Chemotherapy

Chemotherapy side effects affecting nutritional status include nausea and vomiting (N/V), mucositis, altered taste, xerostomia, dysphagia, myelosuppression, fatigue, and diarrhea. Symptoms can be decreased with pharmacologic interventions such as antiemetic, antidiarrheal, and hematopoietic agents, although many patients who are treated with "dose-intensive" regimens experience significant side effects. In premenopausal women treated with CT, infertility and early menopause causing hot flashes and night sweats may occur. These women are also at risk for osteoporosis due to early menopause. Chemotherapeutic agents commonly used to treat breast cancer (summarized in Table 8.1) include cyclophosphamide (Cytoxan®), docetaxel (Taxotere®), doxorubicin (Adriamycin®), epirubicin (Ellence®), 5-fluorouracil (5-FU), methotrexate, and paclitaxel (Taxol®).

Table 8.1   *Medications Commonly Used to Treat Breast Cancer*

Drug (Route of Administration)	*Mode of Action*	*Potential Side Effects/ Nutrition Implications*
Chemotherapeutic Agents		
Cyclophosphamide (Cytoxan®) (intravenous or oral)	• Alkylating agent • Interferes with RNA transcription, causing growth imbalance and cell death	↑ uric acid; ↓ platelets, hemoglobin, red blood cells, white blood cells; anorexia, nausea and vomiting, stomatitis, mucositis, abdominal pain, cardiotoxicity in high doses
Docetaxel (Taxotere®) (intravenous)	• Inhibits mitosis and leads to cell death	↑ alkaline phosphatase, alanine aminotransferase, aspartate aminotransferase, and bilirubin; ↓ hemoglobin, platelets, white blood cells; stomatitis, nausea and vomiting, diarrhea, myalgia, arthralgia, nail pigmentation
Doxorubicin (Andriamycin®) (intravenous)	• Interferes with DNA-dependent RNA synthesis	↑ uric acid; ↓ platelets and white blood cells; esophagitis common in patients who have also received radiation; nausea and vomiting, diarrhea, stomatitis, anorexia, cardiotoxicity
Epirubicin (Ellence®) (intravenous)	• Inhibits DNA, RNA, and protein synthesis	↓ hemoglobin, neutrophils, platelets, white blood cells; nausea and vomiting, diarrhea, anorexia, mucositis

(continues)

Table 8.1 *Medications Commonly Used to Treat Breast Cancer, Continued*

Drug (Route of Administration)	Mode of Action	Potential Side Effects/ Nutrition Implications
Chemotherapeutic Agents		
5-Fluorouracil (5-FU) (intravenous)	• Inhibits DNA and RNA synthesis	↑ alkaline phosphatase, alanine aminotransferase, aspartate aminotransferase, lactate dehydrogenase, bilirubin; ↓ hemoglobin, platelets, red blood cells, white blood cells, albumin; anorexia, nausea and vomiting, gastrointestinal ulceration; contraindicated in poor nutritional status or following major surgery within previous month
Methotrexate (intravenous)	• Antimetabolite • Reversibly binds to dihydrofolate reductase, blocking the reduction of folic acid to tetrahydrofolate, a cofactor necessary for purine, protein, and DNA synthesis	↑ uric acid; ↓ platelets, red blood cells, white blood cells; gingivitis, stomatitis, diarrhea, abdominal distress, anorexia, gastrointestinal ulceration and bleeding, enteritis, nausea and vomiting. • May alter results of laboratory assay for folate status. Folic acid derivatives antagonize methotrexate effects and should be avoided. • Alcohol may increase heptotoxicity.
Paclitaxel (Taxol®) (intravenous)	• Inhibits normal reorganization of microtubule network needed for mitosis and other vital cellular functions	↑ alkaline phosphatase, aspartate aminotransferase, triglycerides; ↓ neutrophils, white blood cells, hemoglobin, platelets; nausea and vomiting, diarrhea, mucositis peripheral neuropathy, myalgia, arthralgia
Targeted Biologic Therapy		
Bevacizumab (Avastin®) (intravenous)	• Recombinant humanized monoclonal IgG$_1$ antibody • Binds and inhibits the biological activity of vascular endothelial growth factor (VEGF) • Inhibits angiogenesis	↓ white blood cells; ↑ proteinuria; diarrhea, nausea and vomiting, anorexia, stomatitis, abdominal pain, wound healing complications, gastrointestinal perforations, congestive heart failure, hypertension

(continues)

Table 8.1   *Medications Commonly Used to Treat Breast Cancer, Continued*

Drug (Route of Administration)	Mode of Action	Potential Side Effects/ Nutrition Implications
Targeted Biologic Therapy		
Trastuzumb (Herceptin®) (intravenous)	• Recombinant DNA-derived monoclonal antibody that selectively binds to HER-2 • Inhibits proliferation of cells that overexpress HER-2	↓ hemoglobin, white blood cells; anorexia, abdominal pain, diarrhea, nausea and vomiting
Hormonal Therapy		
Anastrozole (Arimidex®) (oral)	• Aromatase inhibitor; aromatase is an enzyme that converts testosterone to estrogen in the peripheral tissue • Significantly decreases estrogen levels • For use in postmenopausal women with ER/PR-positive tumors	↑ liver enzymes, hot flashes, bone pain; ↑ risk of osteoporosis • Ensure adequate calcium and vitamin D for bone health and encourage weight-bearing exercise.
Exemextane (Aromasin®) (oral)	• Aromatase inhibitor • Mechanism and indication the same as for Arimidex®	↑ bilirubin, alkaline phosphatase, creatinine, hot flashes; ↑ risk of osteoporosis • Ensure adequate calcium and vitamin D for bone health and encourage weight-bearing exercise.
Letrozole (Femara®) (oral)	• Aromatase inhibitor • Mechanism and indication the same as for Arimidex®	↑ cholesterol, hot flashes; ↑risk for osteoporosis • Ensure adequate calcium and vitamin D for bone health and encourage weight-bearing exercise. • St. John's wort may decrease effectiveness of the medication.
Tamoxifen (Nolvadex®) (oral)	• Selective estrogen-receptor modulator (SERM) • For use in premenopausal women or women with DCIS or LCIS	↑ BUN, calcium, T_4, liver enzymes; ↑ white blood cells and platelets; ↑ risk of pulmonary embolism, thromboembolism, endometrial cancer, hot flashes • Ensure adequate calcium and vitamin D for bone health and encourage weight-bearing exercise.

Source: Nursing 2007 Drug Handbook. 27th ed. Philadelphia, PA: Lippincott Williams & Wilkins, 2007.

Weight Gain Associated with Chemotherapy and Hormonal Therapy

Patients who experience anorexia or N/V often lose weight and should be referred to a registered dietitian (RD). In contrast, weight gain during CT is common; the typical increase ranges from 2.5 to 6.2 kg, though greater gains are not uncommon. Weight gain also occurs in the first 6 months after completion of CT.

Harvie et al. studied the causes of weight gain in women receiving CT.[55] Women in the study gained significant amounts of weight (5 kg ± 3.8 kg) and body fat (7.1 kg ± 4.5 kg) over the year. Waist circumference increased by 5.1 cm ± 4.5 cm; abdominal skin-fold increased by 16.2 mm ± 10 mm; and fat-free mass decreased by 1.7 kg ± 2.5 kg. Resting energy expenditure (REE) declined by 3% during CT and remained depressed for at least 3 months after treatment. There was no significant change in dietary intake or physical activity over the year, and weight gain was attributed to a decline in REE combined with a failure to decrease caloric intake or increase physical activity.

In another study, sarcopenic obesity (weight gain with lean tissue loss or the absence of lean tissue gain) and decreased physical activity, but not overeating, were determined to be the causes of weight gain in premenopausal women receiving CT.[56] Resistance training, especially that focusing on the lower body, should be encouraged in women undergoing CT to prevent loss of lean body mass, which leads to a decrease in REE and subsequent weight gain. In the Women's Healthy Eating and Living (WHEL) study, all regimens of CT were associated with weight gain and only 10% of study participants returned to their initial weight.[57]

Although women commonly complain of weight gain when they are treated with tamoxifen, use of this hormonal therapy was not associated with weight gain in the WHEL study.[57] Previous studies have reported conflicting results about tamoxifen's role in weight gain. Studies reporting significant weight gains with tamoxifen were limited by short follow-up, small sample size, and lack of a control group.

Menopausal Vasomotor Symptoms

The most common complaints in women with ER-positive tumors are the result of early menopause due to CT-induced ovarian failure, surgical ovarian oblation, or treatment with antiestrogenic drugs including SERMs and AIs.[58] Most women experience hot flashes associated with these kinds of treatments. Although hot flashes can affect the quality of life in survivors, they may also be a strong predictor of breast cancer recurrence in women who are treated with tamoxifen.[59] Data from the WHEL study showed that women who reported hot flashes at baseline were less likely after 7.3 years to develop breast cancer recurrence than those who did not report hot flashes at baseline. Hot flashes were a stronger predictor of recurrence than age, hormone receptor status, or the stage of cancer at diagnosis (stage I versus stage II). Additional research is needed to clarify the relationship between hot flashes and recurrence.

Few studies have addressed the management of menopausal symptoms in breast cancer survivors.[60] HRT is contraindicated in breast cancer survivors, especially those with ER-positive tumors. The use of selective serotonin reuptake inhibitors (SSRIs), the selective serotonin and norepinephrine reuptake inhibitor (SSNRI) venlafaxine, and the anticonvulsant gabapentin has been shown to reduce hot flashes, but the long-term safety of these agents is unknown.[61]

Many women are interested in CAM approaches for the alleviation of their menopausal symptoms. The safety of phytoestrogens from soy, lignans, and supplements of red clover, licorice root, kudzu root, and soy isoflavones has not been established in breast cancer survivors, and it is prudent to advise women to avoid these supplements. Black cohosh (*Cimicifuga racemosa*) has been approved by the German E Commission for the nonprescription treatment of menopausal symptoms. Black cohosh has a relatively good safety profile but research supporting its use for the treatment of hot flashes in women with breast cancer is inconclusive.[62] This herb is not a phytoestrogen, and its mechanism of action is not clear.

The North American Menopause Society (NAMS), in its position paper on the management of hot flashes, suggests lifestyle-related strategies for dealing with mild menopausal symptoms, including keeping the core body temperature cool, using paced respiration, and exercising regularly.[63] NAMS found no benefit with the use of dong quai, evening primrose oil, ginseng, a Chinese herbal mixture, acupuncture, or magnet therapy. Hot flash "triggers" such as alcohol, hot drinks, or spicy foods are a problem for some, but not all, women.

Osteoporosis

Breast cancer survivors are at risk for osteoporosis and fractures because of low estrogen levels caused by early menopause as a result of CT or oophorectomy in premenopausal women or the use of AIs in postmenopausal women.[64] Tamoxifen has been shown to preserve bone mineral density (BMD) in the spine and hip in postmenopausal women, although the extent of the protection is not clear—few studies have directly investigated the net BMD increase.[65] Likewise, few studies have focused on the purported link between tamoxifen and a decreased risk of bone fractures.

Recommendations for preventing and treating bone loss in breast cancer survivors are similar to those for women without breast cancer. Women are advised to undergo an initial dual-energy x-ray absorptiometry (DEXA) bone scan and then an annual or biennial DEXA to assess BMD.

Recommendations have also been made regarding the use of calcium, vitamin D, and exercise to ward off bone loss. In 2006, for example, NAMS issued a position paper supporting the role of calcium and vitamin D in reducing fractures. It recommends 1,200 mg of calcium per day from food and supplements and adequate vitamin D, defined as a serum level of 25 (OH)D of 30 ng/mL (or higher).[66] In clinical practice, supplementation with 800–1,000 IU of vitamin D_3 is typically needed to obtain a level of 30 ng/mL (or more) of 25(OH)D, but some women may need even larger amounts. Women should be advised to engage in regular weight-bearing and muscle-strengthening exercise to prevent and bone loss and to prevent falls. The use of bisphosphonates in combination with AIs may minimize bone loss.[67]

Cardiovascular Disease

The risk of cardiovascular disease (CVD) depends on the type of adjuvant systemic therapy received. Radiation to the left chest wall is associated with an increase in the long-term risk of cardiovascular events. Early menopause also increases the long-term risk of CVD because it results in the loss of the protective effects of estrogen. Some concerns have been raised that the reduction of estrogen associated with use of AIs may also increase CVD risk, but studies to date have been inconclusive. For all these reasons, women should follow the standard guidelines for reducing CVD risk, such as maintaining a healthy weight, avoiding smoking, exercising regularly, and controlling blood pressure, blood sugar, and lipids.

Congestive heart failure can result from CT consisting of anthracyclines or tratuzumab. Tamoxifen increases the risk of deep venous thrombosis and cerebrovascular disease.

Preventing Recurrence

In the United States, the number of breast cancer survivors is estimated to exceed 2 million. Many of these survivors are interested in nutrition and lifestyle interventions beyond conventional treatment to improve their prognosis. Although hundreds of studies have focused on the potential links between diet and etiology of breast cancer, only a few studies to date have addressed diet and survival.[68] The Women's Intervention Nutrition Study (WINS) and the WHEL study are two randomized trials that focused on lifestyle intervention, including diet and exercise (Table 8.2).[69, 70] Both WINS

Table 8.2   *Summary of Intervention Trials on Preventing Breast Cancer Recurrence*

Name of Study/ Year Published/ Country	Size of Cohort/ Years of Follow-up	Findings
Women's Healthy Eating and Living (WHEL), 2007, United States[71]	• 1,490 women with early-stage breast cancer • Mean 6.7 years of follow-up	A combination of consuming five or more servings of vegetables/fruit and accumulating the equivalent of walking 30 minutes 6 days per week was associated with a significant survival advantage (HR = 56). Benefits were observed in both obese and non-obese women.
Women's Intervention Nutrition Study (WINS), 2006, United States[72]	• 2,437 women with early-stage breast cancer • 5 years	Reducing dietary fat to 15–20% of calories was associated with a longer relapse-free survival in women with ER-negative/PR-negative cancers. No benefit was seen in ER-positive/PR positive cancers.

and WHEL enrolled women who had completed primary conventional cancer treatment. In addition to these two studies, at least five ongoing prospective cohort studies are addressing diet and breast cancer survival in women who have undergone conventional therapy and are in remission.

Weight and Risk of Recurrence and Mortality

Weight and elevated body mass index (BMI) have been associated with a poorer prognosis, but more recent data on this subject are mixed. In the Nurses' Health Study, 5,204 participants who were diagnosed with invasive, nonmetastatic breast cancer between 1976 and 2000 were followed for a median of 9 years.[73] High body weight prior to diagnosis was associated with poorer survival. Participants who gained 6 pounds after diagnosis had a RR of death from breast cancer of 1.35; those who gained 17 pounds had a RR of 1.64. Similar findings were seen for breast cancer recurrence and mortality from all causes.

Abrahamson et al., in a large population-based follow-up study, found that breast cancer survival is reduced among younger women aged 20–54 with general or abdominal obesity.[74] Young women who had a BMI of 30 or more or a waist-to-hip ratio (WHR) of 0.80 or more near the time of their diagnosis of breast cancer also had increased mortality. In contrast to these findings, more recent data from the WHEL study revealed that combined healthy lifestyle behaviors, consisting of five servings of vegetables and fruit per day and the equivalent of walking 30 minutes at a moderate pace 6 days per week, was associated with a 50% reduction in mortality rates in both obese and non-obese women with early-stage breast cancer.[70]

The means by which overweight influences survival include increased endogenous production of estrogen by adipose tissue, decreased levels of SHBG, diagnosis at a later stage, larger tumor size at diagnosis, increased insulin and insulin-like growth factors, and poorer response to treatment. Obesity is also associated with reduced immune function, which could indirectly promote recurrence. Elevated WHR is associated with hyperinsulinemia and insulin resistance independent of BMI and may be a contributing factor in mortality. A higher BMI may also be related to increased mortality as a result of incorrect dosing of CT, incomplete removal of the primary tumor, or difficulty in detecting recurrences in large women.

Low-Fat, High-Fiber, High-Vegetable and -Fruit Diet

A low-fat, high-fiber, high-vegetable and -fruit diet does not appear to reduce mortality or recurrence in breast cancer survivors. In the WHEL trial, a diet including 5 vegetable servings plus 16 ounces of vegetable juice, 3 fruit servings, 30 grams of fiber, and 15–20% of calories from fat did not reduce mortality from breast cancer, mortality from any cause, or the combined outcome of invasive breast cancer recurrence or new primary breast cancer during the 7.3-year follow-up period in women with early-stage breast cancer (stage I, stage II, or stage IIIa).[69] Women in the control group consumed 5 servings of vegetables and fruit per day, so it is possible that eating more than 5 servings of vegetables and fruit per day does not confer additional benefit. These results were surprising, as a high-fiber, low-fat diet intervention has been demonstrated to decrease serum bioavailable estradiol levels in women with a history of breast cancer.[70]

Dietary Fat and ER-Negative/PR-Negative Breast Cancer Recurrence

Dietary fat intake may influence the recurrence or the diagnosis of a new breast cancer in women with early-stage breast cancer, according to interim analyses from the Women's Intervention Nutrition Study (WINS).[72] WINS, a randomized, prospective, multicenter trial involving more 2,400 participants, showed that a reduction in dietary fat to 15–20% of total calories was marginally associated with longer relapse-free survival. The benefit was mainly seen in women with ER-negative/PR-negative cancers. Reduced body weight in the intervention group might be responsible for the improvement in relapse-free survival. Although additional research is needed to confirm the relationship between dietary fat and relapse, women with ER-negative/PR-negative breast cancers should be advised to reduce their dietary fat intake to 20% of calories. The expertise of a registered dietitian should be utilized to help women achieve this goal.

Combined Healthy Lifestyle Behaviors

Healthy lifestyle behaviors, when combined, have been demonstrated to have a beneficial effect on mortality in breast cancer survivors. Combined healthy lifestyle behaviors, consisting of 5 servings of vegetables and fruit per day, and the equivalent of walking 30 minutes at a moderate pace 6 days per week, were associated with a 50% reduction in mortality rates in a prospective study of 1,490 women diagnosed with early-stage breast cancer. The women in this study had completed primary therapy, although the majority of them were still taking tamoxifen.[71] Women who were physically active and consumed 5 servings of vegetables and fruit per day had an estimated 10-year mortality rate of 7%, or approximately half of the rate in women with lower levels of physical activity and lower vegetable and fruit consumption. The effect was seen in both obese and non-obese women; it was stronger in women with ER-positive or PR-positive cancers.

Green Tea

Epidemiologic research in Japan suggests that Asian women who have been treated for stage I or stage II breast cancer and who drink 3–5 cups of green tea per day reduce their risk of recurrence compared to women who drink 0–2 cups of green tea per day (HR stage I = 0.37; HR stage II = 0.80).[75] No benefit was found for stage III and IV breast cancer. This study suggests regular green tea consumption may protect against recurrence of breast cancer when patients are diagnosed with and treated for early-stage cancer, though the results need to be confirmed with randomized trials. Nevertheless, women with early-stage breast cancer may want to consider drinking 3–5 cups of green tea per day, as there are no known harmful effects and some potential benefit.

Vitamin D

Low vitamin D levels at the time of diagnosis may be associated with a poor prognosis. In a prospective study involving 512 women with newly diagnosed breast cancer, vitamin D deficiency at the time of breast cancer diagnosis was associated with an increased risk of distant recurrence and death.[76]

Vitamin D levels were deficient (< 50 nmol/L or <20 ng/mL) in 37.5% of these patients, insufficient (50–72 nmol/L or 20–28.8 ng/mL) in 38.5%, and adequate (> 72 nmol/L or 28.8 ng/mL) in 24%. Low vitamin D levels were associated with premenopausal status, high BMI, high insulin levels, high tumor grade, and low dietary intake of retinol, vitamin E, grains, and alcohol. Distant disease-free survival (DDFS) was significantly worse in women with deficient (versus adequate) vitamin D levels (HR = 1.94), as was overall survival (HR = 1.73). There was no survival difference between women with insufficient versus adequate vitamin D levels. Associations with DDFS were independent of age, BMI, insulin, tumor stage and nodal status (T and N in the TNM system), ER status (positive or negative), and tumor grade. The data suggested a small but not statistically significant increased risk of metastasis with high levels of vitamin D.

Epidemiological studies suggest that the season in which diagnosis is made may also affect survival. Diagnosis of breast cancer in the summer is associated with greater survival than diagnosis in the winter. Women of all ages in Norway who were diagnosed in the summer had 25% better survival after standard treatment compared with women who were diagnosed in the winter.[77] Women younger than age 50 had 40% better survival if they were diagnosed in the summer versus the winter. Although no conclusions about the biological mechanism could be made based on this epidemiological study, the authors theorized that women diagnosed in the summer had higher circulating vitamin D levels, which may have modulated cell signaling, induced apoptosis, regulated cell-cycle progression, and reduced angiogenic activity and invasiveness. Similar findings have been reported in the United Kingdom.[78]

Women with a history of breast cancer should have their serum 25(OH) levels measured. Additional research identifying the optimal serum level to prevent recurrence is needed, but the study results suggest that women should take enough vitamin D to maintain an adequate serum level.

Cruciferous Vegetables

A clinical trial seeking to determine whether cruciferous vegetables are protective against breast cancer recurrence is now under way.[79] In the meantime, it is reasonable to encourage women to increase consumption of cruciferous vegetables because of these foods' proposed anticarcinogenic properties and ability to modulate estrogen metabolites. Currently, there is no evidence to support the use of supplements of I3C, the component of cruciferous vegetables thought to modulate estrogen levels.

Table 8.3 provides a summary of the recommendations for prevention of recurrence for breast cancer survivors.

Table 8.3   *Nutrition Recommendations for Breast Cancer Survivors*

1. Engage in the equivalent of brisk walking 6 days per week for ½ hour per session. Eat 5 servings of vegetables and fruits per day. Select colorful vegetables that are yellow, orange, and deep green. Increase consumption of broccoli, cabbage, cauliflower, and other cruciferous vegetables, which should be either uncooked or lightly steamed to ensure maximum benefit.

2. Maintain a healthy weight. Avoid sweetened beverages such as soda, lemonade, and sports drinks. Consume energy-dense foods sparingly. Avoid fast foods.

3. Limit red meat to 3 servings per week or less, and avoid processed meats. If processed meat (including turkey breast) is consumed, select brands that are nitrate- and preservative-free. These foods can be found in many health food supermarkets.

4. Avoid charbroiled and overcooked foods (burnt or charred), including beef, chicken, lamb, pork, or fish. Cook these foods at a temperature below 325° F—the surface temperature at which heterocyclic amines (HCAs) form—whether grilling, pan-frying, or oven-roasting the foods. When grilling, marinating the meat prior to cooking can reduce the formation of HCAs. Avoid cooking over a direct flame, as fat or marinade drippings can cause flare-ups that deposit HCAs and other carcinogens on the surface of food. Flip food once a minute. Microwaving the meat for 1–2 minutes at a medium setting prior to grilling can inhibit HCAs formation. Use other methods of food preparation such as stewing, poaching, or slow-cooking in a Crock-Pot.

5. Aim for 1,400–1,500 mg of calcium per day and 1,100 IU of vitamin D_3 as cholecalciferol. Measure serum 25(OH) vitamin D levels to determine vitamin D sufficiency. Low levels of vitamin D are associated with increased risk of recurrence and death. Increase vitamin D supplementation as necessary to achieve a sufficient serum level of vitamin D, currently thought to be 30 ng/mL or more. Optimal serum ranges of vitamin D for the prevention of breast cancer recurrence are not known.

6. Drink 3–5 cups of green tea per day.

7. Avoid alcoholic drinks. Even small amounts of alcohol increase breast cancer risk, regardless of the type of alcohol. Women who drink alcohol should take a multivitamin supplement with the RDA for folic acid.

8. For ER-negative/PR-negative breast cancer, dietary fat should be decreased to 15–20% of total daily calories. Recommend consultation with a registered dietitian to achieve this goal.

9. Breast cancer survivors should receive nutritional care from a registered dietitian for diet and supplement advice. A registered dietitian can help with weight management and the prevention and treatment of the metabolic syndrome. In general, a multivitamin supplement should not provide more than the RDA for nutrients, with the exception of vitamin D. Calcium supplementation is often necessary to meet the recommendations for this nutrient. Nutrients and phytochemicals should come from food, not from supplements. Excess amounts of some nutrients, such as folic acid, may increase breast cancer risk in some individuals.

(continues)

Table 8.3 *Nutrition Recommendations for Breast Cancer Survivors, Continued*

10. Women with ER-positive/PR-positive breast cancers who experience hot flashes due to endocrine therapy or early menopause should avoid taking supplements containing phytoestrogens from soy or lignans, or supplements of red clover, licorice root, kudzu root, or soy isoflavones. The safety of these supplements has not been established for the management of hot flashes in breast cancer survivors. Diets high in soy from food should also be avoided. Black cohosh, which is not a phytoestrogen, has a relatively good safety profile, but research supporting its use for the treatment hot flashes in women with breast cancer is inconclusive. No benefit has been found for dong quai, evening primrose oil, or ginseng. Lifestyle strategies such as keeping the core body temperature cool, using paced respiration, and exercising regularly may help for managing mild hot flashes. Spicy foods, hot drinks, or alcohol may be hot flash triggers in some women.

Future Directions for Research

Nutrition's part in the etiology, treatment, prevention, and recurrence of breast cancer continues to unfold. Although strong evidence is lacking about the relationship between diet and breast cancer, women should continue to embrace healthy eating and lifestyle behaviors for their potential overall health benefits. Additional research is needed about the role of diet during fetal development, infancy, childhood, and adolescence as part of the etiology of breast cancer. Diet during these periods of development may be an important predictor of breast cancer risk, but as yet data are lacking in this area. Areas for additional exploration include how diet influences subgroups of women characterized by certain tumor subtypes and genetic, epigenic, or hormonal status. Similarly, research is needed on breast cancer risk and chemicals that act as endocrine disruptors. Additionally, studies addressing survivorship and diet are essential, especially those geared toward finding the optimal levels of vitamin D to prevent recurrence.

REFERENCES

1. American Cancer Society. *Cancer Facts and Figures 2008*. Atlanta, GA: American Cancer Society; 2008.
2. Nguyen PL, Taghian AG, Katz MS, et al. Breast cancer subtype approximated by estrogen receptor, progesterone receptor, and HER-2 is associated with local and distant recurrence after breast-conserving therapy. *J Clin Oncol*. 2008;26:2373–2378.
3. Yager JD, Davidson NE. Estrogen carcinogenesis in breast cancer. *N Engl J Med*. 2006;354:270–282.
4. Armstrong K, Eisen A, Weber B. Assessing the risk of breast cancer. *N Engl J Med*. 2000; 342:564–571.

5. Estimating breast cancer risk: Questions and answers. National Cancer Institute website. http://www.cancer.gov/cancertopics/factsheet/estimating-breast-cancerrisk. Accessed November 11, 2007.

6. Barlow WE, White E, Ballard-Barbash R, et al. Prospective breast cancer risk prediction model for women undergoing screening mammography. *J Natl Cancer Inst.* 2006;98:1204–1214.

7. Modan B, Chetrit A, Alfandary E, Katz L. Increased risk of breast cancer after low-dose radiation. *Lancet.* 1989;333:629–631.

8. Smith RA, Saslow D, Sawyer KA, et al. American Cancer Society guidelines for breast cancer screening: Update 2003. *CA Cancer J Clin.* 2003;54:141–169.

9. Saslow D, Boetes C, Burke W, et al. American Cancer Society guidelines for breast screening with MRI as an adjunct to mammography. *CA Cancer J Clin.* 2007; 57:75–89.

10. National Comprehensive Cancer Network. Clinical practice guidelines in oncology: Breast cancer. V.2. 2007. http://www.nccn.org/professionals/physician_gls/PDF/breast.pdf. Accessed December 5, 2007.

11. Brenton JD, Carey LA, Ahmed AA, Caldas C. Molecular classification and molecular forecasting of breast cancer: Ready for clinical application? *J Clin Oncol.* 2005;23:7350–7360.

12. Harris EE, Correa C, Hwang WT, et al. Late cardiac mortality and morbidity in early stage breast cancer patients after breast-conservation treatment. *J Clin Oncol.* 2006;24:4100–4106.

13. Smedira H. Practical issues in counseling healthy women about their breast cancer risk and use of tamoxifen citrate. *Arch Intern Med.* 2000;160:3034–3042.

14. FDA approves new uses for Evista. US Food and Drug Administration website. http://fda.gov/bbs/topics/NEWS/2007/NEW01698.html. Accessed December 5, 2007.

15. Bundred NJ. The effects of aromatase inhibitors on lipids and thrombosis. *Br J Cancer.* 2005;93:S23–S27.

16. Mouridsen H, Keshaviah A, Coates AS, et al. Cardiovascular adverse events during adjuvant endocrine therapy for early breast cancer using letrozole or tamoxifen: Safety analysis of BIG 1-98 trial. *J Clin Oncol.* 2007;25:5715–5722.

17. World Cancer Research Fund/American Institute for Cancer Research. *Food, Nutrition, Physical Activity, and the Prevention of Cancer: A Global Perspective.* Washington DC: AICR; 2007.

18. Michels KB, Mohllajee AP, Roset-Bahmanyar E, et al. Diet and breast cancer: A review of the prospective observational studies. *Cancer.* 2007;109(12)(suppl): 2712S–2749S.

19. Collaborative Group on Hormonal Factors in Breast Cancer. Breast cancer and breastfeeding: Collaborative reanalysis of individual data from 47 epidemiological studies in 30 countries, including 50302 women with breast cancer and 96973 women without the disease. *Lancet.* 2002;360:187–195.

20. Hilakivi-Clarke L, Cho E, deAssis S, et al. Maternal and prepubertal diet, mammary development and breast cancer risk. *J Nutr.* 2001;131:154S–157S.

21. Eliassen AH, Colditz GA, Rosner B, Willett WC, Hankinson SE. Adult weight change and risk of postmenopausal breast cancer. *JAMA.* 2006;296:193–201.

22. Smith-Warner SA, Spiegelman D, Yaun SS, et al. Alcohol and breast cancer in women: A pooled analysis of cohort studies. *JAMA.* 1998;279:535–540.

23. Hamajima N, Hirose K, Tajima K, et al. Alcohol, tobacco and breast cancer—collaborative reanalysis of individual data from 53 epidemiological studies including

58,515 women with breast cancer and 95,067 women without the disease. *Br J Cancer.* 2002;87:1234–1245.

24. Suzuki R, Ye W, Rylander-Rudqvist T, et al. Alcohol and postmenopausal breast cancer risk defined by estrogen and progesterone receptor status: A prospective cohort study. *J Natl Cancer Inst.* 2005;97:1601–1608.

25. Stolzenberg-Solomon R, Chang SC, Leitzmann M, et al. Folate intake, alcohol use, and postmenopausal breast cancer risk in the Prostate, Lung, Colorectal, and Ovarian Cancer Screening. *Am J Clin Nutr.* 2006;83:895–904.

26. Thiébaut AC, Kipnis V, Chang SC, et al. Dietary fat and postmenopausal invasive breast cancer in the National Institutes of Health–AARP Diet and Health Study cohort. *J Natl Cancer Inst.* 2007;99:451–462.

27. Prentice RL, Caan B, Chlebowski RT, et al. Low-fat dietary pattern and the risk of invasive breast cancer: The Women's Health Initiative randomized controlled dietary modification trial. *JAMA.* 2006;295:629–642.

28. Cho E, Chen WY, Hunter DJ, et al. Red meat intake and risk of breast cancer among premenopausal women. *Arch Intern Med.* 2006;166:2253–2259.

29. Taylor E, Burley V, Greenwood D. Meat consumption and risk of breast cancer in the UK Women's Cohort Study. *Br J Cancer.* 2007;96:1139–1146.

30. van der Hel OL, Peeters PH, Hein DW, et al. *GSTM1* null genotype, red meat consumption and breast cancer risk. *Cancer Causes Control.* 2004;3:295–303.

31. Key T, Fraser G, Thorogood P, et al. Mortality in vegetarians and nonvegetarians: Detailed findings from a collaborative analysis of 5 prospective studies. *Am J Clin Nutr.* 1999;70(suppl):516S–524S.

32. Willet W. Lessons from dietary studies in Adventists and questions for the future. *Am J Clin Nutr.* 2003;78(suppl):539S–543S.

33. Kushi, P. What is macrobiotics? Kushi Institute website. http://www.kushi institute.org/html/what_is_macro.html. Accessed December 10, 2007.

34. Higdon JV, Delage B, Williams DE, et al. Cruciferous vegetables and human cancer risk: Epidemiologic evidence and mechanistic basis. *Pharmacol Res.* 2007;55: 224–236.

35. Lampe J, Peterson S. Brassica biotransformation and cancer risk: Genetic polymorphisms alter the preventive effects of cruciferous vegetables. *J Nutr.* 2002;132: 2991–2994.

36. Fowke JH, Longcope C, Herbert JR. Brassica vegetable consumption shifts estrogen metabolism in healthy postmenopausal women. *Cancer Epidemiol Biomarkers Prev.* 2000;9:773–779.

37. Indole-3-carbinol in preventing breast cancer in nonsmoking women who are at high risk for breast cancer. National Institutes of Health website. http://www.clinical trials.gov/ct2/show/record/NCT00033345. Accessed December 16, 2007.

38. Fink B, Steck S, Wolff M, et al. Dietary flavonoid intake and breast cancer risk among women on Long Island. *Am J Epidemiol.* 2006;165:514–523.

39. Carlson JR, Bauer B, Vincent A, et al. Reading the tea leaves: Anticarcinogenic properties of (–)-epigallocatechin-3-gallate. *Mayo Clin Proc.* 2007;82:725–732.

40. Wu A, Tseng CC, van den Berg D, et al. Tea intake, *COMT* genotype, and breast cancer in Asian-American women. *Cancer Res.* 2003;63:7526–7529.

41. Wuttke W, Hubertus J, Seidlova-Wuttke D. Isoflavones: Safe food additives or dangerous drugs? *Ageing Res Rev.* 2007;6:150–188.

42. Messina M, Loprinzi C. Soy for breast cancer survivors: A critical review of the literature. *J Nutr.* 2001;131:3095S–3108S.

43. Brooks J, Ward W, Lewis J, et al. Supplementation with flaxseed alters estrogen metabolism in postmenopausal women to a greater extent than does supplementation with an equal amount of soy. *Am J Clin Nutr.* 2004;79:318–325.
44. Thompson L, Chen J, Li T, et al. Dietary flaxseed alters tumor biological markers in postmenopausal breast cancer. *Clin Cancer Res.* 2005;11:3828–3835.
45. Galeone C, Pelucchi C, Levi F, et al. Onion and garlic use and human cancer. *Am J Clin Nutr.* 2006;84:1027–1032.
46. Holick M. Vitamin D deficiency. *N Engl J Med.* 2007;357:266–281.
47. Lappe J, Travers-Gustafson, Davies K, et al. Vitamin D and calcium supplementation reduces cancer risk: Results of a randomized trial. *Am J Clin Nutr.* 2007;85: 1586–1591.
48. Vasquez A, Manso G, Cannell J. The clinical importance of vitamin D (cholecalciferol): A paradigm shift with implications for all healthcare providers. *Altern Ther.* 2004;10:28–36.
49. Rudel R, Attfield K, Schifano J, et al. Chemicals causing mammary gland tumors in animals signal new directions for epidemiology, chemicals testing, and risk assessment for breast cancer prevention. *Cancer.* 2007;109(12)(suppl):2635S–2666S.
50. Brody J, Moysich K, Humblet O, et al. Environmental pollutants and breast cancer: Epidemiologic studies. *Cancer.* 2007;109(12)(suppl):2667S–2711S.
51. Gartner LM, Morton J, Lawrence RA, et al. Breast feeding and the use of human milk. *Pediatrics.* 2005;115:496–506.
52. Bauer J, Capra S, Ferguson M. Use of the scored Patient-Generated Subjective Global Assessment (PG-SGA) as a nutrition assessment tool in patients with cancer. *Eur J Clin Nutr.* 2002;56:779–785.
53. Read JA, Crockett N, Volker DH, et al. Nutritional assessment in cancer: Comparing the Mini-Nutritional Assessment (MNA) with the Scored Patient-Generated Subjective Global Assessment (PGSGA). *Nutrition and Cancer.* 2005;53:51–56.
54. Henderson J, Donatelle R. Complementary and alternative medicine use by women after completion of allopathic treatment for breast cancer. *Altern Ther Health Med.* 2004;10:52–57.
55. Harvie M, Campbell I, Baildam A, et al. Energy balance in early breast cancer patients receiving adjuvant chemotherapy. *Breast Cancer Res Treat.* 2004;83: 201–210.
56. Denmark-Wahnefried W, Peterson B, Winer E, et al. Changes in weight, body composition, and factors influencing energy balance among premenopausal breast cancer patients receiving adjuvant chemotherapy. *J Clin Oncol.* 2001;19:2381–2389.
57. Saquib N, Flatt S, Natarajan L, et al. Weight gain and recovery of pre-cancer weight after breast cancer treatments: Evidence from the Women's Healthy Eating and Living (WHEL) study. *Breast Cancer Res Treat.* 2007;105:177–186.
58. Hayes, D. Follow-up of patients with early breast cancer. *N Engl J Med.* 2007;356: 2505–2513.
59. Mortimer J, Flatt S, Parker BA, et al. Tamoxifen, hot flashes and recurrence in breast cancer. *Breast Cancer Res Treat.* 2008;108:421–426.
60. Antoine C, Liebens B, Carly B, et al. Safety of alternative treatments for menopausal symptoms after breast cancer: A qualitative systematic review. *Climacteric.* 2007; 10:23–26.
61. Management of menopausal symptoms in patients with breast cancer: An evidence-based approach. *Lancet.* 2005;6:687–695. http://www.oncology.thelancet.com. Accessed December 23, 2007.

62. Walji R, Boon H, Guns E, et al. Black cohosh (*Cimicifuga racemosa* [L.]Nutt.): Safety and efficacy for cancer patients. *Support Cancer Care*. 2007;15(8):913–921.
63. Treatment of menopause-associated vasomotor symptoms: Position statement of the North American Menopause Society. *Menopause*. 2004;11:11–33.
64. Winer E, Hudis C, Burstein HG, et al. American Society of Clinical Oncology technology assessment on the use of aromatase inhibitors for early breast cancer for postmenopausal women with hormone receptor-positive breast cancer: Status report. *J Clin Oncol*. 2005;23:619–629.
65. Ding H, Field T. Bone health in postmenopausal women with early breast cancer: How protective is tamoxifen? *Cancer Treat Rev*. 2007;33:506–513.
66. North American Menopause Society. The role of calcium in peri- and post-menopausal women: Position statement of the North American Menopause Society. *Menopause*. 2006;13:859–861.
67. Berry, J. Are all aromatase inhibitors the same? A review of controlled clinical trials in breast cancer. *Clin Ther*. 2005;27:1671–1684.
68. Kushi L, Kwan M, Lee M, et al. Lifestyle factors and survival in women with breast cancer. *J Nutr*. 2007;137:236S–242S.
69. Pierce J, Natarajan L, Caan B, et al. Influence of a diet very high in vegetables, fruit, and fiber and low in fat on prognosis following treatment for breast cancer. The Women's Healthy Eating and Living (WHEL) randomized trial. *JAMA*. 2007; 298:289–298.
70. Rock CL, Flatt SW, Thomson CA, et al. Effects of a high-fiber, low-fat diet intervention on serum concentrations of reproductive steroid hormones in women with a history of breast cancer. *J Clin Oncol*. 2004;22:2379–2387.
71. Pierce J, Stefanick M, Flatt S, et al. Greater survival after breast cancer in physically active women with high vegetable–fruit intake regardless of obesity. *J Clin Oncol*. 2007;25:2345–2351.
72. Chlebowski R, Blackburn G, Thomson C, et al. Dietary fat reduction and breast cancer outcome: Interim efficacy results from the Women's Intervention Nutrition Study. *J Natl Cancer Inst*. 2006;98:1767–1776.
73. Kroenke C, Chen W, Rosner B, et al. Weight, weight gain, and survival after breast cancer diagnosis. *J Clin Oncol*. 2005;23:1370–1378.
74. Abrahamson P, Gammon M, Lund M, et al. General and abdominal obesity and survival among young women with breast cancer. *Cancer Epidemiol Biomarkers Prev*. 2006;15:1871–1877.
75. Inoue M, Tajima K, Mitzutani M, et al. Regular consumption of green tea and the risk of breast cancer recurrence: Follow-up study from the Hospital-based Epidemiologic Research Program at Aichi Cancer Center (HERPACC), Japan. *Cancer Letters*. 2001;167:175–182.
76. Goodwin PJ, Ennis M, Pritchard I, et al. Frequency of vitamin D deficiency at breast cancer diagnosis and association with risk of distant recurrence and death in a prospective cohort study of T1-3, NO-0, MO BC. *J Clin Oncol*. 2008;26(May 20 suppl; abstr 511).
77. Porojnicu A, Lagunova Z, Robsahm T, et al. Changes in risk of death from breast cancer with season and latitude. *Breast Cancer Res Treat*. 2007;102:323–328.
78. Lim, HS, Roychoudhuri R, Peto J, et al. Cancer survival is dependent on season of diagnosis and sunlight exposure. *Int J Cancer*. 2006;119:1530–1506.
79. Thomson CA, Rock CL, Caan BJ, et al. Increase in cruciferous vegetables intake in women previously treated for breast cancer participating in a dietary intervention trial. *Nutr Cancer*. 2007;57:11–19.

Chapter 9

Reproductive Cancers

Heather Hendrikson, RD, CSP, LD

INTRODUCTION

Cancers of the female reproductive system include ovarian, endometrial, cervical, uterine sarcoma, vaginal, and vulvar types. Uterine cancer is the most common female reproductive cancer (RC) in the United States.[1] Ovarian cancer is the second most common gynecologic cancer and the leading cause of death from reproductive malignancies.[1-3] Table 9.1 presents the projected new cases and deaths from RC in 2008 in the United States.

The largest body of evidence in nutrition therapy and RC relates to patients with ovarian cancer, especially advanced stages that can lead to bowel obstruction. Most RC, including ovarian, endometrial, cervical, uterine, and vaginal types, can lead to abdominal bowel obstruction and fluid accumulation as a result of tumor advancement. The management of bowel obstruction is usually similar regardless of the underlying type of gynecologic cancer.

Table 9.1 *Estimated New Reproductive Cancer Cases and Deaths in the United States, 2008*

Type of Reproductive Cancer	New Cases	Deaths
Uterus	40,100	7,470
Ovary	21,650	15,520
Cervix	11,070	3,870
Vulva	3,460	870
Vagina	2,210	760

Source: American Cancer Society, *Cancer Facts and Figures 2008.*

Prevention

Ovarian Cancer

One of the risk factors for ovarian cancer is age: Approximately half of these cancers are diagnosed in women who are older than 63 years of age. Obesity appears to increase the risk of ovarian cancer, and the rate of death is 50% higher in obese women. Other risk factors include estrogen replacement therapy or hormone replacement therapy; a family history of ovarian, breast, or colorectal cancer; and a personal history of breast cancer.[1]

Limited evidence suggests that a diet characterized by non-starchy vegetables, moderate alcohol consumption, and low fat, when followed for at least four years, lowers the risk for ovarian cancer. Birth control pills used for greater than five years, bearing children, and lactation protect against ovarian cancer, as do late menarche, early menopause, and tubal ligation or hysterectomy. More compelling evidence shows the factors leading to, or the consequences of, greater adult-attained height are a probable cause of ovarian cancer. Adult-attained height is a marker for genetic, environmental, hormonal, and nutritional factors affecting growth during the period from preconception to completion of linear growth. Adult height increases as populations become less vulnerable to undernutrition, infestations, and infections, and as food supplies become more secure and abundant. This trend has now slowed or even stopped in most high-income countries.[1-5]

Ovarian cancer has no signs and symptoms during its early stages. As a consequence, the disease is usually in an advanced stage when diagnosed. Noticeable signs and symptoms may include swelling of the stomach, pelvic pressure or stomach pain, trouble eating or feeling full quickly, and having to urinate often or with increased sense of urgency. It is important to see a doctor if these symptoms persist for greater than two weeks. Regular women's health exams, which include a pelvic exam and a Pap smear, are used as a screening device.[1]

Endometrial Cancer

It is unknown what causes endometrial cancers. Nevertheless, most are hormone-driven, and an imbalance toward increased estrogen production increases the risk for endometrial cancer. Risk factors include total number of menstrual cycles, history of not being able to become pregnant or having never given birth, estrogen replacement therapy, treatment with tamoxifen (a hormonal drug used for breast cancer treatment and risk reduction), and a history of other ovarian diseases. Convincing data suggest that obesity—and especially fat accumulation in the abdominal region—is a risk factor for endometrial cancer. Although most women's estrogen is made in the ovaries, fat tissue can change some other hormones into estrogens. A diet high in animal fat, often leading to obesity, and diabetes, which is more common in overweight individuals, are also risk factors. Other factors that may play a role in the development of endometrial cancer include smoking; a family history, especially of certain types of colon, breast, or ovarian cancer; and previous pelvic radiation therapy.[1]

Physical activity, bearing children, birth control pills, and early menopause are probably protective against the development of endometrial cancer. Limited evidence suggests non-starchy vegetables protect against endometrial cancer, whereas red meat and the factors that result in greater adult-attained height, or its consequences, can lead to cancer of the endometrium.[1–3]

Possible signs and symptoms of endometrial cancer include unusual bleeding, spotting, or discharge. Pelvic pain, a pelvic mass, and weight loss are symptoms of more advanced endometrial cancer.[1]

Cervical Cancer

No strong evidence is available linking any aspect of food, nutrition, or physical activity to the risk of cervical cancer.[2, 3] The most important risk factor for cancer of the cervix is infection with human papillomavirus (HPV).[1]

The most common symptom of cervical cancer is abnormal vaginal bleeding, but early cervical pre-cancers or cancers often have no signs or symptoms. Therefore, two preventive measures, which can sometimes even prevent pre-cancers, are important for women: avoiding HPV infection and receiving regular Pap tests.

Steps to avoid HPV consist of delaying sex, using condoms, and being immunized with the HPV vaccine (Gardasil). The HPV vaccine, which consists of a series of three shots given over six months, is administered before sexual activity begins. The American Cancer Society (ACS) recommends the vaccine for females aged 11–12 years and as early as age 9 years in some individuals if recommended by a physician. The ACS also suggests that women aged 13–18 years receive the vaccine for "catch-up" purposes and that women aged 19–26 years speak with their physician to determine if the vaccine is indicated. The vaccine does not protect individuals from all cancer-causing types of HPV, however, so Pap tests are still needed.[1]

The Pap test, using either conventional or liquid-based cytology, is the most common screening form for pre-cancers. The majority of cervical cancers are found in women who have not had Pap tests at the recommended intervals. Initiation and timing of tests depend on the patient's age and risk factors. The ACS recommends working closely with a women's health professional to determine commencement and frequency of testing. An HPV DNA test, which includes a sampling of the cells of the cervix, can be used in conjunction with a Pap test. Administration of the HPV DNA test also depends on age and risk factors. Patients are advised to consult with their physicians to determine the necessity for this test.[1]

Uterine Cancer

Risk factors for uterine cancer include prior pelvic radiation therapy and race—this disease is twice as common in African Americans as in whites or Asian Americans. Hormone balance plays a large role in uterine cancer, with risks including obesity, estrogen replacement therapy, treatment with tamoxifen, infertility, diabetes, early menstruation (before age 12), and menopause after age 52.[1]

Most uterine sarcomas are asymptomatic and cannot be prevented. Their signs and symptoms may include unusual bleeding or discharge and pelvic pain and/or mass. There are no recommended screening tests or examinations to detect uterine sarcomas. The Pap test can occasionally find some early uterine cancers, but most cases are not detected by this test.[1]

Vaginal Cancer

Risk factors for vaginal cancer include age (most cases appear in women older than age 60), vaginal irritation, cervical or pre-cervical cancer, and smoking. Another risk is vaginal adenosis: Vaginal walls are normally lined with squamous cells, but in adenosis the vagina may contain one or more areas of the types of cells lining the uterus. Also, 65–80% of vaginal cancers have been found to contain HPV. Lastly, human immunodeficiency virus (HIV) infection can increase the risk of vaginal cancer because immunosuppression can increase the risk of HPV, thereby increasing the risk of cancer development.[1]

The exact cause of vaginal cancer is unknown. Prevention measures include avoiding HPV infection and receiving regular Pap tests to detect pre-cancers. Signs and symptoms include abnormal vaginal bleeding, often after intercourse; abnormal vaginal discharge; a mass that can be felt; and pain during intercourse. In advanced stages of the disease, painful urination, constipation, and continuous pain in the pelvis may occur.[1]

Vulvar Cancer

Risks of vulvar cancer include age (85% of women diagnosed are older than age 50 and 50% are older than age 70), HPV infection, smoking, HIV infection, vulvar intraepithelial neoplasia (VIN), lichen sclerosis, other genital cancers, and melanoma or atypical moles on nonvulvar skin. Regular gynecologic checkups are essential to assist in detection of this disease. Usually, vulvar cancer is characterized by persistent itching and a growth or ulcer in the vulvar area.[1]

Treatment Options

Most cases of RC are treated with surgery. The surgical interventions will vary depending on disease type, stage, and presence of metastatic disease. Surgery is often followed by chemotherapy and/or radiation therapy. For non-disease-specific nutrition care during medical, radiological, and surgical oncology treatments, refer to Chapters 4 and 5. The following sections detail the treatments for each type of RC.

Ovarian Cancer

Surgery in ovarian cancer is important for staging and tumor removal. Staging assists in determining the treatment plan but often requires removing the uterus, both ovaries, and the fallopian tubes, along with the omentum (a layer of fatty tissue over the abdomen) and lymph nodes in the pelvic and abdominal areas. Also, surgery typically includes tumor removal and/or debulking, so as to eliminate as much of the tumor as possible. Chemotherapy, which can be delivered either intravenously or directly into the abdomen for advanced-stage disease, is also used as treatment for ovarian cancer.[1] Chemotherapy medications commonly used to treat ovarian cancer and their nutrition-related side effects are listed in Table 9.2. Radiation therapy is not routinely used in ovarian cancer.[1, 6] Recurrent cancer may require hematopoietic stem cell transplantation.[1]

Endometrial Cancer

Surgical intervention for endometrial cancer most commonly involves a radical hysterectomy, which includes the removal of the uterus, cervix, upper part of the vagina, and other tissues next to the uterus, along with laparoscopic lymph node sampling. Radiation therapy is used and can include either brachytherapy, in which radioactive pellets are placed via the vagina, or external radiation. Hormone therapy with progesterone-like drugs is administered to slow the growth of the cancer and is more often used in cases of advanced or recurrent endometrial cancer. Chemotherapy may be given depending on the stage of disease,[1] with this treatment typically being offered to women with more advanced stages of disease. The chemotherapy

Table 9.2   *Chemotherapy Agents Used in Ovarian Cancer and Their Nutritional Side Effects*

Chemotherapy Agent	Nausea and/or Vomiting	Anorexia	Dysgeusia	Stomatitis or Esophagitis	Diarrhea	Constipation	Abdominal Pain
Cisplatin	X	X	X				
Carboplatin	X	X	X (metallic taste)				
Docetaxel	X				X		
Doxorubicin	X			X			
Etoposide	X	X		X	X		
Gemcitabine	X				X	X	
Paclitaxel	X			X	X		
Topotecan	X			X	X		X
Vinorelbine	X	X		X		X	

Source: www.cancer.about.com.

agents typically employed in endometrial cancer are cisplatin, carboplatin, doxorubicin, and paclitaxel.

Cervical Cancer

Several types of surgery are performed to treat cervical cancer. Some involve removing the uterus; others do not. Cryosurgery, which kills abnormal cells on the cervix by freezing them, and laser surgery, which burns cells or removes small pieces of tissue, are used in treating pre-invasive cervical cancer (stage 0) only. Conization involves the removal of a cone-shaped piece of tissue from the cervix. This surgical technique can be used to find the cancer or treat early cancers, especially in women who want to have children. Depending on staging and treatment plans, a simple hysterectomy (uterus only is removed) or radical hysterectomy including a pelvic lymph node dissection can be done.

Trachelectomy may allow young women who have an early stage of cervical cancer to be treated and still be able to have children. This procedure entails removal of the cervix and upper part of the vagina and the placement of a "purse-string" stitch to act as an artificial opening of the cervix in the uterus. Women who have undergone a trachelectomy have a 50% pregnancy rate after five years, but have a higher than normal rate of miscarriage; a caesarean section is required to deliver their children.

Pelvic exenteration, besides removing the reproductive organs mentioned previously, includes removal of the bladder, vagina, rectum, and part of the colon. This procedure is used more often in the presence of a recurrent cancer occurring after initial treatment and remission.[1]

Radiation therapy for cervical cancer can take the form of either external radiation or internal radiation.[1] Chemotherapy is not commonly used in cervical cancer. although it may be employed in select cases.[1, 6] If chemotherapy is required, the agents used more commonly are carboplatin, cisplatin, paclitaxel, 5-fluorouracil, cyclophosphamide, and ifosfamide.

Uterine Cancer

Surgery to remove uterine cancer typically includes a radical hysterectomy, which entails the removal of the uterus, cervix, upper part of the vagina, and other tissues next to the uterus, and can include lymph node removal in the pelvis and lower abdominal back. Radiation therapy for this type of cancer may consist of either brachytherapy, in which radioactive pellets are inserted via the vagina, or external radiation therapy. Chemotherapy (doxorubicin combined with either Platinol® or paclitaxel) and hormone therapy are also used in the treatment of uterine cancer, typically if surgery and radiation therapy have failed.[1]

Vaginal Cancer

The two main treatments for vaginal cancer are surgery and radiation therapy. Surgery generally includes laser surgery in which a high-energy beam of light vaporizes the abnormal tissues. A wide local excision or partial vaginectomy are performed rarely, but may be needed if other treatment options fail. Topical chemotherapy applied directly to the vaginal lining or intravenous chemotherapy (cisplatin, carboplatin, 5-fluorouracil, paclitaxel, etoposide, capecitabine, bleomycin, mitomycin C, vincristine or ifosfamide) may be used to treat advanced stages.[1]

Vulvar Cancer

Laser surgery, in which a focused laser beam is employed to vaporize the layer of vulvar skin containing the abnormal cells, is used in the treatment of pre-invasive cancer. Excision—that is, removal of the cancer and a margin of the normal-appearing skin around it—is sometimes called a local excision; if the area removed is more extensive, the procedure is called a simple partial vulvectomy. A vulvectomy can be simple or radical. It can include inguinal node dissection and sentinel lymph node biopsy. In advanced stages, pelvic exenteration is performed; this procedure involves a vulvectomy and removal of the pelvic lymph nodes, as well as one or more of the following structures: the lower colon, rectum, bladder, uterus, cervix, and vagina.[1]

External-beam radiation is often used in conjunction with chemotherapy in cases of vulvar cancer. Radiation therapy can also be used to treat the groin nodes and pelvic nodes alone. Chemotherapy can be given intravenously for more invasive cancer, or it can be applied as a topical cream directly to the skin in less invasive cancers.[1]

Primary Surgery and Nutritional Issues

Early postoperative oral intake in patients with RC has been debated and studied for many years. In the late 1990s, clinicians realized that traditional feeding protocols, which avoided oral intake in the early postoperative period, were not based on scientific literature, but instead were passed down from surgical mentors. Traditional management included nasogastric suction, awaiting the return of bowel sounds, and the passage of flatus or bowel movement before initiating oral intake.[7]

While research has not identified the cause of postoperative ileus, fear of this complication has prompted many surgeons to continue with traditional postoperative management. Scientific data demonstrate that small intestinal function returns almost immediately after surgery, gastric emptying returns by the second postoperative day, and colonic function is normal in two to three days.[7] Studies have concluded early postoperative oral intake results in decreased length of hospitalization and is well tolerated when compared with traditional dietary management in patients undergoing abdominal surgery.[7, 8] These studies utilized clear liquid diets on postoperative day 1 and advanced to a regular diet once liquids were tolerated.[7, 8] Patients also receiving irradiation, neurotoxic chemotherapy, or extensive abdominal surgery may need a more individualized diet; more research is currently needed in these specific areas.[7]

The disease stage and patient condition at time of surgery may influence which type of surgical intervention is appropriate. The use of a nutrition laboratory value, prealbumin, has also been proposed as a predictor of patient outcomes. In a study by Geisler and colleagues, prealbumin level and complications were used to establish which patients would not be good candidates for primary radical cytoreductive surgery for ovarian cancer.[9] The prospective study was carried out at one institution and included patients with advanced epithelia ovarian cancer (stage III or IV). The study participants had a mean age of 59 years, had a mean BMI of 32 kg/m^2, and were operated on by two staff surgeons over a two-year period. Although 114 patients met the criteria for inclusion, 6 patients were deemed too ill to undergo surgery regardless of their prealbumin levels. Ultimately, 108 patients underwent primary surgical debulking with optimal cytoreduction. Of these individuals, 88 had a prealbumin level less than 18 mg/dL and 24 had a level less than 10 mg/dL.

Following the surgeries, the investigators found that postoperative complications increased with lower prealbumin levels. Postoperative complications included estimated blood loss greater than 2,000 mL; death within 30 days; unplanned intensive care unit admission; unplanned readmission to the hospital; significant vascular, gastrointestinal, or genitourinary injury; and hospital stay greater than 14 days. All complications occurred in patients with prealbumin levels of less than 18 mg/dL, and a significantly larger number of complications occurred in patients with prealbumin levels of less than 10 mg/dL. All postoperative mortality occurred in patients with prealbumin less than 10 mg/dL.

In this study, the patients with a prealbumin level less than 10 mg/dL were given nutrition support in the form of parenteral nutrition (PN) for greater than 10 days prior to surgery. After this period of PN, only 50% of the patients had improved prealbumin levels; the other 13 patients' prealbumin level remained less than 10 mg/dL. All 24 patients underwent surgery, and all 13 of the PN patients whose prealbumin remained less than 10 mg/dL preoperatively experienced postoperative complications.

Due to the increased risk of postoperative complications, it appears that patients with extremely poor nutrition status—in this study, characterized by a prealbumin level of less than 10 mg/dL—may be better served by neoadjuvant chemotherapy with interval cytoreductive surgery once their nutritional status improves. The researchers suggest providing nutrition support to all patients with a prealbumin level of less than 10 mg/dL prior to surgery in the form of nutrition supplements, enteral nutrition (EN), or PN.

Nutrition Management During Aggressive Therapy

Malnutrition in gynecological cancer patients is a significant problem, especially among patients who have been diagnosed with ovarian cancer.[10] Laky and colleagues used the Patient-Generated Subjective Global Assessment (PG-SGA) to establish this point. The PG-SGA, which has been previously validated,[11] is an easy-to-use nutrition assessment tool that allows for quick identification and prioritization of malnutrition in patients with cancer. It classifies patients into one of three categories: well nourished, moderately or suspected of being malnourished, and severely malnourished. The Laky et al. study included 145 patients with gynecologic cancer, aged 20–91 years. Using the PG-SGA, 67% of the patients with ovarian cancer were classified as moderately or suspected of being malnourished, which was higher than the rate for all other gynecologic cancers combined.[10]

Deterioration in the nutritional status of patients with ovarian cancer has multifactoral roots. Both the derangements in cytokine levels and the bowel obstruction associated with an enlarging tumor can lead to cachexia and malnutrition. Very few agents have proven to have true anticachectic activity in patients with advanced cancer, although research is now underway to identify medications targeted at blocking the activity of cancer-related catabolic factors.[12] Patients with ovarian cancer should undergo routine nutrition screening and assessment, preferably with a validated tool such as the PG-SGA, to enable their healthcare providers to detect and treat nutritional issues.

Providing adequate nutrition by mouth is often challenging in the presence of advanced disease, gastrointestinal side effects associated with chemotherapy, or radiation enteritis symptoms. The results of a small study conducted by Dillon and associates[13] could lead to more promising research in this area, however. Their study included 6 patients with stage IIIC ovarian cancer and a mean age of 47 years. The patients were either undergoing primary therapy or therapy for recurrence and were classified as cachectic based on a weight loss of more than 10% of their premorbid weight. All participants were on a 21-day chemotherapy cycle and were studied on day 20 of the cycle. Study participants were given a balanced oral amino acid supplement containing 40 g of amino acids and 166 calories. Phenylalanine concentration in the blood and muscle were analyzed both before and after consumption of the amino acid supplement. The amino acid supplement led to increased protein synthesis and a stable protein breakdown. The researchers concluded that, despite the patients' advanced cancer, ongoing therapy, and enhanced inflammatory burden, amino acids were capable of acutely stimulating muscle protein synthesis.[13] Further research, including studies focusing on important outcomes such as quality of life and survival, is required to establish the role of an amino acid supplement in this patient population.

Oral supplementation and nutrient-dense foods are key elements in managing patients with gynecologic cancer who experience weight loss and eating difficulties. Determining the individual nutrient needs of these patients is challenging and, unfortunately, not well studied. The only study in this area to date was done by Dickerson and colleagues.[14] It included 61 hospitalized patients with biopsy-proven cervical or ovarian carcinoma who were followed by the Nutrition Support Service. Resting energy expenditure was measured by indirect calorimetry and compared to predicted energy expenditure as determined by the Harris–Benedict equation for females. Measured resting energy expenditure varied between 53% and 157% of predicted energy expenditure. This study demonstrated the Harris–Benedict equation for females provides an unreliable estimate of caloric expenditure in patients with cervical or ovarian cancer receiving specialized nutrition support.[14] Therefore, it is important to monitor patients' weight and nutrition status closely, provide counseling regarding food and supplement selections, and, if aggressive therapy is desired, provide nutrition support during times of hypermetabolic stress and prolonged periods of inadequate oral intake.

Nutrition Management in Advanced Reproductive Cancer

Intestinal obstruction is a well-recognized complication of advanced ovarian cancer. It significantly affects survival, influences quality of life,[15] and occurs in approximately 45% of patients.[8] Bowel obstruction may present at diagnosis or with recurrent disease following anticancer therapy.[16] Malignant bowel obstruction is particularly common and is the most frequent cause of death in patients with ovarian cancer.[15, 16]

Hospitalization and conservative measures, which include nasogastric suction, bowel rest, and intravascular fluids, constitute the initial treatment approach for intestinal obstruction.[15] If this approach fails, surgical intervention or drainage gastrostomy is considered. More than half of all patients with ovarian cancer and intestinal obstruction can benefit from a definitive surgical procedure, a therapeutic approach that is associated with a low perioperative mortality rate and a mean survival rate of 6.8 months following surgical intervention.[17] The decision to offer palliative surgery must be balanced against the potential morbidity and mortality and the ability to improve the quality of life for a patient with a limited life expectancy. Data suggest that patients undergoing repeat surgery for recurrent bowel obstruction have a low likelihood of achieving successful palliation and experience significant morbidity, including enterocutaneous fistula, wound infection, rapid development of subsequent bowel obstructions, and limited survival.[18]

Patients with advanced unresectable disease and/or inoperable bowel obstruction, as a result of carcinomatosis and intestinal encasement with tumor, have a worse prognosis and require palliation with drainage gastrostomy, intravenous fluid supplementation, and an oral liquid diet.[15, 17, 18] Gastrostomy tube placement in ovarian carcinoma is technically feasible and safe in the palliative setting.[19] Additionally, it plays an important role in the treatment of women with obstructive gynecological cancer, allowing for gastric drainage and decompression without the disadvantages of nasogastric tubes.[20] One 7-year retrospective review, which included 94 patients with ovarian cancer requiring drainage gastrostomy tube placement due to malignant bowel obstruction, demonstrated that gastrostomy drainage tubes, as compared to nasogastric tube drainage, allowed the majority of patients to receive end-of-life care either at home or in an inpatient hospice setting.[19]

Since the early 1970s, studies have supported the use of PN in gynecologic oncology patients during aggressive treatment of gastrointestinal obstruction due to the morbidities and mortalities associated with preoperative and postoperative malnutrition and overall quality of life.[21] Nutrition support is used in the inpatient or home setting, often in conjunction with gastrostomy drainage tubes. However, research has yielded conflicting data on the use of PN in patients with nonoperative bowel obstruction. In the seven-year retrospective review mentioned previously, no survival benefit was found with the use of PN.[19] Another study by Abu-Rustum and associates[17] demonstrated a median survival of 84 days for all patients post-gastrostomy drainage tube placement. The median survival for patients with obstructive ovarian cancer who received salvage chemotherapy and PN was 89 days, compared to median survival of 71 days for patients who received salvage chemotherapy alone. The researchers concluded chemotherapy alone is ineffective in restoring bowel function in heavily pretreated patients with recurrent disease.[17] A recent study by Brard and colleagues[15] concluded that terminally ill ovarian cancer patients with intestinal obstruction receiving PN have a median survival benefit of 4 weeks. This survival benefit decreased when patients were treated with concurrent chemotherapy. The researchers concluded, contrary to previous research that terminally ill ovarian cancer patients should not receive PN, a subgroup of patients benefited from PN and found it life-sustaining.[15]

Issues of cost, quality of life, and human values need to be investigated to assess the full impact of PN in this patient population, especially given the variable outcomes described in the literature.[15] The value of PN in patients with advanced- or end-stage ovarian cancer remains debatable.[15, 17] Conversely, PN may be justified for selected patients[9] and should be carefully considered by the medical team and the patient.

One study, which was conducted prior to the establishment of palliative care programs, suggested that care given to ovarian cancer patients at the end of life might be inadequate.[22] In more recent times, the combination of gastrostomy drainage tubes, PN use, and palliative care programs has enabled many patients to meet their end-of-life wishes. In particular, home PN and gastrostomy drainage tubes often give patients freedom from the hospital setting. A study of home PN in patients with malignant bowel obstruction demonstrated a low complication rate and found PN was usually perceived by patients and care providers as beneficial. In this study, home PN was found to have palliative benefits and to facilitate compassionate home care for carefully selected patients with malignant bowel obstruction.[23] Nutrition intervention and care of patients with reproductive cancers must include an individualized approach, taking into account patient and family end-of-life wishes.

SUMMARY

Limited data are available to guide nutrition management during the treatment of reproductive cancers. Research suggests that most of these patients are in a hypermetabolic state and, therefore, are at risk for becoming malnourished. Assessment and intervention tools, including aggressive initiation of oral diet postoperatively, monitoring of prealbumin levels, use of high-protein oral supplements, employing gastrostomy drainage tubes, and initiation of nutrition support as needed should be implemented to prevent and treat nutritional issues. The use of PN in the palliative care process is controversial, and the patient's end-of-life goals must be considered when deciding whether to pursue this option.

REFERENCES

1. American Cancer Society. http://www.cancer.org.
2. Kushi LH, Byers T, Doyle C, et al; The American Cancer Society 2006 Nutrition and Physical Activity Guidelines Advisory Committee, American Cancer Society guidelines on nutrition and physical activity for cancer prevention: Reducing the risk of cancer with healthy food choices and physical activity. *CA Cancer J Clin*. 2006;56(5):254–281.
3. World Cancer Research Fund/American Institute for Cancer Research. *Food, Nutrition, Physical Activity, and the Prevention of Cancer: A Global Perspective*. Washington, DC: AICR; 2007.
4. Bandera EV. Nutritional factors in ovarian cancer prevention: What have we learned in the past 5 years? *Nutr Cancer*. 2007;59(2):142–151.
5. Schulz M, Nothlings U, Allen N, et al. No association of consumption of animal foods with risk of ovarian cancer. *Cancer Epidemiol Biomarkers Prev*. 2007;16(7):1527.
6. Penn State Milton S. Hershey Medical Center College of Medicine. Health and disease information: Reproductive cancers. www.hmc.psu.edu/healthinfo/r/reprocancers.htm. Accessed October 31, 2006.

7. Keely DG, Stanhope CR. Postoperative enteral feeding: Myth or fact? *Gynecol Oncol*. 1997;67:233–234.

8. Schilder JM, Hurteau JA, Look KY, et al. A prospective controlled trial of early postoperative oral intake following major abdominal gynecologic surgery. *Gynecol Oncol*. 1197;67(3):235–240.

9. Geisler JP, Linnemeier GC, Thomas AJ, Manahan KJ. Nutritional assessment using prealbumin as an objective criterion to determine whom should not undergo primary radical cytoreductive surgery for ovarian cancer. *Gynecol Oncol*. 2007;106 (1):128–131.

10. Laky B, Janda M, Baur J, et al. Malnutrition among gynaecological cancer patients. *Eur J Clin Nutr*. 2007;61(5):642–646.

11. Bauer J, Capra S, Ferguson M. Use of the scored Patient-Generated Subjective Global Assessment (PG-SGA) as a nutrition assessment tool in patients with cancer. *Eur J Clin Nutr*. 2002;56:779–785.

12. Gadducci A, Cosio S, Fanucchi A, Genazzani AR. Malnutrition and cachexia in ovarian cancer patients: Pathophysiology and management. *Anticancer Res*. 2001; 21(4B):2941–2947.

13. Dillon EL, Volpi E, Wolfe RR, et al. Amino acids metabolism and inflammatory burden in ovarian cancer patients undergoing intense oncological therapy. *Clin Nutr*. 2007;26(6):736–743.

14. Dickerson RN, White KG, Curcillo PG, et al. Resting energy expenditure of patients with gynecologic malignancies. *J Am Coll Nutr*. 1995;14(5):448–454.

15. Brard L, Weitzen S, Strubel-Lagan SL, et al. The effect of total parenteral nutrition on the survival of terminally ill ovarian cancer patients. *Gynecol Oncol*. 2006; 103:176–180.

16. Ripamonti C, Bruera E. Palliative management of malignant bowel obstruction. *Intl J Gynecol Cancer*. 2002;12:135–143.

17. Abu-Rustum NR, Barakat RR, Venkatraman E, Spriggs D. Chemotherapy and total parenteral nutrition for advanced ovarian cancer with bowel obstruction. *Gynecol Oncol*. 1197;64:493–495.

18. Pothuri B, Meyer L, Gerardi M, Barakat RR, Chi DS. Reoperation for palliation of recurrent malignant bowel obstruction in ovarian carcinoma. *Gynecol Oncol*. 2004; 95:193–195.

19. Pothuri B, Montenarano M, Gerardi M, et al. Percutaneous endoscopic gastrostomy tube placement in patients with malignant bowel obstruction due to ovarian carcinoma. *Gynecol Oncol*. 2005;96(2):330–334.

20. Tsahalina E, Woolas RP, Carter PG, et al. Gastrostomy tubes in patients with recurrent gynaecological cancer and intestinal obstruction. *BJOG: Intl J Obstetr Gynaecol*. 1999;106(9):964–968.

21. Ford JH Jr, Dudan RC, Bennett JS, Averette HE. Parenteral hyperalimentation in gynecologic oncology patients. *Gynecol Oncol*. 1972;1:70–75.

22. Herrinton LJ, Neslund-Dudas C, Rolnick SJ, et al. Complications at the end of life in ovarian cancer. *J Pain Symp Manage*. 2007;34(3):237–243.

23. August DA, Thorn D, Fisher RL, Welcheck CM. Home parenteral nutrition for patients with inoperable malignant bowel obstruction. *J Parenteral Enteral Nutr*. 1991;15(3):323–327.

Chapter 10

Prostate Cancer

Natalie Ledesma, MS, RD, CSO

INTRODUCTION

Prostate cancer is the most commonly diagnosed malignancy in men in Western countries.[1] Nearly 219,000 men were expected to be diagnosed with prostate cancer in 2007 in the United States. By race, incidence rates are much higher in African American men than in Caucasian men. Cancer death rates due to prostate cancer have been declining since 1990. In 2007, 27,000 men were expected to die from prostate cancer.

The cause of prostate cancer is unknown, but the hormone androgen, acting via the androgen receptor, appears to spur the development of prostate cancer.[2] Researchers are also devoting considerable effort to identifying the genetic role in prostate cancer incidence.

Established risk factors for prostate cancer include age, race, nationality, family history, and diet.[3] Other potential risk factors include obesity, physical activity, infection and inflammation of the prostate, and vasectomy. The risk of prostate cancer increases considerably after the age of 50. It is estimated that nearly 2 of 3 prostate cancer patients are older than age 65. While diet has been implicated as a reason for the variations in prostate cancer rates observed worldwide, epidemiologists have determined that men in Western countries, including North America, northwestern Europe, Australia, and the Caribbean Islands, have a higher rate of prostate cancer. The disease is less common in Asia, South America, Central America, and Africa. Finally, there appears to be an inherited or genetic component that increases the risk of prostate cancer: The risk of prostate cancer is more than doubled for a man who has a father or brother with prostate cancer.

Since 1996, the 5-year survival rate for prostate cancer (for men with local or regional stages) has remained an impressive 100% in white men and 98% in African American men.[1] The survival rate continues to stay high with time: The 10-year and 15-year survival rates are 93% and 77%, respectively. While only 5% of men are diagnosed with metastatic (i.e., distant-stage) disease, the 5-year survival rate for these men is 33%.

Medical Treatment

Treatment of prostate cancer depends on a variety of factors, including the patient's age, cancer stage, and any other medical conditions. Surgery, external-beam radiation therapy (EBRT), and active surveillance are strategies that are typically used for men with early-stage prostate cancer. Some men may also receive hormone therapy. Aggressive surveillance, formerly called "watchful waiting," may be appropriate for older men or for men with less aggressive tumors, as determined by cell type.

Healthy men with localized disease and no lymphatic involvement are good candidates for surgery to remove the prostate cancer cells.[4] The goal of radiation therapy is to kill the cancer cells where they reside. Current techniques include EBRT, three-dimensional conformal radiation therapy, intensity-modulated radiation therapy, and radioactive seed implants, or brachytherapy. Radiation therapy may also be indicated for advanced disease, including palliative therapy. For men with metastatic disease, chemotherapy, radiation, hormone therapy, or a combination of these methods may be used.

Most patients complete their prostate cancer treatment with limited impact. The most common side effects of prostate cancer therapies include urinary, bowel, and erectile dysfunction, as well as infertility[5] (Table 10.1). Improved surgical techniques have decreased the side effect of urinary incontinence. The predominant nutrition-related issue in prostate cancer

Table 10.1 *Treatment Side Effects in Prostate Cancer*

Treatment	*Side Effect*
Surgery	• Urinary dysfunction • Erectile dysfunction—less with nerve-sparing surgery • Infertility
Radiation	• Urinary dysfunction—less with IMRT, worse with brachytherapy initially • Erectile dysfunction • Bowel dysfunction—worse with EBRT, less with IMRT and brachytherapy • Infertility
Hormone therapy	• Hot flashes • Loss of bone mineral density (osteoporosis) • Weight gain

EBRT = external-beam radiation therapy.
IMRT = intensity-modulated radiation therapy.

treatment is diarrhea when patients are undergoing radiation therapy; this side effect is primarily observed with full pelvic radiation therapy.

Nearly all men will experience some sort of erectile dysfunction for the first year following treatment. However, nerve-sparing surgery can substantially decrease the risk that significant dysfunction will continue. Current surgical techniques estimate that sexual potency will fully return by 1 year following surgery in 50% of men who undergo a radical prostatectomy. At 2 years, sexual function increases to 75%. Although fewer effects on sexual function are apparent immediately following radiation therapy, the improvement in sexual function in the 2 years after this kind of treatment is minimal. Only 25% and 50% of men who have brachytherapy and EBRT, respectively, experience erectile dysfunction.

Both surgery and radiation therapy will, unfortunately, likely result in infertility. Men who wish to father children after surgery or radiation therapy are advised to use sperm banking. Additionally, patients on hormone therapy may face other challenges, including hot flashes, loss of bone mass, and oftentimes weight gain. Researchers have recently established that loss of bone mineral density (BMD) and related fractures are significantly associated with hormone therapy or androgen deprivation therapy (ADT).[6] Continuous ADT further increases the risk of osteoporosis.[7]

Nutrition Issues

Research suggests that differences in diet and lifestyle may largely account for the variability of prostate cancer rates observed in different countries.[8] Following a healthy diet may reduce the incidence of prostate cancer and the risk of prostate cancer progression. It is estimated that more than one-third of cancer deaths in the United States can be attributed to diet in adulthood.[9]

Many studies indicate that a plant-based diet may help lower the risk of developing prostate cancer and may beneficially affect the progression of the disease. In preliminary results in one study, dietary and lifestyle changes led to a 4% decrease in prostate-specific antigen (PSA), a protein marker for prostate cancer growth, and significantly decreased prostate cancer cell growth.[10] PSA levels increased 6% in the control group. Another study assessing the recurrence of prostate cancer reported that a plant-based diet, in combination with stress reduction, may significantly slow disease progression.[11] PSA doubling time—the value monitored to assess for prostate cancer recurrence—increased from 11.9 months (prestudy) to 112.3 months (intervention). Additionally, individuals who made comprehensive lifestyle changes had an improved quality of life.[12]

Fruits and Vegetables

Fruits and vegetables are great dietary sources of vitamins, minerals, fiber, and cancer-fighting phytonutrients. Extensive research indicates that diets rich in fruits and vegetables are associated with a lower risk of many cancers[10–14]; evidence specific to prostate cancer is inconsistent, but appears promising.[10–16] In a study of men who were followed via active surveillance, the risk of prostate cancer was reduced significantly in men who consumed 2–3 kg (50% lower risk) and more than 3 kg (60% lower risk) of fruits and vegetables per week compared with men who consumed less than 2 kg per week.[12] In many of the studies reporting no significant effect between fruits and vegetables and prostate cancer, men may not have consumed adequate amounts of these foods to lower their risk.

Furthermore, some evidence suggests that certain components in fruits and vegetables, such as phytonutrients, may have a particularly strong anticancer effect. A key indicator of phytonutrient content is the vibrant, intense color of many fruits and vegetables. For example, the benefits of fruits and vegetables in regard to cancer protection may be related to high amounts of carotenoids (a family of phytonutrients) in certain fruits and vegetables.[17–20] In particular, lycopene appears to exert protective effects against prostate cancer. Higher plasma lycopene levels are generally associated with lower risk of prostate cancer[19–23] and/or advanced prostate cancer.[24] One possible explanation for this relationship is the inverse association between the consumption of cooked tomato products, the richest source of lycopene, and insulin-like growth factor (IGF-1), a peptide hormone that has been implicated in the risk of various cancers, including prostate cancer.[25] In Western countries, tomato-based products typically account for 85% of dietary lycopene.[26] As with many nutrients and phytonutrients, it is best to obtain lycopene from foods—tomatoes contain other compounds that have beneficial properties.[27] In one study, higher tomato sauce intake resulted in a clear statistically significant inverse association with overall incident prostate cancer.[20] Additionally, lycopene-rich foods are best absorbed in the presence of fat, such as a small amount of olive oil.[28]

A growing body of evidence suggests that cruciferous vegetables and their phytonutrients are associated with a reduced risk of prostate cancer[17, 29–31] and risk of aggressive prostate cancer.[32] The anticancer properties of cruciferous vegetables may be attributable to indole-3-carbinol (I3C), its metabolite diindolylmethane (DIM), and/or isothiocyanates. I3C consistently inhibits prostate tumor growth in vitro and in vivo[33] and induces apoptosis in prostate cancer cells.[30] DIM may reduce the risk of prostate cancer recurrence.[27] Sulforaphane[34] (one of the isothiocyanates), I3C, and DIM may also function by upregulating phase II detoxifying enzymes, thereby suggesting another explanation for the anticancer effects of cruciferous vegetables.[35] Cruciferous vegetables include arugula, broccoli, bok choy, Brussels sprouts, cabbage, cauliflower, collard greens, horseradish, kale, kohlrabi, mustard greens, radishes, rutabagas, turnips, and watercress.

When these various food components are combined, they likely act synergistically. One study illustrating this effect found a significantly reduced rate of tumor growth when rats were fed a diet rich in tomatoes and/or broccoli. The tumors decreased 34% in rats fed a tomato-rich diet, 42% in rats fed a broccoli-rich diet, and 52% in rats fed a diet rich in both tomatoes and broccoli.[31]

In the fruit category, research suggests that components in pomegranates exhibit strong anti-inflammatory and antioxidant effects.[36] Preliminary studies have found that pomegranate and its components inhibit tumor growth, decrease PSA levels, induce apoptosis,[36–38] and inhibit angiogenesis.[39] Patients with prostate cancer significantly increased their PSA doubling time (mean of 54 months compared to 15 months) by consuming 8 ounces of pomegranate juice daily.[40]

While research is inconclusive, a minimum of 8–10 servings of fruit and vegetables per day may be necessary to provide the greatest protection against cancer.[41] See Table 10.2 for fruit and vegetable recommendations.

Table 10.2   *Food/Nutrient Recommendations for Protection Against Prostate Cancer*

Food or Nutrient	Summary	Recommendation
Fruits and vegetables	One serving = • ½ cup fruit or vegetable • 1 cup raw leafy greens • ¼ cup dried fruit or vegetable • 6 oz fruit or vegetable juice Eat 1 cup or more vegetables with lunch and dinner.	8–10 total servings daily • 5 or more vegetable servings • 3 fruit servings • 12 oz tomato-based juice
Fiber	• Choose breads with 3 g (or more) fiber per slice. • The first ingredient on the label should be whole or sprouted grain flour, not white flour, unbleached white flour, or enriched wheat flour. • Whole grains include, among others, oats, barley, brown rice, quinoa, amaranth, bulgur, millet, buckwheat, spelt, wild rice, and teff.	30–45 g daily • This goal can be achieved by meeting your fruit and vegetable goal plus 1 serving of legumes or at least 2 servings of whole grains.

(continues)

Table 10.2   *Food/Nutrient Recommendations for Protection Against Prostate Cancer, Continued*

Food or Nutrient	Summary	Recommendation
Refined carbohydrates and sugars	Dietary sources include products made with refined flours (examples: white bread, white rice, white pasta); or refined grains, alcohol, and sweets, such as candy, cookies, cakes, and pastries.	Limit or avoid consumption of refined carbohydrates and sugars.
Meat	Dietary sources include beef, pork, and lamb.	• Reduce meat consumption. • Avoid grilled or fried meats.
Dairy	Dietary sources include milk, butter, yogurt, cheese, and ice cream.	Reduce dairy consumption.
Soy	Dietary sources include soybeans, edamame, tofu, soymilk, tempeh, miso, and soy nuts.	1 or more servings daily
Green tea	• Green tea contains does contain caffeine, albeit much less than coffee or black tea. • If opting for decaffeinated green tea, choose naturally decaffeinated teas with water, as the typical caffeine extraction results in a significant loss of phytonutrients.	1–4 cups daily
Saturated fat	Dietary sources include meats, baked goods, and whole-milk dairy products, including butter, cheese, and ice cream.	Reduce consumption of meat and dairy products.
Trans-fatty acids	Dietary sources include margarine, fried foods, commercially made peanut butter, salad dressings; and processed foods, including breads, crackers, cereals, and cookies.	Avoid *trans*-fats.
Omega-6 fatty acids	• Dietary sources of arachidonic acid include meats, butter, egg yolks, whole milk, and whole-milk dairy products. • Dietary sources of linoleic acid include common vegetable oils, such as corn oil, safflower oil, sunflower oil; and cottonseed oil; and processed foods made with these oils.	• Reduce consumption of meat and dairy products. • Limit consumption of linoleic acid-rich oils.

Table 10.2   *Food/Nutrient Recommendations for Protection Against Prostate Cancer, Continued*

Food or Nutrient	Summary	Recommendation
Omega-3 fatty acids	• Dietary sources of EPA and DHA include cold-water fish (examples: salmon, sardines, black cod, trout, herring). • Dietary sources of ALA include flaxseeds, chia seeds, walnuts, hempseeds, and pumpkin seeds. • Flaxseeds can have a laxative-like effect; thus it is wise to gradually increase consumption, aiming to achieve 2 tbsp ground flax daily.	Include these healthy fats daily through diet and/or supplements.
Omega-9 fatty acids	Dietary sources include extra-virgin olive oil, canola oil, macadamia nut oil, almonds, and avocados.	Include these healthy fats daily.
Selenium	• Dietary sources include Brazil nuts, seafood, enriched brewer's yeast, and grains. • Two Brazil nuts provide 200 mcg selenium.	200 mcg selenium daily through diet and/or supplements
Vitamin E	Dietary sources include vegetable oils, wheat germ, sweet potatoes, nuts, seeds, and avocados.	Although more research is necessary, studies to date suggest that men at risk or with prostate cancer should take 50–200 IU alpha-tocopherol with 400 mg gamma-tocopherol.
Calcium	Dietary sources include dairy products, beans, leafy greens, and fortified products, such as soy milk, cereal, and orange juice.	• 1,000–1,200 mg daily • Avoid ≥ 2000 mg per day.
Vitamin D	• Dietary sources include cold-water fish, eggs, and fortified products, such as milk, soy milk, and cereals. • Generally, our dietary intake is not adequate to meet the normal daily requirements. More often, vitamin D is generated through skin synthesis of sunlight (ultraviolet rays).	• 400–2,000 IU daily • Maintain serum 25(OH)-vitamin D > 35 ng/mL.

Dietary Fiber

A plant-based diet is naturally high in fiber. A diet rich in natural fiber obtained from fruits, vegetables, legumes, and whole grains may reduce the risk and/or progression of prostate cancer. Dietary fiber intake and the consumption of cereals, nuts, and seeds have been inversely associated with prostate cancer[42, 43] and prostate cancer mortality.[44] Fiber binds to toxic compounds and carcinogens, which are then later eliminated from the body.[45]

Various mechanisms have been proposed to explain the protective effects of dietary fiber against prostate cancer. These hypotheses include: increased fecal bulk and decreased intestinal transit time, which allow less opportunity for mutagens to interact with the intestinal epithelium[46]; fiber binding to bile acids, which are thought to promote cell proliferation[47]; fermentation in the gut, producing short-chain fatty acids, which improves the gut environment[46, 47]; and the antioxidants in whole grains, which have been linked to disease prevention.[47] Moreover, a high-fiber diet decreases circulating hormone levels that may promote prostate cancer and/or its progression.[43, 46] Refer to Table 10.2 for dietary fiber recommendations.

Refined Carbohydrates and Sugar

Refined carbohydrates and high-sugar foods are generally low in both nutrient value and dietary fiber. Evidence suggests that refined cereals (primarily breads and pasta)[48] and desserts[16] have been associated with prostate cancer. Additionally, these foods appear to increase serum insulin and serum IGF-1 levels, which lead to the development and promotion of cancer.[49–52] IGF-1 may speed tumor development by inhibiting apoptosis, enhancing cell proliferation, promoting synthesis of sex steroids, and inhibiting the synthesis of sex hormone-binding globulin (SHBG).[53] In a recent study, consumption of a diet high in refined carbohydrates led to hyperinsulinemia and increased tumor growth.[54] Another study established that mice fed a no-carbohydrate ketogenic diet (84% fat, 0% carbohydrate, 16% protein kcal) had decreased insulin and IGF-1 levels and smaller tumors compared with mice fed either a low-fat diet (12% fat, 72% carbohydrate, 16% protein kcal) or a Western diet (40% fat, 44% carbohydrate, 16% protein kcal).[55] See Table 10.2 for refined carbohydrate/sugar sources and recommendations.

Meat

Many studies have suggested an association between meat intake and prostate cancer, and there exist plausible mechanisms to explain why the two may be related. The benefits of phytonutrients were noted earlier in this chapter, but animal products contain none of these nutrients. One of the original theories linking meat to prostate cancer focused on fat content and, in particular, the larger amount of saturated fat found in meat. Strong correlations have been observed in which meat-based dietary fat has been linked with prostate cancer mortality.[56] Additionally, consumption of animal protein increases IGF-1 levels.[49]

More recent theories have examined the relationship between genotoxins, such as heterocyclic amines (HCAs) and polycyclic aromatic hydrocarbons (PAHs), and the risk of prostate cancer.[57–60] These carcinogenic compounds form when meat is cooked at high temperatures by dry-heat methods, including frying, grilling, broiling, and barbecuing. Intake of well-done or very-well-done meat increased the risk of prostate cancer by 26% and nearly doubled the risk of advanced prostate cancer when the highest tertile was compared with the lowest, although no association was observed between meat type and cancer risk.[60] HCAs, and specifically PhIP (2-amino-1-methyl-6-phenylimidazo(4,5-*b*)pyridine), appear to significantly elevate PSA levels.[61] Additionally, consumption of even one cooked meat meal can result in PhIP activating estrogen receptor-mediated signaling pathways, which in turn increases prostate cancer risk.[62] See Table 10.2 for meat sources and recommendations regarding meat consumption.

Dairy Products

Various studies suggest a relationship between dairy foods and prostate cancer. In one study, men who consumed 21 dairy servings weekly, compared with those who consumed 5 or fewer servings weekly, more than doubled their risk of prostate cancer.[63] Dietary calcium and total milk intake, particularly low-fat milk, significantly increased the men's risk of prostate cancer. In a prospective study, greater intake of dairy products (more than 2.75 servings versus 0.98 or fewer servings of total dairy per day), and particularly low-fat dairy products, was weakly associated with increased risk of prostate cancer.[64] Similarly, consumption of low-fat and nonfat milk was related to an increased risk of prostate cancer; this relationship was strongest for men with localized or low-grade tumors.[65]

Interestingly, whole milk was associated with a decreased risk of prostate cancer. A recent cohort study reported that skim milk, but not other dairy foods, was associated with increased risk of advanced prostate cancer (two or more servings versus zero servings per day).[66] Of note, low-fat dairy products often contain slightly higher calcium content than whole-milk dairy products. The association between dairy foods and prostate cancer may be related to the calcium content and/or the animal fats in dairy.[67, 68] Additionally, milk and dairy products appear to increase IGF-1 levels.[69] See Table 10.2 for dairy sources and recommendations.

Soy

Soy and its components are dietary factors that may play a role in the lower rates of prostate cancer observed in Asian countries. A Japanese case-control study found that men who consumed the largest amounts of dietary soy isoflavones (≥ 89.9 mg/day) compared with men who consumed the small amounts of these substances (< 30.5 mg/day) reduced their risk of prostate cancer by 58%.[70] This finding was further supported by a meta-analysis, which reported an inverse association between soy foods and prostate cancer risk.[71]

Several plausible mechanisms may explain soy's anticancer benefits, most of which have some hormonal relationship: decreased blood androgen levels, increased SHBG, inhibited 5-alpha reductase, and/or a favorable effect on estrogen metabolism.[72, 73] Additionally, although research findings are not consistent on this point, a review noted that PSA values in patients with prostate cancer decreased significantly with greater consumption of soy isoflavones in four of eight trials.[74] See Table 10.2 for soy sources and recommendations.

Green Tea

Green tea is rich in the phytonutrients known as polyphenols (flavonoids), which exhibit several anticancer properties.[75] Laboratory studies[76-79] and animal studies[80] indicate that green tea catechins may inhibit tumor growth and induce apoptosis. Nonetheless, the Ohsaki Cohort study reported no association between green tea and the risk of prostate cancer.[81]

Of great interest, however, is green tea's ability to either blunt or enhance other components' effects. Green tea catechins inhibit carcinogenesis when combined with HCAs, thereby lessening the latter substances' detrimental effects.[82] The combination of soy and green tea synergistically inhibits tumor weight and metastasis and significantly reduces plasma concentrations of both testosterone and dihydrotestosterone.[83] Moreover, a synergistic effect has been observed between green tea consumption and dietary lycopene.[84] See Table 10.2 for green tea recommendations.

Dietary Fat

Dietary fat has been implicated as a risk factor for prostate cancer. A comprehensive review reported that 20 of 30 studies found positive—albeit not all statistically significant—associations between dietary fat and risk of prostate cancer.[85] Prostate cancer mortality has also been associated with dietary fat.[56] Strong correlations were noted for meat, added fats and oils, ice cream, margarine, salad/cooking oil, and vegetable shortening.

Most researchers agree that the dietary goal should be to consume approximately 20% of total calories in the form of fat.[86] Ultimately, however, the *type* of fat may be of greater significance than the total *amount* of fat.

Saturated Fat

Saturated fats from meat and dairy products have been identified as risk factors for prostate cancer[87–90] and metastatic prostate cancer.[91–93] See Table 10.2 for saturated fat sources and recommendations.

Trans-Fat

Trans-fats, like those found in hydrogenated oils, have been connected with prostate cancer.[94–96] A recent prospective study reported that men with the highest plasma *trans*-fats level had a 116% increase in nonaggressive prostate tumors; no association was observed with aggressive prostate tumors.[94] See Table 10.2 for *trans*-fat sources and recommendations.

Essential Fatty Acids: Omega-6 and Omega-3 Fatty Acids

Current research suggests that levels of essential fatty acids and the balance between them may play a critical role in the prevention and treatment of cancer, including prostate cancer.[97] The optimal ratio appears to be a 1:1 to 4:1 ratio of omega-6 (Ω-6) to omega-3 (Ω-3) fatty acids.

Although not all studies have observed an association between prostate cancer and Ω-6 fatty acids (e.g., linoleic acid, which can be converted to arachidonic acid), a high intake of Ω-6 fatty acids may increase tumor growth.[97–99] Furthermore, studies are now linking the effects of Ω-6 fatty acids in the diet to stimulation of growth-related genes.[99, 100] See Table 10.2 for Ω-6 fatty acid sources and recommendations.

In contrast to other types of fats, Ω-3 fatty acids [e.g., alpha-linolenic acid (ALA), eicosapentaenoic acid (EPA), and docosahexanaenoic acid (DHA)] may actually reduce the risk of prostate cancer and its progression.[15, 97–99, 101] These fats are also known to strengthen the immune system and to have anti-inflammatory effects. Mechanisms underlying Ω-3 fats' protective effects may potentially focus on their ability to induce apoptosis, suppress cancer cell initiation, compete with arachidonic acid, and modify gene expression. In one study, men who consumed fatty fish rich in Ω-3 fats once or more per week, compared to men who never consumed fish, reduced their risk of prostate cancer by 43%.[101] The researchers also observed that this effect was modified by a variation in the COX-2 gene. An older study reported that men who consumed fish two or more times per week reduced their risk of prostate cancer progression.[102] See Table 10.2 for Ω-3 fatty acid sources and recommendations.

Fish and plant-based foods contain different types of Ω-3 fatty acids. Fish contain EPA and DHA, two specific fatty acids that have shown the most promising anticancer effects.[103] In contrast, plant-based foods contain Ω-3 fatty acids in the form of ALA. In an ideal environment, ALA is converted to EPA and DHA, although this process is notably inefficient.[104, 105] However, the conversion process is enhanced with a diet low in saturated fats and a more balanced Ω-6/Ω-3 fat ratio.[106]

The purported association between ALA and prostate cancer is controversial because study results on this subject are mixed. Note, however, that the primary sources of ALA in these studies were red meat, milk, butter, mayonnaise, and margarine.[93, 107, 108] Results from studies assessing the effects of flaxseed—the richest plant source of Ω-3 fatty acids—on prostate cancer risk appear much more promising.[109–111] The beneficial effects of flax may be due to its high concentration of lignans; these substances are known to lower circulating levels of testosterone.[109, 112] In one study, patients with prostate cancer who consumed 30 g flax daily (2½ tablespoons) and a diet containing 20% of total calories from fat reduced their rate of tumor growth.[109] Ground flaxseeds are preferred for their greater bioavailability relative to whole seeds and for their greater lignan content relative to flaxseed oil.

Other fats, all derived from plant sources, that appear to be neutral[15, 113, 114] or possibly protective[115, 116] against prostate cancer are the Ω-9 fatty acids, also known as monounsaturated fats. See Table 10.2 for Ω-9 fatty acid sources and recommendations.

Selenium

Selenium, an antioxidant, appears to inhibit cellular changes that may lead to prostate cancer,[117] hinder angiogenesis,[117] and induce apoptosis.[118] Research has consistently observed an inverse association between selenium and prostate cancer risk,[119–122] although no statistically significant association was observed in the Vitamins and Lifestyle (VITAL) study.[123] The VITAL study was specifically designed to examine whether supplemental vitamin E and selenium might alter future cancer risk. In this prospective, cohort study involving 35,242 men, no association was found between selenium supplementation and prostate cancer risk (HR = 0.90; 95% CI = 0.62–1.3 for 10-year average intake of more than 50 mcg/day versus non-use; p for trend = 0.97). It is possible that consumption of 50 mcg/day may not be enough to demonstrate an effect; thus, in future studies, it may be beneficial to compare supplementation with 200 mcg/day to 0–50 mcg/day.

Another study found low plasma selenium levels to be associated with a fourfold to fivefold increased risk of prostate cancer.[124] Other research has shown a 63% reduction in prostate cancer recurrence in men taking selenium supplements.[119]

Vitamin E

Although the research is mixed, studies continue to show vitamin E may have promise in lowering the risk of prostate cancer and/or advanced disease. In a recent meta-analysis of randomized controlled trials, vitamin E was associated with a significant reduction in the incidence of prostate cancer.[125] While no statistically significant effect was observed between supplemental vitamin E (greater than or equal to 400 IU/day versus no supplementation) and prostate cancer risk, risk for advanced prostate cancer decreased significantly with greater intake of supplemental vitamin E.[123] Furthermore, higher serum alpha-tocopherol, a type of vitamin E, was associated with reduced risk of prostate cancer[126, 127] and advanced disease.[127]

The optimal type of vitamin E is also being debated. Although the majority of vitamin E studies have used a synthetic form (dl-alpha-tocopherol), research indicates that the natural forms of vitamin E (gamma-tocopherol and d-alpha-tocopherol) have greater bioavailability.[128, 129] Large doses of alpha-tocopherol suppress levels of gamma-tocopherol,[130, 131] and gamma-tocopherol may offer greater protection against prostate cancer.[130, 132–134] In a recent prospective trial, despite the lack of effect demonstrated for supplemental vitamin E in terms of prostate cancer risk, dietary gamma-tocopherol was significantly inversely related to the risk of advanced prostate cancer.[132] A supplement containing mixed tocopherols (d-alpha, gamma, beta) and tocotrienols may offer more protection than a supplement containing only alpha-tocopherol.[135] Additionally, vitamin E succinate has been shown to inhibit prostate cancer growth.[136]

Calcium

Calcium has been implicated in increasing the risk of prostate cancer. A recent large, prospective trial observed that a higher dietary intake of calcium (more than 2,000 mg/day versus less than 1,000 mg/day) was associated with an increased risk for nonaggressive prostate cancer, though higher supplementary calcium intake did not appear to be related to this risk.[85] No relationship was observed between calcium intake and aggressive disease. A meta-analysis also supported the association between high intake of calcium and risk of prostate cancer.[137] Men who consumed 1,329–2,250 mg calcium/day had a 39% greater risk of prostate cancer compared to men who consumed 228–802 mg calcium/day.

Conversely, total and supplemental calcium consumption were weakly associated with advanced (≥ 2,000 mg/day versus 500–750 mg/day) and fatal (≥ 1,000 mg/day versus 500–750 mg/day) prostate cancer, though neither factor was found to be related to nonaggressive prostate cancer.[66] Whereas calcium from skim milk increased the risk of prostate cancer, nondairy calcium sources (≥ 600 mg/day versus < 250 mg/day) were associated with a lower risk of nonaggressive prostate cancer. Similarly, consuming 1,500 mg/day or more of calcium increased the risk of advanced and fatal prostate cancer.[138] Moreover, high calcium intake significantly increased the risk for fatal, but not incident, prostate cancer.[20] Results from this line of research are not entirely consistent, however, as some research shows no association between calcium and prostate cancer.[65]

Vitamin D

Although not all studies agree,[65] vitamin D appears to offer at least some protection against prostate cancer.[139–141] Epidemiological studies indicate that sunlight exposure—which is a significant source of vitamin D—has an inverse relationship with prostate cancer mortality and that prostate cancer risk is greater in men with lower levels of vitamin D.[142, 143] Increasing serum 25(OH)-vitamin D levels by 25 nmol/L was associated with a 17% reduction in total cancer incidence and a 29% decrease in total cancer mortality.[144]

Vitamin D absorption declines with age, and vitamin D deficiency is not uncommon among older adults.[145–148] Men with, and at risk for, prostate cancer—especially those on hormone therapy—may benefit from a serum 25(OH)-vitamin D test. Optimal serum 25(OH)-vitamin D levels have not been established, although research suggests a level in the range of 90–100 nmol/L (36–40 ng/mL) may be ideal.[149]

Body Weight and Physical Activity

Recent studies have consistently found that overweight and obesity are associated with progressive prostate cancer disease and increased overall mortality.[150] Research suggests that obesity is associated with a decline in the risk of nonaggressive disease and increased risk of aggressive prostate cancer.[151] A recent cohort study reported higher body mass index (BMI) was significantly associated with higher plasma volume and lower PSA concentrations.[152] Hemodilution may explain the lower serum PSA concentrations found among obese men with prostate cancer. Thus it may be that obese men are not being diagnosed as early as normal-weight men. In another study, men who maintained a healthy body weight were less likely to have a recurrence of prostate cancer,[153] whereas obese men had a 30% increased risk of cancer recurrence compared with those with lower body weights. Very obese men (BMI > 35) had a definitely heightened risk of recurrence, with this risk increasing by 69%.

A prospective study suggested that men who engage in the largest amounts of exercise reduce their risk of advanced prostate cancer by 36% compared to the non-exercisers[154]; their risk of fatal prostate cancer appears to be reduced by 33%. This finding was further supported by results from a recent study showing that vigorous physical activity is associated with a lower risk of dying from prostate cancer.[20] While there are many benefits of physical activity, research indicates exercise training alters IGF-1 levels, thereby lowering the individual's risk of prostate cancer.[155, 156] Furthermore, evidence affirms that individualized exercise programs are effective means of enhancing muscular function and improving the quality of life of cancer survivors.[157] Healthy weight control is encouraged through consumption of a healthful plant-based diet and regular exercise to maintain or increase lean muscle mass.

SUMMARY

Surgical and radiation techniques for prostate cancer continue to advance at a rapid pace. With more men using hormone therapy, the long-term side effects of this type of treatment need to be managed effectively in more patients. The loss of bone mineral density and related fractures are real risks for which patients should be monitored for both prevention and management purposes.

Emphasis on the role played by nutrition in prostate cancer will likely continue to grow, as has clearly been the case in recent years. Research has begun to examine the effect of diet on gene expression, and the field of nutrigenomics will grow exponentially in the upcoming years. Diet and lifestyle modifications are strongly encouraged to prevent and/or possibly inhibit the disease. Patients' use of complementary therapies and dietary supplements should be included in a comprehensive nutrition assessment and discussed with the healthcare team. As with all cancers, management of survivorship issues and optimization of quality of life are essential concerns.

REFERENCES

1. American Cancer Society. *Cancer Facts & Figures 2007*. Atlanta, GA: Author; 2007.
2. National Cancer Institute. What you need to know about prostate cancer. http://www.cancer.gov/cancertopics/wyntk/prostate/page4. Accessed January 4, 2009.

3. American Cancer Society. *Cancer reference information: Detailed guide: Prostate cancer.* http://www.cancer.org/docroot/CRI/CRI_2_3x.asp?dt=36. Accessed June 27, 2007.

4. Lagomarcino Ledesma N, Myers JS. Prostate cancer. In: Kogut VJ, Luthringer SL, eds. *Nutritional Issues in Cancer Care.* Pittsburgh, PA: Oncology Nursing Society; 2005:153–186.

5. Carroll PR, Carducci MR, Zietman AL, Rothaermal JM. *Report to the Nation on Prostate Cancer: A Guide for Men and Their Families.* Santa Monica, CA: Prostate Cancer Foundation; 2005.

6. Israeli RS, Ryan CW, Jung LL. Managing bone loss in men with locally advanced prostate cancer receiving androgen deprivation therapy. *J Urol.* 2008;179(2): 414–423.

7. Malcolm JB, Derweesh IH, Kincade MC, et al. Osteoporosis and fractures after androgen deprivation initiation for prostate cancer. *Can J Urol.* 2007;14(3):3551–3559.

8. Heber D, Fair W, Ornish D. *Nutrition and Prostate Cancer: A Monograph from the CaP CURE Nutrition Project.* 2nd ed. Capcure; January 1999. http://www.capcure .org.il/abstracts/pub-pdf/nutrition.pdf.

9. Byers T, Nestle M, McTiernan A, et al.; American Cancer Society 2001 Nutrition and Physical Activity Guidelines Advisory Committee. American Cancer Society guidelines on nutrition and physical activity for cancer prevention: Reducing the risk of cancer with healthy food choices and physical activity. *CA: Cancer J Clin.* 2002;52(2):92–119.

10. Ornish D, Weidner G, Fair WR, Marlin R, Pettengill EB. Intensive lifestyle changes may affect the progression of prostate cancer. *J Urol.* 2005;174(3): 1065–1069.

11. Saxe GA, Major JM, Nguyen JY, Freeman KM, Downs TM. Potential attenuation of disease progression in recurrent prostate cancer with plant-based diet and stress reduction. *Integr Cancer Ther.* 2006;5(3):206–213.

12 Dubenmier JJ, Weidner G, Marlin R, Crutchfield L, Dunn-Emke S. Lifestyle and health-related quality of life of men with prostate cancer managed with active surveillance. *Urol.* 2006;67(1):125–130.

13. Sunny L. A low fat diet rich in fruits and vegetables may reduce the risk of developing prostate cancer. *Asian Pac J Cancer Prev.* 2005;6(4):490–496.

14. Nguyen JY, Major JM, Knott CJ, Freeman KM, Downs TM. Adoption of a plant-based diet by patients with recurrent prostate cancer. *Integr Cancer Ther.* 2006; 5(3):214–223.

15. Hodge AM, English DR, McCredie MR, et al. Foods, nutrients and prostate cancer. *Cancer Causes Control.* 2004;15(1):11–20.

16. Deneo-Pellegrini H, De Stefani E, Ronco A, Mendilaharsu M. Foods, nutrients and prostate cancer: A case-control study in Uruguay. *Brit J Cancer.* 1999;80(3–4): 591–597.

17. Kolonel LN, Hankin JH, Whittemore AS, et al. Vegetables, fruits, legumes and prostate cancer: A multiethnic case-control study. *Cancer Epidemiol Biomarkers Prev.* 2000;9(8):795–804.

18. Norrish AE, Jackson RT, Sharpe SJ, Skeaff CM. Prostate cancer and dietary carotenoids. *Am J Epidemiol.* 2000;151(2):119–123.

19. Wu K, Erdman JW Jr, Schwartz SJ, et al. Plasma and dietary carotenoids, and the risk of prostate cancer: A nested case-control study. *Cancer Epidemiol Biomarkers Prev.* 2004;13(2):260–269.

20. Giovannucci E, Liu Y, Platz EA, Stampfer MJ, Willett WC. Risk factors for prostate cancer incidence and progression in the Health Professionals Follow-up Study. *Int J Cancer.* 2007;121(7):1571–1578.

21. Hwang ES, Bowen PE. Can the consumption of tomatoes or lycopene reduce cancer risk? *Integr Cancer Ther.* 2002;1(2):121–132.

22. Lu QY, Hung JC, Heber D, et al. Inverse associations between plasma lycopene and other carotenoids and prostate cancer. *Cancer Epidemiol Biomarkers Prev.* 2001;10(7):749–756.

23. Zhang J, Dhakal I, Stone A, et al. Plasma carotenoids and prostate cancer: A population-based case-control study in Arkansas. *Nutr Cancer.* 2007;59(1):46–53.

24. Key TJ, Appleby PN, Allen NE, et al. Plasma carotenoids, retinol, and tocopherols and the risk of prostate cancer in the European Prospective Investigation into Cancer and Nutrition Study. *Am J Clin Nutr.* 2007;86(3):672–681.

25. Mucci LA, Tamimi R, Lagiou P, et al. Are dietary influences on the risk of prostate cancer mediated through the insulin-like growth factor system? *BJU Intl.* 2001;87(9):814–820.

26. Fraser ML, Lee AH, Binns CW. Lycopene and prostate cancer: Emerging evidence. *Expert Rev Anticancer Ther.* 2005;5(5):847–854.

27. Boileau TW, Liao Z, Kim S, et al. Prostate carcinogenesis in *N*-methyl-*N*-nitrosourea (NMU)-testosterone-treated rats fed tomato powder, lycopene, or energy-restricted diets. *J Natl Cancer Inst.* 2003;95(21):1578–1586.

28. Weisburger JH. Evaluation of the evidence on the role of tomato products in disease prevention. *Proc Soc Exp Biol Med.* 1998;218(2):140–143.

29. Wang L, Liu D, Ahmed T, et al. Targeting cell cycle machinery as a molecular mechanism of sulforaphane in prostate cancer prevention. *Intl J Oncol.* 2004;24(1):187–192.

30. Chinni SR, Li Y, Upadhyay S, Koppolu PK, Sarkar FH. Indole-3-carbinol (I3C) induced cell growth inhibition, G_1 cell cycle arrest and apoptosis in prostate cancer cells. *Oncogene.* 2001;20(23):2927–2936.

31. Canene-Adams K, Lindshield BL, Wang S, Jeffery EH, Clinton SK, Erdman JW Jr. Combinations of tomato and broccoli enhance antitumor activity in dunning r3327-h prostate adenocarcinomas. *Cancer Res.* 2007;67(2):836–843.

32. Kirsh VA, Peters U, Mayne ST, et al. Prospective study of fruit and vegetable intake and risk of prostate cancer. *J Natl Cancer Inst.* 2007;99(15):1200–1209.

33. Souli E, Machluf M, Morgenstern A, Sabo E, Yannai S. Indole-3-carbinol (I3C) exhibits inhibitory and preventive effects on prostate tumors in mice. *Food Chem Toxicol.* 2008;46(3):863–870.

34. Brooks JD, Paton VG, Vidanes G. Potent induction of phase 2 enzymes in human prostate cells by sulforaphane. *Cancer Epidemiol Biomarkers Prev.* 2001;10(9):949–954.

35. Li Y, Li X, Sarkar FH. Gene expression profiles of I3C- and DIM-treated PC3 human prostate cancer cells determined by cDNA microarray analysis. *J Nutr.* 2003;133(4):1011–1019.

36. Malik A, Afaq F, Sarfaraz S, Adhami VM, Syed DN, Mukhtar H. Pomegranate fruit juice for chemoprevention and chemotherapy of prostate cancer. *Proc Natl Acad Sci USA.* 2005;102(41):14813–14818.

37. Toi M, Bando H, Ramachandran C, et al. Preliminary studies on the anti-angiogenic potential of pomegranate fractions in vitro and in vivo. *Angiogenesis.* 2003;6(2):121–128.

38. Seeram NP, Aronson WJ, Zhang Y, et al. Pomegranate ellagitannin-derived metabolites inhibit prostate cancer growth and localize to the mouse prostate gland. *J Agric Food Chem*. 2007;55(19):7732–7737.

39. Sartippour MR, Seeram NP, Rao JY, et al. Ellagitannin-rich pomegranate extract inhibits angiogenesis in prostate cancer in vitro and in vivo. *Int J Oncol*. 2008;32 (2):475–480.

40. Pantuck AJ, Leppert JT, Zomorodian N, et al. Phase II study of pomegranate juice for men with rising prostate-specific antigen following surgery or radiation for prostate cancer. *Clin Cancer Res*. 2006;12(13):4018–4026.

41. Pierce JP, Faerber S, Wright FA, et al. A randomized trial of the effect of a plant-based dietary pattern on additional breast cancer events and survival: The Women's Healthy Eating and Living (WHEL) study. *Control Clin Trials*. 2002;23 (6):728–756.

42. Pelucchi C, Talamini R, Galeone C, et al. Fibre intake and prostate cancer risk. *Intl J Cancer*. 2004;109(2):278–280.

43. Tymchuk CN, Barnard RJ, Heber D, Aronson WJ. Evidence of an inhibitory effect of diet and exercise on prostate cancer cell growth. *J Urol*. 2001;166(3): 1185–1189.

44. Hebert JR, Hurley TG, Olendzki BC, et al. Nutritional and socioeconomic factors in relation to prostate cancer mortality: A cross-national study. *J Natl Cancer Inst*. 1998;90(21):1637–1647.

45. Harris PJ, Roberton AM, Watson ME, Triggs CM, Ferguson LR. The effects of soluble-fiber polysaccharides on the adsorption of a hydrophobic carcinogen to an insoluble dietary fiber. *Nutr Cancer*. 1993;19(1):43–54.

46. Slavin JL. Mechanisms for the impact of whole grain foods on cancer risk. *J Am Coll Nutr*. 2000;19(3)(suppl):300S–307S.

47. Slavin J. Why whole grains are protective: Biological mechanisms. *Proc Nutr Soc*. 2003;62(1):129–134.

48. Chatenoud L, La Vecchia C, Franceschi S, et al. Refined-cereal intake and risk of selected cancers in Italy. *Am J Clin Nutr*. 1999;70(6):1107–1110.

49. Dewell A, Weidner G, Sumner MD, et al. Relationship of dietary protein and soy isoflavones to serum IGF-1 and IGF binding proteins in the Prostate Cancer Lifestyle Trial. *Nutr Cancer*. 2007;58(1):35–42.

50. Aksoy Y, Aksoy H, Bakan E, Atmaca AF, Akcay F. Serum insulin-like growth factor-I and insulin-like growth factor-binding protein-3 in localized, metastasized prostate cancer and benign prostatic hyperplasia. *Urol Intl*. 2004;72(1):62–65.

51. Barnard RJ, Ngo TH, Leung PS, Aronson WJ, Golding LA. A low-fat diet and/or strenuous exercise alters the IGF axis in vivo and reduces prostate tumor cell growth in vitro. *Prostate*. 2003;56(3):201–206.

52. Moyad MA. The use of complementary/preventive medicine to prevent prostate cancer recurrence/progression following definitive therapy: Part I—lifestyle changes. *Curr Opin Urol*. 2003;13(2):137–145.

53. Grimberg A. Mechanisms by which IGF-I may promote cancer. *Cancer Biol Ther*. 2003;2(6):630–635.

54. Venkateswaran V, Haddad AQ, Fleshner NE, et al. Association of diet-induced hyperinsulinemia with accelerated growth of prostate cancer (LNCaP) xenografts. *J Natl Cancer Inst*. 2007;99(23):1793–1800.

55. Freedland SJ, Mavropoulos J, Wang A, et al. Carbohydrate restriction, prostate cancer growth, and the insulin-like growth factor axis. *Prostate*. 2008;68(1):11–19.

56. Colli JL, Colli A. Comparisons of prostate cancer mortality rates with dietary practices in the United States. *Urol Oncol.* 2005;23(6):390–398.

57. Nowell S, Ratnasinghe DL, Ambrosone CB, et al. Association of *SULT1A1* phenotype and genotype with prostate cancer risk in African-Americans and Caucasians. *Cancer Epidemiol Biomarkers Prev.* 2004;13(2):270–276.

58. Hu JJ, Hall MC, Grossman L, et al. Deficient nucleotide excision repair capacity enhances human prostate cancer risk. *Cancer Res.* 2004;64(3):1197–1201.

59. Ferguson LR. Meat consumption, cancer risk and population groups within New Zealand. *Mutation Res.* 2002;506–507:215–224.

60. Koutros S, Cross AJ, Sandler DP, et al. Meat and meat mutagens and risk of prostate cancer in the agricultural health study. *Cancer Epidemiol Biomarkers Prev.* 2008; 17(1):80–87.

61. Bogen KT, Keating GA 2nd, Chan JM, et al. Highly elevated PSA and dietary PhIP intake in a prospective clinic-based study among African Americans. *Prostate Cancer Prostatic Dis.* 2007;10(3):261–269.

62. Creton SK, Zhu H, Gooderham NJ. The cooked meat carcinogen 2-amino-1-methyl-6-phenylimidazo(4,5-*b*)pyridine activates the extracellular signal regulated kinase mitogen-activated protein kinase pathway. *Cancer Res.* 2007;67(23): 11455–11462.

63. Tseng M, Breslow RA, Graubard BI, Ziegler RG. Dairy, calcium, and vitamin D intakes and prostate cancer risk in the National Health and Nutrition Examination epidemiologic follow-up study cohort. *Am J Clin Nutr.* 2005;81(5):1147–1154.

64. Ahn J, Albanes D, Peters U, et al. Dairy products, calcium intake, and risk of prostate cancer in the prostate, lung, colorectal, and ovarian cancer screening trial. *Cancer Epidemiol Biomarkers Prev.* 2007;16(12):2623–2630.

65. Park SY, Murphy SP, Wilkens LR, Stram DO, Henderson BE, Kolonel LN. Calcium, vitamin D, and dairy product intake and prostate cancer risk: The Multiethnic Cohort Study. *Am J Epidemiol.* 2007;166(11):1259–1269.

66. Park Y, Mitrou PN, Kipnis V, Hollenbeck A, Schatzkin A, Leitzmann MF. Calcium, dairy foods, and risk of incident and fatal prostate cancer: the NIH–AARP Diet and Health Study. *Am J Epidemiol.* 2007;166(11):1270–1279.

67. Grant WB. An ecologic study of dietary links to prostate cancer. *Altern Med Rev.* 1999;4(3):162–169.

68. Kesse E, Bertrais S, Astorg P, Jauen A, Arnault N. Dairy products, calcium and phosphorus intake, and the risk of prostate cancer: Results of the French prospective SU.VI.MAX (Supplementation en Vitamines et Mineraux Antioxydants) study. *Br J Nutr.* 2006;95(3):539–545.

69. Gunnell D, Oliver SE, Peters TJ, et al. Are diet–prostate cancer associations mediated by the IGF axis? A cross-sectional analysis of diet, IGF-I and IGFBP-3 in healthy middle-aged men. *Br J Cancer.* 2003;88(11):1682–1686.

70. Nagata Y, Sonoda T, Mori M, et al. Dietary isoflavones may protect against prostate cancer in Japanese men. *J Nutr.* 2007;137(8):1974–1979.

71. Yan L, Spitznagel EL. Meta-analysis of soy food and risk of prostate cancer in men. *Intl J Cancer.* 2005;117(4):667–669.

72. Hamilton-Reeves JM, Rebello SA, Thomas W, Slaton JW, Kurzer MS. Soy protein isolate increases urinary estrogens and the ratio of 2:16-alpha-hydroxyestrone in men at high risk of prostate cancer. *J Nutr.* 2007;137(10):2258–2263.

73. Yi MA, Son HM, Lee JS, et al. Regulation of male sex hormone levels by soy isoflavones in rats. *Nutr Cancer.* 2002;42(2):206–210.

74. Messina M, Kucuk O, Lampe JW. An overview of the health effects of isoflavones with an emphasis on prostate cancer risk and prostate-specific antigen levels. *J AOAC Intl*. 2006;89(4):1121–1134.

75. Leone M, Zhai D, Sareth S, Kitada S, Reed JC, Pellecchia M. Cancer prevention by tea polyphenols is linked to their direct inhibition of antiapoptotic Bcl-2-family proteins. *Cancer Res*. 2003;63(23):8118–8121.

76. Bettuzzi S, Rizzi F, Belloni L. Clinical relevance of the inhibitory effect of green tea catechins (GtCs) on prostate cancer progression in combination with molecular profiling of catechin-resistant tumors: An integrated view. *Pol J Vet Sci*. 2007;10 (1):57–60.

77. Gupta S, Hussain T, Mukhtar H. Molecular pathway for (–)-epigallocatechin-3-gallate-induced cell cycle arrest and apoptosis of human prostate carcinoma cells. *Arch Biochem Biophys*. 2003;410(1):177–185.

78. Yu HN, Yin JJ, Shen SR. Growth inhibition of prostate cancer cells by epigallocatechin gallate in the presence of Cu^{2+}. *J Agric Food Chem*. 2004;52(3):462–466.

79. Brusselmans K, De Schrijver E, Heyns W, Verhoeven G, Swinnen JV. Epigallocatechin-3-gallate is a potent natural inhibitor of fatty acid synthase in intact cells and selectively induces apoptosis in prostate cancer cells. *Intl J Cancer*. 2003;106 (6):856–862.

80. Gupta S, Srivastava M, Ahmad N, et al. Lipoxygenase-5 is overexpressed in prostate adenocarcinoma. *Cancer*. 2001;91(4):737–743.

81. Kikuchi N, Ohmori K, Shimazu T, et al. No association between green tea and prostate cancer risk in Japanese men: The Ohsaki Cohort Study. *Br J Cancer*. 2006;95(3):371–373.

82. Eder E. Intraindividual variations of DNA adduct levels in humans. *Mutation Res*. 1999;424(1–2):249–261.

83. Zhou JR, Yu L, Zhong Y, Blackburn GL. Soy phytochemicals and tea bioactive components synergistically inhibit androgen-sensitive human prostate tumors in mice. *J Nutr*. 2003;133(2):516–521.

84. Jian L, Lee AH, Binns CW. Tea and lycopene protect against prostate cancer. *Asia Pac J Clin Nutr*. 2007;16(suppl 1):453–457.

85. Fleshner N, Bagnell PS, Klotz L, Venkateswaran V. Dietary fat and prostate cancer. *J Urol*. 2004;171(2 pt 2):S19–S24.

86. Williams GM, Williams CL, Weisburger JH. Diet and cancer prevention: The fiber first diet. *Toxicol Sci*. 1999;52(2)(suppl):72–86.

87. Kushi L, Giovannucci E. Dietary fat and cancer. *Amer J Med*. 2002;113(suppl 9B): 63S–70S.

88. Meyer F, Bairati I, Fradet Y, Moore L. Dietary energy and nutrients in relation to preclinical prostate cancer. *Nutr Cancer*. 1997;29(2):120–126.

89. Fradet Y, Meyer F, Bairati I, Shadmani R, Moore L. Dietary fat and prostate cancer progression and survival. *Eur Urol*.1999;35(5–6):388–391.

90. Bosetti C, Tzonou A, Lagiou P, et al. Fraction of prostate cancer incidence attributed to diet in Athens, Greece. *Euro J Cancer Prev*. 2000;9(2):119–123.

91. Bairati I, Meyer F, Fradet Y, Moore L. Dietary fat and advanced prostate cancer. *J Urol*. 1998;159(4):1271–1275

92. Michaud DS, Augustsson K, Rimm EB, et al. A prospective study on intake of animal products and risk of prostate cancer. *Cancer Causes Control*. 2001;12(6):557–567.

93. Ramon JM, Bou R, Romea S, et al. Dietary fat intake and prostate cancer risk: A case-control study in Spain. *Cancer Causes Control*. 2000;11(8):679–685.

94. Chavarro JE, Stampfer MJ, Campos H, Kurth T, Willett WC, Ma J. A prospective study of *trans*-fatty acid levels in blood and risk of prostate cancer. *Cancer Epidemiol Biomarkers Prev*. 2008;17:95–101.

95. Liu X, Schumacher FR, Plummer SJ, Jorgenson E, Casey G, Witte JS. *Trans*-fatty acid intake and increased risk of advanced prostate cancer: Modification by RNASEL R462Q variant. *Carcinogenesis*. 2007;28(6):1232–1236.

96. King IB, Kristal AR, Schaffer S, Thornquist M, Goodman GE. Serum *trans*-fatty acids are associated with risk of prostate cancer in beta-Carotene and Retinol Efficacy Trial. *Cancer Epidemiol Biomarkers Prev*. 2005;14(4):988–992.

97. Ritch CR, Wan RL, Stephens LB, et al. Dietary fatty acids correlate with prostate cancer biopsy grade and volume in Jamaican men. *J Urol*. 2007;177(1):97–101.

98. Kelavkar UP, Hutzley J, Dhir R, et al. Prostate tumor growth and recurrence can be modulated by the omega-6:omega-3 ratio in diet: Athymic mouse xenograft model simulating radical prostatectomy. *Neoplasia*. 2006;8(2):112–124.

99. Berquin IM, Min Y, Wu R, et al. Modulation of prostate cancer genetic risk by omega-3 and omega-6 fatty acids. *J Clin Invest*. 2007;117(7):1866–1875.

100. Hughes-Fulford M, Li CF, Boonyaratanakornkit J, Sayyah S. Arachidonic acid activates phosphatidylinositol 3-kinase signaling and induces gene expression in prostate cancer. *Cancer Res*. 2006;66(3):1427–1433.

101. Hedelin M, Chang ET, Wiklund F, et al. Association of frequent consumption of fatty fish with prostate cancer risk is modified by COX-2 polymorphism. *Intl J Cancer*. 2007;120(2):398–405.

102. Chan JM, Holick CN, Leitzmann MF, et al. Diet after diagnosis and the risk of prostate cancer progression, recurrence, and death (United States). *Cancer Causes Control*. 2006;17(2):199–208.

103. Rose DP, Connolly JM. Effects of fatty acids and eicosanoid synthesis inhibitors on the growth of two human prostate cancer cell lines. *Prostate*. 1991;18(3):243–254.

104. Davis BC, Kris-Etherton PM. Achieving optimal essential fatty acid status in vegetarians: Current knowledge and practical implications. *Amer J Clin Nutr*. 2003;78 (3)(suppl):640S–646S.

105. Doughman SD, Krupanidhi S, Sanjeevi CB. Omega-3 fatty acids for nutrition and medicine: Considering microalgae oil as a vegetarian source of EPA and DHA. *Curr Diabetes Rev*. 2007;3(3):198–203.

106. Gerster H. Can adults adequately convert alpha-linolenic acid (18:3n-3) to eicosapentaenoic acid (20:5n-3) and docosahexaenoic acid (22:6n-3)? *Intl J Vitamin Nutr Res*. 1998;68(3):159–173.

107. Giovannucci E, Rimm EB, Colditz GA, et al. A prospective study of dietary fat and risk of prostate cancer. *J Natl Cancer Inst*. 1993;85(19):1571–1579.

108. De Stefani E, Deneo-Pellegrini H, Boffetta P, Ronco A, Mendilaharsu M. Alpha-linolenic acid and risk of prostate cancer: A case-control study in Uruguay. *Cancer Epidemiol Biomarkers Prev*. 2000;9(3):335–338.

109. Demark-Wahnefried W, Price DT, Polascik TJ, et al. Pilot study of dietary fat restriction and flaxseed supplementation in men with prostate cancer before surgery: Exploring the effects on hormonal levels, prostate-specific antigen, and histopathologic features. *Urol*. 2001;58(1):47–52.

110. Moyad MA. *The ABCs of Nutrition and Supplements for Prostate Cancer*. Ann Arbor, MI: JW Edwards; 2000.

111. Lin X, Gingrich JR, Bao W, et al. Effect of flaxseed supplementation on prostatic carcinoma in transgenic mice. *Urol*. 2002;60(5):919–924.

112. Denis L, Morton MS, Griffiths K. Diet and its preventive role in prostatic disease. *Eur Urol*. 1999;35(5–6):377–387.
113. Hughes-Fulford M, Chen Y, Tjandrawinata RR. Fatty acid regulates gene expression and growth of human prostate cancer PC-3 cells. *Carcinogenesis*. 2001;22(5): 701–707.
114. Norrish AE, Jackson RT, Sharpe SJ, Skeaff CM. Men who consume vegetable oils rich in monounsaturated fat: Their dietary patterns and risk of prostate cancer (New Zealand). *Cancer Causes Control*. 2000;11(7):609–615.
115. Gonzalez CA, Salas-Salvado J. The potential of nuts in the prevention of cancer. *Br J Nutr*. 2006;96(suppl 2):S87–S94.
116. Lu QY, Arteaga JR, Zhang Q, et al. Inhibition of prostate cancer cell growth by an avocado extract: Role of lipid-soluble bioactive substances. *J Nutr Biochem*. 2005; 16(1):23–30.
117. Corcoran NM, Najdovska M, Costello AJ. Inorganic selenium retards progression of experimental hormone refractory prostate cancer. *J Urol*. 2004;171(2 pt 1): 907–910.
118. Sinha R, El-Bayoumy K. Apoptosis is a critical cellular event in cancer chemoprevention and chemotherapy by selenium compounds. *Curr Cancer Drug Targets*. 2004;4(1):13–28.
119. Clark LC, Dalkin B, Krongrad A, et al. Decreased incidence of prostate cancer with selenium supplementation: Results of a double-blind cancer prevention trial. *Brit J Urol*. 1998;81(5):730–734.
120. Giovannucci E, Rimm EB, Wolk A, et al. Calcium and fructose intake in relation to risk of prostate cancer. *Cancer Res*. 1998;58(3):442–447.
121. Yoshizawa K, Willett WC, Morris SJ, et al. Study of prediagnostic selenium level in toenails and the risk of advanced prostate cancer. *J Natl Cancer Inst*. 1998;90(16): 1219–1224.
122. Hartman TJ, Dorgan JF, Woodson K, et al. Effects of long-term alpha-tocopherol supplementation on serum hormones in older men. *Prostate*. 2001;46(1):33–38.
123. Peters U, Littman AJ, Kristal AR, Patterson RE, Potter JD, White E. Vitamin E and selenium supplementation and risk of prostate cancer in the Vitamins and Lifestyle (VITAL) study cohort. *Cancer Causes Control*. 2008;19(1):75–87.
124. Brooks JD, Metter EJ, Chan DW, et al. Plasma selenium level before diagnosis and the risk of prostate cancer development. *J Urol*. 2001;166(6):2034–2038.
125. Alkhenizan A, Hafez K. The role of vitamin E in the prevention of cancer: A meta-analysis of randomized controlled trials. *Ann Saudi Med*. 2007;27(6):409–414.
126. Surapaneni KM, Ramana V. Erythrocyte ascorbic acid and plasma vitamin E status in patients with carcinoma of prostate. *Indian J Physiol Pharmacol*. 2007;51(2): 199–202.
127. Weinstein SJ, Wright ME, Lawson KA, et al. Serum and dietary vitamin E in relation to prostate cancer risk. *Cancer Epidemiol Biomarkers Prev*. 2007;16(6): 1253–1259.
128. Zu K, Ip C. Synergy between selenium and vitamin E in apoptosis induction is associated with activation of distinctive initiator caspases in human prostate cancer cells. *Cancer Res*. 2003;63(20):6988–6995.
129. Jiang Q, Christen S, Shigenaga MK, Ames BN. Gamma-tocopherol, the major form of vitamin E in the US diet, deserves more attention. *Amer J Clin Nutr*. 2001;74(6):714–722.

130. Chopra RK, Bhagavan HN. Relative bioavailabilities of natural and synthetic vitamin E formulations containing mixed tocopherols in human subjects. *Intl J Vit Nutr Res.* 1999;69(2):92–95.

131. Handelman GJ, Epstein WL, Peerson J, Spiegelman D, Machlin LJ, Dratz EA. Human adipose alpha-tocopherol and gamma-tocopherol kinetics during and after 1 y of alpha-tocopherol supplementation. *Amer J Clin Nutr.* 1994;59(5): 1025–1032.

132. Wright ME, Weinstein SJ, Lawson KA, et al. Supplemental and dietary vitamin E intakes and risk of prostate cancer in a large prospective study. *Cancer Epidemiol Biomarkers Prev.* 2007;16(6):1128–1135.

133. Helzlsouer KJ, Huang HY, Alberg AJ, et al. Association between alpha-tocopherol, gamma-tocopherol, selenium, and subsequent prostate cancer. *J Natl Cancer Inst.* 2000;92(24):2018–2023.

134. Huang HY, Alberg AJ, Norkus EP, et al. Prospective study of antioxidant micronutrients in the blood and the risk of developing prostate cancer. *Amer J Epidemiol.* 2003;157(4):335–344.

135. Galli F, Stabile AM, Betti M, et al. The effect of alpha- and gamma-tocopherol and their carboxyethyl hydroxychroman metabolites on prostate cancer cell proliferation. *Arch Biochem Biophys.* 2004;423(1):97–102.

136. Malafa MP, Fokum FD, Andoh J, et al. Vitamin E succinate suppresses prostate tumor growth by inducing apoptosis. *Int J Cancer.* 2006;118(10):2441–2447.

137. Gao X, LaValley MP, Tucker KL. Prospective studies of dairy product and calcium intakes and prostate cancer risk: A meta-analysis. *J Natl Cancer Inst.* 2005;97(23): 1768–1777.

138. Giovannucci E, Liu Y, Stampfer MJ, Willett WC. A prospective study of calcium intake and incident and fatal prostate cancer. *Cancer Epidemiol Biomarkers Prev.* 2006;15(2):203–210.

139. Peehl DM, Krishnan AV, Feldman D. Pathways mediating the growth-inhibitory actions of vitamin D in prostate cancer. *J Nutr.* 2003;133(7)(suppl): 2461S–2469S.

140. Chen TC, Wang L, Whitlatch LW, Flanagan JN, Holick MF. Prostatic 25-hydroxyvitamin D-1-alpha-hydroxylase and its implication in prostate cancer. *J Cell Biochem.* 2003;88(2):315–322.

141. Gross C, Stamey T, Hancock S, Feldman D. Treatment of early recurrent prostate cancer with 1,25-dihydroxyvitamin D$_3$ (calcitriol). *J Urol.* 1998;159(6):2035–2039.

142. Ahonen MH, Tenkanen L, Teppo L, Hakama M, Tuohimaa P. Prostate cancer risk and prediagnostic serum 25-hydroxyvitamin D levels (Finland). *Cancer Causes Control.* 2000;11(9):847–852.

143. Tuohimaa P, Tenkanen L, Ahonen M, et al. Both high and low levels of blood vitamin D are associated with a higher prostate cancer risk: A longitudinal, nested case-control study in the Nordic countries. *Intl J Cancer.* 2004;108(1):104–108.

144. Giovannucci E, Liu Y, Rimm EB, et al. Prospective study of predictors of vitamin D status and cancer incidence and mortality in men. *J Natl Cancer Inst.* 2006;98 (7):451–459.

145. Thomas MK, Lloyd-Jones DM, Thadhani RI, et al. Hypovitaminosis D in medical inpatients. *New Engl J Med.* 1998;338:777–778.

146. Rasmussen LB, Hansen GL, Hansen E, et al. Vitamin D: Should the supply in the Danish population be increased? *Intl J Food Sci Nutr.* 2000;51(3):209–215.

147. Webb AR, Pilbeam C, Hanafin N, Holick MF. An evaluation of the relative contributions of exposure to sunlight and of diet to the circulating concentrations of 25-hydroxyvitamin D in an elderly nursing home population in Boston. *Amer J Clin Nutr.* 1990;51:1075–1081.

148. Silverberg SJ, Shane E, de la Cruz L, et al. Vitamin D hydroxylation abnormalities in parathyroid hormone secretion and 1,25-dihydroxyvitamin D-3 formation in women with osteoporosis. *New Engl J Med.* 1989;320:277–281.

149. Bischoff-Ferrari HA, Giovannucci E, Willett WC, Dietrich T, Dawson-Hughes B. Estimation of optimal serum concentrations of 25-hydroxyvitamin D for multiple health outcomes. *Am J Clin Nutr.* 2006;84(1):18–28.

150. Demark-Wahnefried W, Moyad MA. Dietary intervention in the management of prostate cancer. *Curr Opin Urol.* 2007;17(3):168–174.

151. Freedland SJ, Platz EA. Obesity and prostate cancer: Making sense out of apparently conflicting data. *Epidemiol Rev.* 2007;29:88–97.

152. Bañez LL, Hamilton RJ, Partin AW, et al. Obesity-related plasma hemodilution and PSA concentration among men with prostate cancer. *JAMA.* 2007;298(19): 2275–2280.

153. Bassett WW, Cooperberg MR, Sadetsky N, et al. Impact of obesity on prostate cancer recurrence after radical prostatectomy: Data from CaPSURE. *Urol.* 2005;66(5): 1060–1065.

154. Nilsen TI, Romundstad PR, Vatten LJ. Recreational physical activity and risk of prostate cancer: A prospective population-based study in Norway (the HUNT study). *Int J Cancer.* 2006;119(12):2943–2947.

155. Barnard RJ, Leung PS, Aronson WJ, Cohen P, Golding LA. A mechanism to explain how regular exercise might reduce the risk for clinical prostate cancer. *Eur J Cancer Prev.* 2007;16(5):415–421.

156. Tymchuk CN, Barnard RJ, Heber D, Aronson WJ. Evidence of an inhibitory effect of diet and exercise on prostate cancer cell growth. *J Urol.* 2001;166(3):1185–1189.

157. Schneider CM, Hsieh CC, Sprod LK, Carter SD, Hayward R. Cancer treatment-induced alterations in muscular fitness and quality of life: The role of exercise training. *Ann Oncol.* 2007;18(12):1957–1962.

Chapter 11

Lung Cancer

Jayne M. Camporeale, MS, RN, OCN, APN-C
Susan Roberts, MS, RD, LD, CNSD

INTRODUCTION

One of the most difficult and challenging areas of oncology involves the treatment of lung cancer, which is largely a disease of the twentieth century. Before 1930, there were few reported cases. In the 1930s, however, a sharp rise in mortality from lung cancer was noted. By the mid-1950s, lung cancer had become the leading cause of cancer mortality in men—a dubious distinction that it maintains today. Eventually women caught up to men, with 1986 being the first year that more women died from lung cancer than breast cancer.[1] Today, lung cancer remains the leading cause of cancer mortality in men and women in the United States. Death rates from this cause for 2008 are estimated to be 161,840.[2] Worldwide, in 1990, lung cancer was the most frequently diagnosed cancer in terms of both incidence and mortality, with 1.04 million new cases being identified, accounting for 12.8% of all cancer cases.[3]

Every area of oncology has its own challenges in advancing treatment. Unfortunately, research funding for optimal treatments in lung cancer lags behind other cancer research areas, perhaps because lung cancer is most often attributed to smoking and, therefore, is considered a preventable cancer. As yet, researchers have not found a low-cost, effective screening tool for lung cancer, which poses yet another barrier to research in this area. The disease is usually asymptomatic in the early stages, so most patients are diagnosed at an advanced stage of disease. Fewer than 15% of lung cancers are localized when diagnosed, and only 20% of patients present with lung cancer that makes them candidates for curative treatment.[4] The one-year relative survival rate for lung cancer is 41%, which is 7% higher than the corresponding rate in the 1970s. This improvement is probably related to improved surgical techniques and the use of combined therapies to treat lung cancer.[2] Unfortunately, the five-year survival rate for individuals diagnosed with all stages combined remains a paltry 15%.

Ideally, clinical advances made during the last 20 years will lead to improved outcomes in lung cancer. In the 1990s, the development of low-dose computerized tomography (CT) scanning advanced the treatment of lung cancer.[5] The advent of positron emission tomography/computerized tomography (PET/CT) scanning in the 2000s has further improved lung cancer treatment planning and increased diagnostic accuracy. Finally, a better understanding of the genetic alterations involved in the development of lung cancer is emerging and may result in development of a variety of treatment options.

Background

As the number of lung cancer cases began to increase in the 1930s, speculation about the source of this disease was directed toward two suspected culprits: air pollution and smoking.[6] By 1950, the first definitive epidemiologic studies on smoking and lung cancer were published. These case-controlled studies associated smoking with lung cancer. These studies compared lung cancer patients who smoked with smokers who did not have lung cancer.[6, 7]

In 1964, the office of the U.S. Surgeon General released its landmark report on smoking and health, which concluded that smoking is causally related to lung cancer in men and (despite the availability of fewer data at the time) probably women, too.[8] Since the release of this report, epidemiologic research on lung cancer has been conducted with increased frequency. Although cigarette smoking has remained a central theme in these studies, other causes have been evaluated. After nearly 60 years of research, numerous environmental causes of lung cancer have been identified. Genetics may also play a key role in determining a particular individual's susceptibility to these carcinogens, but the full genomic picture has yet to be identified, and the interplay between genetics and smoking has yet to be fully elucidated.[6]

Incidence of Lung Cancer

Worldwide, lung cancer is the most common and deadly form of cancer, accounting for 1.35 million of the 10.9 million cancer cases expected to be diagnosed in 2008. In 2008, the number of newly diagnosed cancer cases involving the respiratory system, which includes cancers of the larynx, lung, bronchus, and other respiratory organs, was expected to be approximately 232,270 in the United States. Of these new cases, 127,880 were predicted to affect men and 104,390 were predicted to affect women.[2] In the United

States, more people die from lung cancer than from prostate, breast, and colorectal cancer combined.[4]

Although the rate of lung cancer has peaked and is now on the decline in both the United States and the United Kingdom, lung cancer tends to be more common in developed countries. The lowest and highest rates of lung cancer in the United States are found in Utah and Kentucky, respectively, where the lowest and highest smoking prevalence rates are also found.[9] Globally, people in developing countries such as those in East Asia—and especially China—are consuming an increasing proportion of the world's tobacco; by 2010, people in these areas are expected to account for 71% of world tobacco consumption. Two-thirds of all adult Chinese men are smokers by age 25, accounting for one-third of all smokers worldwide.[2, 10] The risk of developing lung cancer is 23 times higher in male smokers and 13 times higher in female smokers compared to lifelong nonsmokers.[2]

Types of Lung Cancer

Lung cancer occurs when normal gene expression goes awry, leading to mutation of an epithelial cell in response to exposure to a carcinogen. The bronchial epithelium of the smoker progresses from squamous metaplasia, to dysplasia, to invasive carcinoma and progressive genomic instability.[1] Many of the genetic defects seen in lung neoplasms are acquired during adult life and are related to exposures to environmental carcinogens. Other genetic events are inherited. Interactions of genes and outside agents likely reflect the activity of environmental agents that alter expression of genes involved in cell cycle regulation, intercellular signaling, cell-cycle arrest, and apoptosis. Susceptible individuals may be at increased risk of lung cancer when they are exposed to even low-dose levels of tobacco smoke or other mutagens.[1] The genetic alterations that occur most commonly are p53 mutations and deletions on chromosomes 3p, 5q, 9p, 11p, and 17p.[4]

The lungs are divided into right and left sides; the right lung is divided into three lobes and the left lung has two lobes. The right and left bronchus arise from the trachea and ultimately branch into smaller airways. A rich network of lymphatic vessels weaves throughout the loose interstitial connective tissues of the lungs, ultimately draining into various lymph node stations (Figure 11.1). This network of lymph vessels, while designed for prevention of illness, makes it possible for lung cancer to metastasize elsewhere, as the lymph drainage may transport the cancer to other body sites.[11] Common sites of metastases in lung cancer include the brain, bones, adrenal glands, and liver.[12]

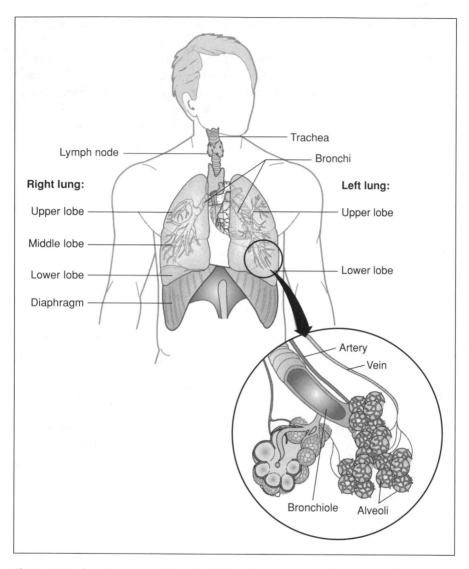

Figure 11.1 *Lung Anatomy and Lymphatic Network*

Four major histologic types of lung cancer are distinguished: squamous cell cancer, adenocarcinoma, and large-cell carcinoma—which are collectively termed non-small-cell lung cancer (NSCLC)—plus small-cell undifferentiated carcinoma, which is also known as small-cell lung cancer (SCLC). Other less commonly occurring lung cancers include undifferentiated cancers, carcinoids, and bronchial gland tumors.[4]

Squamous cell carcinoma is closely correlated with smoking and is more common in men. This type of tumor generally occurs in the larger, more central bronchi, tends to spread locally, and metastasizes later than other patterns.[11] Its pathologic hallmark is the presence of keratin pearls produced by tumor cells with intercellular bridges.[11]

Adenocarcinoma is the most common type of lung cancer in women, young adults, and nonsmokers. Pathologically, intracytoplasmic mucin production is seen with this type of cancer.[11] Adenocarcinoma accounts for the largest subset of NSCLC cases in Western countries and Japan. These lesions are usually more peripheral, smaller, and more slowly growing than squamous cell cancers. Bronchoalveolar carcinoma (BAC) is a subtype of adenocarcinoma whose pattern of neoplastic growth occurs along preexisting alveolar structures without evidence of stromal, vascular, or pleural invasion.[11]

Large-cell carcinomas probably represent squamous cell carcinomas that are so undifferentiated they can no longer be recognized. These tumors are usually found as large peripheral masses with necrosis. On pathology, sheets of round to polygonal cells with prominent nucleoli and pale-staining cytoplasm without differentiating features are seen.[11]

Small-cell carcinoma—the classic oat-cell cancer—is strongly correlated with cigarette smoking, occurring most often in the hilar or central chest, and metastasizing widely.[11] Small-cell cancer pathologically reveals populations of small cells with variable amounts of cytoplasm.[11]

The incidence rates for lung cancer histology have changed over time. Today, NSCLC is the most common lung cancer, accounting for 85–90% of all lung cancers in the United States. Adenocarcinoma accounts for 49% of all NSCLC cases,[4, 7, 13] likely related to changes in smoking habits. The introduction of low-tar cigarettes has been correlated with the increase in adenocarcinoma incidence. It is speculated that filter-cigarette users take larger puffs and retain smoke longer to compensate for the lower nicotine yield. Low-tar cigarettes also enhance the delivery of smoke to the peripheral regions of the lung, where adenocarcinoma is most often found. Additionally, many non-filter-cigarette users who switch to lower-tar cigarettes with filters actually increase their daily cigarette consumption.[14] Filter cigarettes also have a higher nitrate content, and nitrate has been proven to produce adenocarcinoma in lab studies.[4]

SCLC accounts for 15% of all lung cancer cases diagnosed.[15] It is staged in one of two ways: as limited or extensive disease. Only 25% of all SCLC patients will have disease that is truly limited. The World Health Organization classifies SCLC into three cell types: pure or classic, variant cell, or mixed. The subtypes do not have any notable differences in terms of outcome, however. Indeed, the most important prognostic factor for SCLC is stage of disease at time of diagnosis.[4]

Etiology of Lung Cancer

Cigarette Smoke

Trends in population prevalence of cigarette smoking strongly predict lung cancer incidence and mortality. Worldwide, smoking is the main cause of lung cancer.[6] During the period 1997–2001, cigarette smoking and exposure to tobacco smoke resulted in approximately 438,000 premature deaths in the United States and led to $92 billion in productivity losses annually.[16] Multiple economic, political, and social factors impede progress toward elimination of smoking. Smoking dates back to the ancient Mayan civilization. Tobacco's medicinal qualities, addictive properties, and use throughout the years in rituals and ceremonies have made acceptance of its harmful properties more difficult.[17]

In the United States, cigarette smoking decreased in males from 1964, when the U.S. Surgeon General's report was published, until 1990, when the prevalence leveled at 25%; female prevalence reached a plateau shortly after male prevalence entered a steady state.[7] An estimated 45 million Americans currently smoke cigarettes.[2]

The historic smoking trends in the United States offer an explanation for past trends in lung cancer rates and current rates, while also providing predictions for future occurrence. Mortality rates are expected to decrease until 2020, assuming a 30-year lag between population patterns and subsequent incidence, and then to remain constant. By 2030, lung cancer incidence is predicted to be divided equally between males and females.[7] However, smoking does not explain the whole picture of lung cancer: Not all persons who smoke get lung cancer, and 10% of lung cancer cases occur in people who have never smoked.

Other Sources of Nicotine

Second-hand smoke (SHS), also known as environmental tobacco smoke (ETS), is a mixture of sidestream smoke—the smoke given off by the burning end of a tobacco product—and mainstream smoke—the smoke exhaled by smokers.[18] It is primarily emitted from cigarettes, with smaller amounts being given off by pipes and cigars, and contains more than carcinogens.[18] More than 126 million nonsmoking Americans are believed to be exposed to SHS in homes, vehicles, workplaces, and public areas.[2] The U.S. Surgeon General's report entitled *The Health Consequences of Involuntary Exposure to Tobacco Smoke* reported that 3,000 people, or 1.6% of all nonsmoking adults, die annually from breathing SHS.[18] The carcinogens most commonly found in ETS include arsenic, cadmium, benzopyrenes, nitrosamines, and vinyl chloride.[19]

Multiple epidemiologic studies have been conducted on ETS and the development of lung cancer in nonsmokers, mostly involving women.[19] For example, Asomaning and colleagues[20] focused on the effects of SHS exposure relevant to lung development from birth to age 25. This case-controlled study involved 1,669 participants and 1,263 controls at Massachusetts General Hospital. The study participants were required to be age 18 or older and to have a diagnosis of primary lung cancer. The control cases were friends or spouses of other patients visiting Massachusetts General Hospital. The study concluded that individuals who were first exposed to SHS before age 25 have a higher risk of lung cancer development than do persons who were older when first exposed to SHS. While there are some flaws in this study with respect to SHS exposure, it appears that, if anything, exposures to environmental tobacco smoke are underreported.[20]

Environmental Factors

Radon

Radon is a colorless, odorless, inert, radioactive gas found in soil, water, and air. Radon is known to cause lung cancer in humans through the inhalation of radon decay products, which emit alpha particles that damage the respiratory epithelium.[21, 22] Radon and smoking are also known to act synergistically, so there is an absolute increased risk for lung cancer due to radon exposure for a smoker versus a never-smoker.[22]

Radon and its effects were first discovered in underground uranium miners. The miners who worked where concentrations of radon were higher because of confined air space were found to have higher rates of lung cancer.[21, 23] Indoor radon was first recognized as a danger several decades ago, when initial measurements were made and revealed that levels in some homes were as high as those in the uranium mines.[23] Multiple case-controlled studies were then performed, and their results supported the introduction of radon monitoring in homes.[21]

Air Pollution

Outdoor air pollution is a complex mixture of different gaseous and particulate components, whose composition varies both by locality and by time.[22] The biologic rationale for the carcinogenic potential of air pollution focuses on the numerous components of air pollution, which may include benzopyrene, benzene, fine particles, metals, and possibly ozone.[22] Overall, the evidence for an increased risk of lung cancer from exposure to air pollution is strong.[22, 24]

Indoor air pollution may also play a role in lung cancer development. Very high rates of lung cancer have been discovered in some regions in China among women who spend much time at home. Exposure to combustion-based sources of heating and cooking as well as oil vapors from some styles of cooking have been studied.[22] Although the results of many studies have been inconclusive, a persistent, significant increase in risk of lung cancer has been associated with air pollution from combustion or cooking oil vapors, which merits further research.[22]

Asbestos

Another contributor to the current burden of lung cancer is widespread asbestos exposure, which occurred in the United States from the 1940s to the 1960s. Asbestos and asbestiform fibers are naturally occurring fibrous silicates with commercial use in thermal insulation and acoustics. They are classified into two types: chrysotile and amphiboles. Chrysotile is the most widely used type of asbestos.[22] All commercial forms of asbestos are carcinogenic in mice, rats, hamsters, and rabbits.[25] In humans, occupational exposure to chrysotile, amosite, anthophyllite, and mixed fibers containing crocidolite has resulted in a high incidence of lung cancer.[25] Owing to this link with cancer, use of asbestos has been restricted or banned in many countries.[22]

Few studies have examined the health effects of household and residential exposure to asbestos. Household sources include installation, degradation, removal, and repair of asbestos-containing products. Cigarette smoking and asbestos exposure, when present together, act in a synergistic fashion to increase lung cancer incidence.[25]

Nonenvironmental Factors

Socioeconomics

In the United States and many other countries, smoking rates—and thus incidence of lung cancer—are higher in individuals of lower socioeconomic status. Socioeconomic status is an important determinant of health and is associated with many interacting lung cancer risk factors, such as smoking, diet, and exposure to inhaled carcinogens at work and in the environment.[7]

For women, poorer females are more likely affected by these risk factors than their wealthier counterparts.[16] The Norwegian Women and Cancer Study included 96,638 women and evaluated cancer risk and educational level. The study concluded the risk of lung cancer was strongly related to education, explained mostly by differences in smoking habits.[26]

Gender

Women appear to be overrepresented in terms of lung cancer patients who are nonsmokers. At the same time, women have better relative survival rates compared to men for each disease stage.[13, 26] Women who develop lung cancer are more likely to have never smoked than men. However, women who do smoke tend to have less education, start smoking earlier, and have a higher number of packs per year consumption.[26] Hormones—specifically estrogen—may promote bronchial cell proliferation, which may play a role in lung cancer by influencing the metabolism of carcinogens or precipitating the development of lung disease.[27]

Race and Ethnicity

Lung cancer incidence is much higher among African American men than among white American men, whereas the rates are similar for African American and white American women.[7] African American men are diagnosed at a 37% higher rate and die at a 43% higher rate than white men.[2] The risk of lung cancer is significantly lower among white smokers than among African American smokers who smoke no more than 10 cigarettes per day and among those who smoke 11–20 cigarettes per day.

The Multi Ethnic Cohort Study enrolled 215,000 men and women from 5 self-reported racial and ethnic classes (Japanese American, African American, white, Native Hawaiian, and Latino) who were living in Hawaii and California from 1993 to 1996. Among both men and women in this study, the mean age of smoking initiation was similar among African Americans, Latinos, and Native Hawaiians. In an age-adjusted analysis, African American males and Native Hawaiian males had the highest incidence of lung cancer.[28] It is unknown why these differences exist, but variations in the metabolism of nicotine among different ethnic and racial populations may underlie the differences in the uptake of carcinogens.[28]

Genetics

Our understanding of the role played by genetic mutations in lung cancer is evolving. If a gene modifies lung cancer susceptibility, it must do so by inhibiting or facilitating tumorigenesis.[19] Tobacco-smoke-induced tumorigenesis is believed to occur when tobacco-smoke carcinogens bind to epithelial cells in lung DNA to form DNA adducts. Adduct formation initiates tumorigenesis through DNA repair processes that may lead to mutations in genes that start or aid tumor growth.[19]

A number of genetic mutations and molecular alterations have been studied, such as those involving p53, *K-ras* proto-oncogene mutations, and chromosomal abnormalities, such as loss or inactivation of material on the short arm of chromosome 3.[19] The *K-ras* gene is the most often mutated gene in lung cancer, representing approximately 90% of the mutations identified as linked to this disease.[29] *K-ras* mutation is particularly common in patients with an extensive smoking history and is found in 20% of all lung cancer tumors.[29]

Other Risk Factors

Other carcinogens known to be involved in the pathogenesis of lung cancer are inorganic arsenic, chromium VI compounds, and silica and polycyclic aromatic hydrocarbons, which are formed during incomplete combustion of inorganic material. These substances have a very widespread distribution, being found in tobacco smoke, engine exhaust, and diesel exhaust.[22] Additionally, individuals with a previous history of radiation therapy to the chest, as might be administered in the setting of breast cancer and Hodgkin's disease, have an increased risk of developing lung cancer.

Prevention of Lung Cancer

Non-nutritional Factors

Most lung cancers could be prevented by the elimination of smoking. Smoking remains the leading preventable cause of premature death.[30] Clearly, not starting smoking is the best way to avoid lung cancer. For those individuals who do smoke, identifying effective mechanisms for smoking cessation is essential. Smoking cessation has clearly been shown to reduce the likelihood of future morbidity.[30] Also, for those persons who do not smoke, it is imperative to avoid exposure to SHS. The American Cancer Society's collaborative effort with national groups on tobacco control focuses on achieving reductions in advertising of tobacco, increasing funding for research, reducing SHS by support of clean indoor air laws, providing access to smoking-cessation programs, increasing tobacco taxes, and supporting global partnerships to reduce tobacco-related deaths.[2]

Nutritional Factors

Epidemiologic studies have yielded insight into the nature of dietary deficiencies that influence the risk of lung cancer. Consistently, research has demonstrated increased consumption of fresh vegetables and fruits lower the risk in both men and women, in both current and former smokers, and among never-smokers, for all lung cancer histologies.[1] A major focus has been on the pro-vitamin A carotenoids, particularly beta-carotene. Collectively, the Alpha-Tocopherol, Beta Carotene (ATBC) cancer prevention study, the Beta-Carotene and Retinol Efficacy Trial (CARET), and the Physicians' Health Study have studied more than 69,000 persons. These studies, in which the beta-carotene dose ranged from 20 mg per day to 50 mg every other day, have all found that supplementation with beta-carotene is not effective in preventing lung cancer and, in fact, may increase the risk.[31–34] Smokers should be cautioned against taking vitamin supplements containing large doses (similar to the amounts used in the randomized trials mentioned earlier) of beta-carotene, as this practice appears to increase their risk of developing lung cancer. By contrast, beta-carotene from food sources is not linked to an increase in risk, and foods containing carotenoids are actually thought to be protective against lung cancer.[35] Research has also failed to find to a beneficial effect with alpha-tocopherol (vitamin E) supplementation at 50 mg/day on the incidence or mortality of lung cancer.[34]

An increased risk of lung cancer has been associated with high dietary intake of foods rich in fat and cholesterol, or with elevated indices of abdominal adiposity. However, the positive association between dietary cholesterol and lung cancer risk has not been reflected in studies of serum cholesterol. Lung cancer risk is also not associated with increasing body mass.[1]

A 2007 study by Galeone and colleagues studied dietary intake of vegetables and fruits in northeast China, where one of the leading causes of death in both sexes is lung cancer. An inverse relationship was found between vegetable and fruit intake and lung cancer risk. The most protective foods were Chinese cabbage, chives, carrots, and celery. This study, while not population or histologically based, provides some credence to the fact that increased consumption of fruits and vegetables is inversely associated with lung cancer incidence.[36]

Selenium has also been suggested to be a chemopreventive agent for lung cancer. Selenium is a trace element that may assist in the repair and prevention of oxidative damage. Thus far, studies are inconclusive on selenium's effects. If there is any benefit to supplementation for lung cancer prevention, it may occur only in those persons with initially low selenium levels.[37, 38]

Table 11.1 summarizes the current evidence for nutrients that do or may influence lung cancer risk.[35]

Table 11.1   *Association Between Various Nutrients and Lung Cancer Risk*

Strength of Evidence	Associated with Increased Risk	Associated with Decreased Risk
Convincing	Beta-carotene supplements	
Probable		• Fruits • Foods containing carotenoids (e.g., carrots, apricots, mangoes, squash, sweet potatoes, spinach, kale, collard greens, tomatoes, grapefruit)
Limited (suggestive)	• Red and processed meats • Butter • Retinol supplements	• Non-starchy vegetables • Selenium and foods containing selenium (e.g., nuts, fish, shellfish, poultry) • Foods containing quercetin (e.g., citrus fruits, apples, onions, parsley, green and black tea, red wine, olive oil, dark cherries, blueberries)
Limited (no conclusion)		• Grains, fiber, legumes, poultry, fish, eggs, milk and dairy products, animal and total fats • Vitamins A, C, and E, the B vitamins, multivitamins, calcium, copper, iron, zinc, pro-vitamin carotenoids, lycopene, flavonoids

Source: World Cancer Research Fund/American Institute for Cancer Research. *Food, Nutrition, Physical Activity, and the Prevention of Cancer: A Global Perspective.* Washington, DC: American Institute for Cancer Research; 2007.

Symptoms and Therapy of Lung Cancer

Lung cancer is commonly diagnosed when the disease is at a more advanced stage and symptoms have appeared.[4] Symptoms may include persistent coughing, hemoptysis, shortness of breath, wheezing, hoarseness, recurring pneumonia or bronchitis, weakness, and anorexia.

The stage of lung cancer at diagnosis is determined by the Tumor, lymph Node, Metastasis (TNM) classification system and directs the care that will be rendered. The TNM classification system is the accepted system for staging many cancers, including lung cancer (see Table 11.2). It was adopted by the American Joint Committee on Cancer (AJCC) and the International Union Against Cancer in 1986 as a means of unifying variations in definitions

Table 11.2 *Staging of Lung Cancer*

Stage Grouping			
Occult carcinoma	TX	N0	M0
Stage 0	Tis	N0	M0
Stage IA	T1	N0	M0
Stage IB	T2	N0	M0
Stage IIA	T1	N1	M0
Stage IIB	T2	N1	M0
	T3	N0	M0
Stage IIIA	T1	N2	M0
	T2	N2	M0
	T3	N1	M0
	T3	N2	M0
Stage IIIB	Any T	N3	M0
	T4	Any N	M0
Stage IV	Any T	Any N	M1

Definition of TNM

Primary Tumor (T)

TX: Primary tumor cannot be assessed, or tumor proven by the presence of malignant cells in sputum or bronchial washings but not visualized by imaging or bronchoscopy

T0: No evidence of primary tumor

Tis: Carcinoma in situ

T1: Tumor 3 cm or less in greatest dimension, surrounded by lung or visceral pleura, without bronchoscopic evidence of invasion more proximal than the lobar bronchus (i.e., not in the main bronchus)

T2: Tumor with any of the following features of size or extent:
• More than 3 cm in greatest dimension
• Involves main bronchus, 2 cm or more distal to the carina
• Invades the visceral pleura
• Associated with atelectasis or obstructive pneumonitis that extends to the hilar region
• Does not involve the entire lung

T3: Tumor of any size that directly invades any of the following: chest wall (including superior sulcus tumors), diaphragm, mediastinal pleura, parietal pericardium; or tumor in the main bronchus less than 2 cm distal to the carina but without involvement of the carina; or associated atelectasis or obstructive pneumonitis of the entire lung

(continues)

Table 11.2   *Staging of Lung Cancer, Continued*

Definition of TNM
Primary Tumor (T), *continued*
T4: Tumor of any size that invades any of the following: mediastinum, heart, great vessels, trachea, esophagus, vertebral body, carina; separate tumor nodule(s) in the same lobe; or tumor with a malignant pleural effusion
Regional Lymph Nodes (N)
All regional lymph nodes are above the diaphragm. They include the intrathoracic, scalene, and supraclavicular nodes.
NX: Regional lymph nodes cannot be assessed
N0: No regional lymph node metastasis
N1: Metastasis to ipsilateral peribronchial and/or ipsilateral hilar lymph nodes, and intrapulmonary nodes including involvement by direct extension of the primary tumor
N2: Metastasis to ipsilateral mediastinal and/or subcarinal lymph node(s)
N3: Metastasis in contralateral mediastinal, contralateral hilar, ipsilateral or contralateral scalene or supraclavicular lymph node(s)
Distant Metastasis (M)
MX: Distant metastasis cannot be assessed
M0: No distant metastasis
M1: Distant metastasis present; this includes separate tumor nodule(s) in a different lobe (ipsilateral or contralateral)
Source: Reprinted with permission from Greene FL, Page DL, Fleming ID, et al. *AJCC Cancer Staging Manual.* 6th ed. New York, NY: Springer; 2002.

and providing consistent meaning and interpretation among clinicians and scientists throughout the world.[4]

In the staging process, the treating professional will also take into account comorbid diseases and general patient condition. In addition to stage, the most important prognostic indicators affecting survival are performance status and weight loss.[4] Patients who have never smoked and patients with a remote smoking history have an increased probability of partial response to chemotherapy compared to patients with a recent smoking history.[39] Patients who cease smoking do gain an advantage in time to progression and survival over those who continue to smoke.[39]

Generally, treatment options include surgery, radiation, and chemotherapy. Depending on the stage of disease at diagnosis, two or more modalities may be recommended.

Sputum cytology is the only noninvasive method available to evaluate patients with suspected lung cancer and determine pathologic classification. Sputum cytology has a positive predictive value near 100% but sensitivity of only 10–15%.[4] Other more common and standard evaluation techniques include fiber-optic bronchoscopy, which can determine the endobronchial extent of disease, identify occult lesions, and measure tumor distance to the carina,[4] and CT-guided percutaneous fine-needle aspiration, which can be used to sample areas that are poorly accessible in the lung and mediastinum. Mediastinoscopy is best for evaluating upper, middle paratracheal and subcarinal lymph nodes. Video-assisted thorascopy (VATS) is usually performed as an adjunct to mediastinoscopy.

Once the invasive procedure is performed and the sample is obtained, the tumor is measured for size, lymph nodes are studied, and other staging studies are performed. PET/CT or CT of the chest, abdomen, and adrenal glands and PET scan will be performed to determine the extent of disease and subsequent treatment.[9] Four stages of NSCLC are distinguished, with the various subdivisions within each stage being based on tumor size and nodal involvement. By comparison, SCLC is staged as limited or extensive only.

Non-Small-Cell Lung Cancer

Surgical Treatment

For many years, surgery has been the standard mode of treatment in patients with stage I–IIIA NSCLC.[39] Surgery is the most consistent and successful option for patients, but a cure by this means is possible only when the cancer is completely resectable and the patient is able to tolerate the extent of resection.[9] Only 20% of patients presenting with lung cancer are candidates for curative surgery.[4] Unfortunately, even with complete resection, relapse often occurs at distant sites.[39]

Surgical procedures that may be performed include pneumonectomy, lobectomy, or limited resection, usually called wedge resection. Lobectomy is the standard of care for surgical management.[9] The local recurrence rate is three times higher in patients who undergo wedge resection over lobectomy; thus lobectomy is recommended for most patients who are able to tolerate the surgery.[4] Minimal-access surgical procedures are gaining ground, and video-assisted lobectomy is being offered more often because it represents a less invasive method to accomplish the same resection as lobectomy.[9]

The average 5-year survival rate following surgery for NSCLC ranges from 23% to 65% for stage IA–IIIA disease.[40] Adjuvant chemotherapy is not recommended for patients with completely resected stage IA NSCLC. Postoperative thoracic radiation is also not recommended for patients with completely resected stage I or II NSCLC.[39] Only 5% of all patients will present with stage II disease, which is further subdivided into stages IIA and IIB. The average 5-year survival rate for stage II disease is 41.2%.[4] In patients with completely resected stage IIIA NSCLC, postoperative radiation is controversial and not routinely recommended due to the lack of randomized clinical trial data evaluating its efficacy.[39]

Chemotherapy and Radiation

Chemotherapy for NSCLC generally consists of platinum-based agents; carboplatin and paclitaxel are the most frequently used chemotherapeutic drugs. Platinum-based chemotherapy prolongs survival, improves symptom control, and yields superior quality of life compared to supportive care.[4] Adjuvant cisplatin-based chemotherapy is often recommended for patients with completely resected stage II–IIIA NSCLC, but is under active investigation for patients with stage IB–IIIA NSCLC who have undergone complete resection. The preferred timing, regimen, and patient selection for use of this therapy has yet to be determined.[41] In patients with unresectable stage III NSCLC, 2 to 8 cycles of platinum-based chemotherapy in association with definitive thoracic irradiation is considered appropriate treatment.[42]

Chemotherapy with concurrent radiation improves local control by sensitizing the tumor to radiation and treating systemic disease.[42] Approximately 25–40% of patients with NSCLC have stage III disease, which is further subdivided into stages IIIA and IIIB. Stage IIIB disease is generally not resectable.[4] Currently, the role of surgery following induction chemotherapy or chemoradiotherapy for patients with initially unresectable cancer is being explored; the 5-year survival rate is 9–15%.[4,41]

Chemotherapy is also appropriate for selected patients with stage IV NSCLC and good performance status, as this type of treatment prolongs survival. The chemotherapy plan should include a 2-drug combination regimen, and non-platinum-based chemotherapy may be used as an alternative to platinum-based agents.[41] Initial treatment with investigational agents or regimens is appropriate for selected patients with stage IV NSCLC, provided they are crossed over to an active treatment regimen if they do not respond after two cycles of chemotherapy.[42] With best supportive care, the 1-year survival rate for stage IV lung cancer is 10%. Platinum-based chemotherapy can improve this rate to 30–35%.[43]

Docetaxol is recommended as second-line therapy for patients with locally advanced or metastatic NSCLC, adequate performance status, and progressive disease after first-line platinum-based therapy. Gefitinib, an orally active inhibitor of the epidermal growth factor receptor (EGFR) tyrosine kinase, was the first targeted therapy to be approved for use in lung cancer and was originally recommended for the treatment of patients with locally advanced or metastatic NSCLC after failure of both platinum-based and doc-etaxol chemotherapy.[41] Unfortunately, a Southwest Oncology Group phase III randomized trial in patients with stage IIIB lung cancer showed no survival benefit with its use.[9] Erlotinib, another EGFR tyrosine kinase inhibitor (TKI), has shown some promise and is approved for second- or third-line treatment of NSCLC in patients who have not responded to one previous round of therapy.[9] Furthermore, cetuximab, another EGFR inhibitor, has demonstrated the ability to extend survival when combined with platinum-based chemotherapy.

Studies have also focused on cancer angiogenesis, which is induced by vascular endothelial growth factor (VEGF). Bevacizumab, a monoclonal antibody against VEGF, has been found to offer a survival benefit when added to a paclitaxel–carboplatin regimen. This agent is associated with a small but significant risk of serious bleeding, so it is not used in patients with squamous cell histology, brain metastases, or hemoptysis, or in those patients who are receiving anticoagulation therapy.[9]

Small-Cell Lung Cancer

SCLC accounts for 15% of all diagnosed lung cancers in the United States. At presentation, two-thirds of patients will have extensive disease.[15] SCLC is defined as limited disease when the tumor is confined to one hemithorax and its regional lymph nodes. Extensive disease means the tumor is more widespread.[44] For patients with stage I SCLC, complete resection via lobectomy with mediastinal nodal dissection or sampling is considered if the disease is very limited. Nevertheless, a mediastinoscopy should be performed prior to surgery to rule out occult disease in the lymph nodes.[4] If nodes are found to be positive after resection, postoperative chemotherapy and radiation should be offered.

SCLC is highly chemosensitive; therefore, combination chemotherapy is the cornerstone of treatment for most patients. Unfortunately, median survival despite treatment is only 9–11 months.[15] In the 1970s, a survival benefit of combination chemotherapy over single-agent therapy was discovered. As in NSCLC, platinum-based chemotherapy is used. In SCLC, cisplatin is combined with etoposide—a standard of care that has been in place for the last 2 decades. Many physicians substitute carboplatin for cisplatin due to the former agent's equally efficacious but more favorable toxicity profile. Other trials continue to study chemotherapy agents for the treatment of SCLC. Some success has been achieved with irinotecan and cisplatin in terms of response rate and median survival. Adding radiation therapy to chemotherapy for treating limited-stage SCLC improves median survival to 14–18 months.[45]

The risk of brain metastases in SCLC is correlated with length of survival. Given this relationship, prophylactic cranial irradiation (PCI) is often offered for complete responders as they face a 50–60% risk of developing brain metastases within 2–3 years after diagnosis.[4, 45]

Complementary and Alternative Therapies

The use of complementary and alternative medicine (CAM) by persons with lung cancer is relatively common.[46, 47] One study, which included 189 women with NSCLC in the United States, found that 44% of these patients used CAM.[46] Women with a younger age, those with more symptoms, and those living in the western or southern regions of the United States were more likely to implement CAM therapies. CAM options included prayer, meditation, tea, herbs, massage and acupuncture. More frequent symptoms—such as pain, dyspnea, and fatigue—led to increased use of CAM.[46] Prayer was practiced more frequently than any other therapy.

Another study examined CAM use in 111 lung cancer patients from 8 European countries.[47] Approximately 24% of those studied used some type of CAM; herbal medicine, teas, homeopathy, animal extracts, and spiritual therapies were the most popular options. In this study, CAM users were more likely to be younger and to have a higher education level than non-users.

Jatoi and colleagues reported that 63% of 1,129 patients with NSCLC were users of multivitamins or other individual vitamin or mineral supplements.[48] As this and the other studies illustrate, because of the prevalence of CAM in lung cancer patients, clinicians must query patients about CAM use and be aware of potential interactions between conventional therapies and CAM.

Several investigators have studied the use of CAM's effectiveness, along with other conventional treatments, against lung cancer. Two studies (one in patients with NSCLC and the other in patients with SCLC), conducted by Jatoi and colleagues,[48, 49] evaluated the association between patient-directed vitamin and mineral supplementation and quality of life and survival. Study participants were classified as users or non-users based on a mailed questionnaire. After adjustments for other prognostic factors, including tumor stage, vitamin/mineral supplementation was associated with improved survival in both studies, and with improved quality of life in the NSCLC cohort. Nevertheless, because of the study methodology and potential confounding reasons for the survival benefit, the investigators do not advise clinicians to recommend vitamin/mineral supplements to patients until prospective clinical trials are conducted.

Astragalus, a Chinese herbal medicine, has been combined with platinum-based chemotherapy to treat NSCLC. *Astragalus*'s proposed immune-enhancing actions include promotion of macrophage and natural-killer cell activity and inhibition of T-helper cell type 2 cytokines. McCulloch and associates performed a meta-analysis of 34 randomized trials evaluating outcomes (survival, tumor response, performance status, chemotherapy toxicity) with *Astragalus* plus platinum-based chemotherapy versus platinum-based chemotherapy alone. The combination of *Astragalus* and platinum-based chemotherapy lowered the risk of death at 1 year in 12 studies and increased tumor response in 30 studies. However, the studies located for the meta-analysis were of poor quality, such that further investigation with high-quality prospective, randomized trials is needed to confirm *Astragulus*'s role (combined with chemotherapy) in the treatment of in lung cancer.[50]

Hydrazine sulfate (HS) has been, and still is, promoted as being able to improve survival when combined with standard chemotherapy regimens and treat symptoms associated with cancer cachexia.[51] However, several randomized trials have demonstrated that HS, when combined with chemotherapy, does not improve tumor response, survival, quality of life, or nutritional status.[52–54] Therefore, HS cannot be recommended in lung cancer patients.

Clearly, more research is needed to confirm the claims that specific CAM therapies can assist in treatment of lung cancer. Refer to Chapter 16 for more detailed information on CAM therapies.

Nutritional Implications of Lung Cancer

The nutritional status of patients with lung cancer is affected by a multitude of factors, including adequacy of nutrient intake, weight loss, presence of treatment-related symptoms, and cancer-related cachexia. Nutritional status at diagnosis and during management of lung cancer has been shown to affect outcomes.

Weight Loss and Outcomes

Studies conducted prior to 2000 strongly support the idea that weight loss and nutritional status play key roles in outcomes for patients with lung cancer. An early study by Lanzotti and colleagues evaluated the use of a regression analysis model to determine clinical factors influencing survival in patients with inoperable lung cancer.[55] The study evaluated 129 patients with limited disease and 187 with extensive disease. Survival was 36 weeks in patients with limited disease and 14 weeks in those with extensive disease. In patients with limited disease, the proposed model found weight loss to be the major factor for prediction of survival, followed by symptom status, supraclavicular metastases, and age.[55]

Dewys and colleagues reported on the prognostic effect of weight loss before initiation of chemotherapy in a variety of cancer diagnoses, including lung cancer.[56] More than 1,000 patients with SCLC and NSCLC were included in the analysis. The percentages of patients who lost weight—defined as more than 10%, 5–10%, 0–5%, or 0% of body weight—in the previous 6 months in the lung cancer group were approximately 15%, 20%, 24%, and 40%, respectively. The effect of weight loss on survival in the lung cancer patients was significant. SCLC patients with no weight loss survived a median of 34 weeks versus 27 weeks for those patients with weight loss ($p < 0.05$). NSCLC patients with no weight loss survived a median of 20 weeks, whereas patients with weight loss had a median survival of 14 weeks ($p < 0.01$).[56]

A third study, by Espinosa and colleagues, also found a relationship between weight loss and survival in advanced nonoperable NSCLC patients undergoing chemotherapy treatment.[57] Those without weight loss (69%) survived a median of 2 more months compared to patients with weight loss (31%). This study also reported a normal serum albumin (more than 4 g/dL) was associated with better response to chemotherapy and survival.[57]

More recent studies provide a less consistent picture of the incidence of weight loss and the effect of nutritional status and weight loss on outcomes. Jagoe and colleagues published two studies in 2001 that included lung cancer patients referred for lung cancer surgery.[58, 59] One study focused on the nutritional status of patients undergoing surgery for lung cancer; the other examined the role of nutritional status on complications after surgery.

In the first study, Jagoe et al. assessed a variety of nutritional indices in 60 patients, including BMI, percent weight loss, albumin, prealbumin, energy and protein intake for 5 days prior to hospital admission, and Subjective Global Assessment (SGA) score.[58] The mean BMI was 25.4; 8 patients (13.3%) had BMI < 20 and 9 patients (15%) were obese (BMI > 30). Fourteen patients (23%) reported weight loss of more than 5% of total body weight; of these, only 3 patients experienced weight loss more than 10% of total body weight. The mean serum albumin level was 44.7 g/dL and the mean prealbumin was 0.28 g/dL; 2 patients had low albumin levels and 7 had low prealbumin levels. The majority of patients were able to consume adequate calories and protein intake (70% and 87%, respectively). The SGA scored 29 patients as mildly to moderately depleted and 1 patient as severely depleted. Therefore, a minority of patients in this study population were nutritionally deficient upon presentation for surgical intervention.

In the second study, Jagoe et al. evaluated essentially the same cohort of patients ($n = 52$) to determine how nutritional status affected the incidence of surgical complications.[59] A univariate analysis found patients with a lower BMI, percent usual body weight, and fat-free mass index to be more likely to die or to require reventilation. A multivariate analysis also found BMI and percent usual body weight to be significant factors for predicting surgical complications. Overall, this series of patients was less nutritionally depleted than those in earlier studies and generally had a less advanced disease stage. Even so, the investigators do conclude nutritional status may be a prognostic indicator of postoperative outcomes.

Ross and colleagues evaluated whether patients with weight loss who undergo chemotherapy experience worse outcomes.[60] Approximately 700 patients with SCLC and NSCLC were included in this study, and some 58% of patients experienced weight loss. Patients with weight loss had a significantly shorter survival time. Patients with SCLC and weight loss survived 8 months compared to 11 months in those without weight loss. NSCLC patients with weight loss lived an average of 6 months versus 9 months for patients without weight loss.

Win and others investigated the incidence and impact of BMI on outcomes in 109 patients with operable lung cancer.[61] In this cohort, the mean BMI was 25.7, and 7 patients had BMI > 19. Most study participants were either at ideal body weight (44 patients) or overweight (58 patients). This study found no association between BMI and postoperative deaths or other surgical outcomes. These same investigators found that both diabetes and a low serum albumin level are predictors of survival.[62]

Tewari and colleagues analyzed the relationship between nutritional status and long-term survival in 642 patients with lung cancer who underwent lobectomy. Twenty-eight percent of patients were classified as having poor nutritional status (BMI < 18.5, preoperative albumin < 30 g/dL, or history of weight loss). Twenty-four percent experienced weight loss, 9% had BMI < 18.5, and 21% presented with an albumin level of less than 30 g/dL. Nutritional status did not affect short-term outcomes but did influence long-term survival. Those patients with a depleted nutritional status had a median survival of 36 months, whereas those with a normal nutritional status had median survival of 58 months.[63]

Overall, the evidence supports paying close attention to the nutritional status of patients with lung cancer at the time of diagnosis and/or when planning surgical intervention.

Nutritional Assessment and Interventions

Patients with lung cancer should undergo nutritional screening by a healthcare professional to determine if weight loss, underweight status, low serum albumin, or gastrointestinal symptoms are present. If any of these conditions are present, it is optimal to refer the patient for further assessment to a registered dietitian (RD) with experience in the field of oncology nutrition. Refer to Chapter 2 for more detailed information related to nutrition screening and assessment in the oncology patient.

Like other cancer patients, patients with lung cancer often experience cancer cachexia.[64, 65] (See Chapters 1 and 15 for more details about cancer cachexia and its treatment.) Cachexia has been defined by Morley et al. as the combination of the following in the setting of ongoing disease: unintentional weight loss ($\geq$ 5% of total body weight); BMI < 20 in patients younger than 65 years or < 22 in patients 65 years or older; albumin < 3.5 g/dL; low fat-free mass (lowest 10 percentile); and evidence of cytokine excess (elevated C-reactive protein).[66] Nutrition therapy alone is usually not sufficient or effective in treating cancer-related cachexia.

A small 8-week study, which included both pancreatic and NSCLC patients, utilized weekly counseling by a dietitian along with an oral nutritional supplement to treat cachexia.[67] The patients' protein and energy intake increased significantly (p < 0.02) over the 8-week period. Weight and lean body mass also increased by 2.5 kg and 1 kg, respectively, although these gains were not statistically significant. In addition, significant improvements were seen in SGA nutritional score, Karnofsky performance status, and quality of life. While this study is limited by its small sample size, it does suggest that intensive nutritional intervention can affect important outcomes in a very difficult-to-treat patient population.

Vitamin D has been promoted as a significant nutrient in cancer prevention. Notably, according to recent research in patients with lung cancer, vitamin D status may also be an important factor in their outcomes. Zhou and colleagues studied the effect of circulating 25-hydroxyvitamin D—25(OH) vitamin D—levels and vitamin D intake on overall survival and recurrence-free survival in 447 patients with NSCL.[68] The data suggest that patients with both a high 25(OH) vitamin D level and high vitamin D intake have improved overall survival and recurrence-free survival, and that this effect is most pronounced in stage IB–IIB patients compared to stage IA patients.[68] In the future, nutrition assessment may routinely include evaluation of vitamin D status. For now, however, the authors recommend further observational studies and randomized trials to confirm vitamin D's role in improving outcomes in patients with lung cancer.

Limited study results are available on the use of nutrition support in patients with lung cancer. Overall, their findings have not shown any nutritional or clinical benefit from the use of adjuvant parenteral nutrition support in this population.[69, 70] Nevertheless, if a patient is responding well to therapy and has a good prognosis but is unable to maintain adequate intake through nutritional counseling, oral diet, and nutritional supplements, enteral nutrition should be considered. Also, if enteral nutrition cannot be tolerated because of prolonged gastrointestinal side effects related to oncologic therapies, parenteral nutrition is an option. The use of parenteral nutrition in cancer patients continues to be controversial, however, and clinicians must weigh all the pros and cons carefully before initiating this therapy. See Chapter 3 for more detailed information related to nutrition support in oncology patients.

Future Novel Options

The research focusing on lung cancer continues to evolve, especially in the area of lung cancer detection. A large number of potential molecular markers are being identified, and this line of research could eventually enhance the scientist's ability to predict relapse and chemosensitivity for treatment. For example, biomarkers in the epithelium of the cheek are currently under investigation. Thus molecular events in higher-risk patients may be monitored for development of changes that are usually evident only via bronchoscopy. Additionally, blood RNA is being studied to detect lung cancer.

In the past, screening attempts for lung cancer with sputum cytology and, to a smaller extent, chest x-ray have failed to demonstrate a reduction in lung cancer mortality. The newest hope for lung cancer screening, low-dose CT, is now under evaluation. As yet, no prospective data have been published regarding how CT might affect long-term outcomes. While the CT may be able to detect earlier-stage lung cancers, it is unknown whether its use would improve mortality.

Celecoxib, a cyclooxygenase 2 (COX-2) inhibitor, is also being studied for its chemoprevention potential. This drug appears to reduce Ki-67, a protein that promotes cell proliferation in premalignant lesions in bronchial epithelia.

SUMMARY

Lung cancer remains a devastating disease that leaves few long-term survivors. Despite research that is aimed toward elucidating the roles played by racial disparities, socioeconomics, and air pollution as factors in its incidence, one cannot escape the fact that lung cancer was virtually nonexistent two centuries ago. Improving the health of the general population through smoking cessation would be a major accomplishment throughout the world. Healthcare expenditures would be markedly decreased and general health status improved. Healthcare professionals are the voice of those who have no voice. It is our job to be role models for our patients by adopting healthy lifestyles and advocating for tighter smoking laws on second-hand smoke. It is also our job to educate our patients on the dangers of smoking and to offer smoking-cessation strategies for our smoking patients who wish to quit.

REFERENCES

1. Schottenfeld D, Searle JG. The etiology and epidemiology of lung cancer. In: Pass HI, Carbone DP, Johnson DH, Minna JD, Turrisi AT III, eds. *Lung cancer: Principles and Practice*. 3rd ed. Philadelphia, PA: Lippincott Williams & Wilkins; 2005:4–24.

2. American Cancer Society. Cancer facts and figures. Available at: http://www .cancer.org. Accessed July 22, 2008.

3. Parkin DM, Pisani P, Ferlay J. Global cancer statistics. *CA Cancer J Clin*. 1999;49:33–64.

4. Chang JY, Bradley JD, Govindan R, Komaki, R. Lung. In: Halperin EC, Perez GA, Brady LW. *Principles and Practices of Radiation Oncology*. 5th ed. Philadelphia, PA: Lippincott Williams & Wilkins; 2008:1076–1108.

5. Houlihan NG. Overview. In: Houlihan N, ed. *Lung Cancer*. Pittsburgh, PA: Oncology Nursing Society; 2004:1–5.

6. Samet JM. Environmental causes of lung cancer: What do we know in 2003? *Chest*. 2004;125:80S–82S.

7. Alberg AJ, Brock MV, Samet JM. Epidemiology of lung cancer: Looking to the future. *J Clin Oncol*. 2005;23:3175–3185.

8. U.S. Department of Health Education and Welfare. *Smoking and Health: Report of Advisory Committee to the Surgeon General*. DHEW Publication No. 1103. Washington, DC: U.S. Government Printing Office; 1964.

9. Molina JR, Yang P, Cassivi SD, et al. Non small cell lung cancer: Epidemiology, risk factors, treatment and survivorship. *Mayo Clinic Proc*. 2008;83:584–594.

10. Office of the Leading Small Group for Implementation of the Framework Convention on Tobacco Control, Ministry of Health, People's Republic of China. *China Tobacco Control Report: Create a Smoke Free Environment, Enjoy a Healthy Life*. Beijing: Author; 2007.

11. Kobzik L, Schoen FJ. The lung. In: Cotran RS, Kumar V, Robbins SL, eds. *Pathologic Basis of Disease*. 5th ed. Philadelphia, PA: WB Saunders; 1994:673–734.

12. Tyson LB. Patient assessment. In: Houlihan N, ed. *Lung Cancer*. Pittsburgh, PA: Oncology Nursing Society; 2004:35–44.

13. Belani CP, Marts S, Schiller J, Socinski MA. Women and lung cancer: Epidemiology, tumor biology, and emerging trends in clinical research. *Lung Cancer*. 2007; 55:15–23.

14. Burns DM, Major JM, Shanks TG, et al. Smoking lower yield cigarettes and disease risks. *Smoking and Tobacco Control Monograph* No. 13, 2001:65–158.

15. Witta SE, Kelly K. Chemotherapy for small cell lung cancer. In: Pass HI, Carbone DP, Johnson D, et al, eds. *Lung Cancer: Principles and Practice*. 3rd ed. Philadelphia, PA: Lippincott Williams & Wilkins; 2005:657–673.

16. Centers for Disease Control and Prevention. *MMWR Weekly*. 2005;54:625–628. Available at: www.cdc.gov. Accessed July 28, 2008.

17. Ingle RJ. Lung cancers. In: Yarbro CH, Frogge MH, Goodman M, et al, eds. *Cancer Nursing: Principles and Practice*. 5th ed. Sudbury, MA: Jones and Bartlett; 2000: 1298–1328.

18. U.S. Department of Health and Human Services. *The Health Consequences of Involuntary Exposure to Tobacco Smoke: A Report of the Surgeon General: Executive Summary*. Washington, DC: U.S. Department of Health and Human Services, Centers for Disease Control and Prevention, Coordinating Center for Health Promotion, National Center for Chronic Disease Prevention and Health Promotion, Office on Smoking and Health; 2006.

19. Brownson RC, Figgs LW, Caisley LE. Epidemiology of environmental tobacco smoke exposure. *Oncogene*. 2002;21:7341–7348.
20. Asomaning K, Miller DP, Liu G, et al. Second hand smoke, age of exposure and lung cancer risk. *Lung Cancer*. 2008;61:13–20.
21. Bochicchio F. Radon epidemiology and nuclear track detectors: Methods, results and perspectives. *Radiation Measurements*. 2005;40:177–190.
22. Boffetta P. Epidemiology of environmental and occupational cancer. *Oncogene*. 2004;23:6392–6403.
23. International Agency for Research on Cancer. *Man-Made Mineral Fibres and Radon: Monographs on the Evaluation of Carcinogenic Risks to Humans, Vol. 43*. Lyon, France: Author; 1988.
24. Lewtas J. Air pollution combustion emissions: Characterization of causative agents and mechanisms associated with cancer, reproductive, and cardiovascular effects. *Mutation Res*. 2007;636:95–133.
25. International Agency for Research on Cancer. *Asbestos: Monographs on the Evaluation of Carcinogenic Risks to Humans, Vol. 14*. Lyon, France: Author; 1977.
26. Braaten T, Weiderpass E, Kumle M, Lund E. Explaining the socioeconomic variation in cancer risk in the Norwegian Women and Cancer Study. *Cancer Epidemiol Biomarkers Prev*. 2005;14:2591–2597.
27. Davies M, Houlihan NG, Joyce M. Lung cancer control. In: Houlihan N, ed. *Lung Cancer*. Pittsburgh, PA: Oncology Nursing Society; 2004:17–34.
28. Haiman CA, Stram DO, Wilkens LR, et al. Ethnic and racial differences in the smoking-related risk of lung cancer. *N Engl J Med*. 2006;354:333–342.
29. Mao L. Recent advances in the molecular diagnosis of lung cancer. *Oncogene*. 2002;21:6960–6969.
30. Wu P, Wilson K, Dimoulas P, Mills EJ. Effectiveness of smoking cessation therapies: A systematic review and meta-analysis. *BMC Public Health*. 2006;6:1–16.
31. Omenn GS, Goodman GE, Thornquist MD, et al. Effects of a combination of beta carotene and vitamin A on lung cancer and cardiovascular disease. *N Engl J Med*. 1996;334:1150–1155.
32. Hennekens CH, Buring JE, Manson JE, et al. Lack of effect of long-term supplementation with beta carotene on the incidence of malignant neoplasms and cardiovascular disease. *N Engl J Med*. 1996;334:1145–1149.
33. Willett WC, Stampfer MJ. What vitamins should I be taking, doctor? *N Engl J Med*. 2001;345:1819–1824.
34. The Alpha-Tocopherol, Beta Carotene Cancer Prevention (ABTC) Study Group. The effect of vitamin E and beta carotene on the incidence of lung cancer and other cancers in male smokers. *N Engl J Med*. 1994;330:1029–1035.
35. World Cancer Research Fund/American Institute for Cancer Research. *Food, Nutrition, Physical Activity, and the Prevention of Cancer: A Global Perspective*. Washington, DC: Author; 2007.
36. Galeone C, Negri E, Pelucchi C, et al. Dietary intake of fruit and vegetable and lung cancer risk: A case-control study in Harbin, northeast China. *Ann Oncol*. 2006;18:388–392.
37. Zhou H, Smith AH, Steinmaus C. Selenium and lung cancer: A quantitative analysis of heterogeneity in the current epidemiological literature. *Cancer Epidemiol Biomarkers Prev*. 2004;13:771–778.
38. Reid ME, Duffield-Lillico AJ, et al. Selenium supplementation and lung cancer incidence: An update of the nutritional prevention of cancer trial. *Cancer Epidemiol Biomarkers Prev*. 2002;11:1285–1291.

39. Pisters KMW, Evans WK, Azzoli CG, et al. Cancer Care Ontario and American Society of Clinical Oncology: Adjuvant chemotherapy and adjuvant radiation therapy for stages I–IIIA resectable non-small cell lung cancer guideline. *J Clin Oncol.* 2007;25:1–13.

40. Mountain CF. Revisions in the international system for staging lung cancer. *Chest.* 1997;111:1710–1717.

41. McGarry R, Turrisi AT. Lung cancer. In: Haffty BG, Wilson LD, eds. *Handbook of Radiation Oncology.* Sudbury, MA: Jones and Bartlett; 2009:375–397.

42. Pfister DG, Johnson DH, Azzoli CG, et al; American Society of Clinical Oncology. American Society of Clinical Oncology treatment of unresectable non-small cell lung cancer guideline: Update 2003. *J Clin Oncol.* 2004;22(2):330–353.

43. Lam WK, Watkins DN. Lung cancer: Future directions. *Respirology.* 2007;12: 471–477.

44. Joyce M. Small cell lung cancer. In: Houlihan N, ed. *Lung Cancer.* Pittsburgh, PA: Oncology Nursing Society; 2004:73–82.

45. Murray N, Erridge S, Turrisi AT. Multimodality therapy for limited stage small cell lung cancer: Combining chemotherapy and thoracic irradiation. In: Pass HI, Carbone DP, Johnson DH, Minna JD, Turrisi AT, eds. *Lung Cancer: Principles and Practice.* 3rd ed. Philadelphia, PA: Lippincott Williams & Wilkins; 2005: 674–691.

46. Wells M, Sarna L, Cooley ME, et al. Use of complementary and alternative medicine therapies to control symptoms in women living with lung cancer. *Cancer Nurs.* 2007;30:45–55.

47. Molassiotis A, Panteli V, Patiraki E, et al. Complementary and alternative medicine use in lung cancer patients in eight European countries. *Complement Ther Clin Pract.* 2006;12:34–39.

48. Jatoi A, Williams B, Nichols F, et al. Is voluntary vitamin and mineral supplementation associated with better outcome in non-small cell lung cancer patients? Results from the Mayo Clinic lung cancer cohort. *Lung Cancer.* 2005;49:77–84.

49. Jatoi A, Williams B, Marks R, et al. Exploring vitamin and mineral supplementation and purported clinical effects in patients with small cell lung cancer: Results from the Mayo Clinic lung cancer cohort. *Nutr Cancer.* 2005;51:7–12.

50. McCulloch M, See C, Xiao-juan S, et al. *Astragalus*-based Chinese herbs and platinum-based chemotherapy for advanced non-small-cell lung cancer: Meta-analysis of randomized trials. *J Clin Oncol.* 2006;24:419–430.

51. Chlebowski RT, Bulcavage L, Grosvenor M, et al. Hydrazine sulfate influence on nutritional status and survival in non-small-cell lung cancer. *J Clin Oncol.* 1990;8:9–15.

52. Kosty MP, Fleishman SB, Herndon JE 2nd, et al. Cisplatin, vinblastine, and hydrazine sulfate in advanced non-small-cell lung cancer: A randomized placebo-controlled, double-blind phase III study of the Cancer and Leukemia Group B. *J Clin Oncol.* 1994;12:1113–1120.

53. Loprinzi CL, Goldberg RM, Su JQ, et al. Placebo-controlled trial of hydrazine sulfate in patients with newly diagnosed non-small-cell lung cancer. *J Clin Oncol.* 1994;12:1126–1129.

54. Hernden JE, Fleishman S, Kosty MP, Green MR. A longitudinal study of quality of life in advanced non-small cell lung cancer: Cancer and Leukemia Group B (CALGB) 8931. *Control Clin Trials.* 1997;18:286–300.

55. Lanzotti VJ, Thomas PR, Boyle LE, et al. Survival with inoperable lung cancer: An investigation of prognostic variables based on simple clinical criteria. *Cancer.* 1977;39:303–313.
56. Dewys WD, Begg C, Lavin PT, et al. Prognostic effect of weight loss prior to chemotherapy in cancer patients. *Am J Med.* 1980;69:491–497.
57. Espinosa E, Felie J, Zamora P, et al. Serum albumin and other prognostic factors related to response and survival in patients with advanced non-small cell lung cancer. *Lung Cancer.* 1995;12:67–76.
58. Jagoe TR, Goodship THJ, Gibson GJ. Nutritional status of patients undergoing lung cancer operations. *Ann Thorac Surg.* 2001;71:929–935.
59. Jagoe TR, Goodship THJ, Gibson GJ. The influence of nutritional status on complications after operations for lung cancer. *Ann Thorac Surg.* 2001;71:936–943.
60. Ross PJ, Ashley S, Norton A, et al. Do patients with weight loss have a worse outcome when undergoing chemotherapy for lung cancers? *Br J Cancer.* 2004;90:1905–1911.
61. Win T, Ritchie AJ, Wells FC, Laroche CM. The incidence and impact of low body mass index on patients with operable lung cancer. *Clin Nutr.* 2007;26:440–443.
62. Win T, Sharples L, Groves A, et al. Predicting survival in potentially curable lung cancer patients. *Lung.* 2008;186:97–102.
63. Tewari N, Martin-Ucar AE, Black E, et al. Nutritional status affects long term survival after lobectomy for lung cancer. *Lung Cancer.* 2007;57:389–394.
64. Johnson G, Sallé A, Lorimier G, et al. Cancer cachexia: Measured and predicted resting energy expenditures for nutritional needs evaluation. *Nutrition.* 2008;24:443–450.
65. Harvie MN, Howell A, Thatcher N, et al. Energy balance in patients with advanced NSCLC, metastatic melanoma and metastatic breast cancer receiving chemotherapy: A longitudinal study. *Br J Cancer.* 2005;92:673–680.
66. Morley JE, Thomas DR, Wilson MG. Cachexia: Pathophysiology and clinical relevance. *Am J Clin Nutr.* 2006;83:735–743.
67. Bauer JD, Capra S. Nutrition intervention improves outcomes in patients with cancer cachexia receiving chemotherapy: A pilot study. *Support Care Cancer.* 2005;13: 270 274.
68. Zhou W, Heist RS, Liu G, et al. Circulating 25-hydroxyvitamin D levels predict survival in early-stage non-small-cell lung cancer patients. *J Clin Oncol.* 2007;25: 479–485.
69. Clamon GH, Feld R, Evans WK, et al. Effect of adjuvant central iv hyperalimentation on the survival and response to treatment of patients with small cell lung cancer: A randomized trial. *Cancer Treat Rep.* 1985;69:167–177.
70. Evans WK, Makuch R, Clamon GH, et al. Limited impact of total parenteral nutrition on nutritional status during treatment for small cell lung cancer. *Cancer Res.* 1985;45:3347–3353.

Chapter 12

Hematologic Malignancies

Kim Robien, PhD, RD, CSO, FADA

INTRODUCTION

The term "hematologic malignancies" refers to cancer of the blood, bone marrow, and lymph nodes. The primary forms of hematopoietic malignancies are leukemias, lymphomas, and multiple myelomas. Several related disorders—namely, myelodysplastic syndromes (MDS), myelofibrosis, amyloidosis, and the myeloproliferative disorders polycythemia vera and essential thrombocytosis—are not cancers, but may eventually evolve into hematologic malignancies. Table 12.1 lists the various types of hematologic malignancies, along with

Table 12.1 *Incidence and Mortality Rates of Hematologic Malignancies in the United States*

Cancer Types	New Cases per Year*	Deaths per Year*
Leukemia		
Acute myelogenous leukemia	5,200	8,990
Chronic myelogenous leukemia	4,570	490
Acute lymphocytic leukemia	5,200	1,420
Chronic lymphocytic leukemia	15,340	4,500
Lymphoma		
Hodgkin's lymphoma	8,190	1,070
Non-Hodgkin's lymphoma	63,190	18,660
Multiple myeloma	19,900	10,790
Myelodysplastic syndrome	10,300[†]	35% 3-year survival[†]

*Unless otherwise noted, data are for 2007 and come from the following source: American Cancer Society. *Cancer Facts and Figures 2007*. Atlanta, GA: American Cancer Society; 2007.
[†]Data are for 2003 and come from the following source: Ma X, Does M, Raza A, Mayne ST. Myelodysplastic syndromes: Incidence and survival in the United States. *Cancer*. 2007;109(8):1536–1542.

incidence and mortality data for the United States. Data on incidence and survival for myelofibrosis, amyloidosis, and the myeloproliferative disorders are not well documented, as these nonmalignant diseases are not reportable to large, population-based cancer monitoring programs.

Leukemias encompass a number of cancers arising from hematopoietic cell lines. Genetic translocations, inversions, or deletions in hematopoietic cells disrupt the normal function of the genes at these locations, altering normal blood cell development.[1] As a result, dysfunctional or nondifferentiated leukemic cells accumulate in the bone marrow space and progressively replace normal hematopoietic cells. Signs and symptoms of leukemia include anemia, fatigue, bleeding, and infections. Leukemias can be either acute or chronic. They can arise from myeloid or lymphoid cell lines, or both, as in the case of myeloid/lymphoid or mixed-lineage leukemia (MLL). The four major forms of leukemia are acute lymphocytic leukemia (ALL), acute myelogenous leukemia (AML), chronic lymphocytic leukemia (CLL), and chronic myelogenous leukemia (CML).[2]

Leukemias are relatively rare cancers, accounting for only 3% of all new cancer cases each year.[3] Approximately 13,290 individuals are diagnosed with AML and 5,430 with ALL annually in the United States.[3] ALL occurs more commonly among children and young adults, with a median age at diagnosis of 10 years, whereas the median age of onset for AML is 65 years.[4] CLL is the most common form of leukemia in adults in Western countries, affecting approximately 15,100 individuals each year in the United States.[3] CML affects approximately 4,500 individuals per year in the United States,[5] with a median age of onset between ages 45 and 55.[6] Leukemia is the most common type of cancer among children, with ALL accounting for 75% of all pediatric leukemia cases, AML for 20% of such cases, and CML for less than 5%.[7]

Advances in the treatment of childhood ALL over the past 50 years have resulted in current 5-year survival rates exceeding 80% for this disease.[8, 9] Adult leukemias are associated with somewhat less optimistic survival statistics. Among adults with AML, 15–25% can be expected to survive 3 or more years, and some may achieve complete remission with appropriate therapy.[10] Among adults with ALL, 35–40% can expect to survive 2 years with appropriate treatment, and some researchers report 3-year survival rates as high as 50%.[11] Overall 5-year survival rates for chronic myelogenous leukemia have increased from 27% in 1990–1992 to 49% in 2002–2004 following the introduction of new tyrosine kinase inhibitors, such as imatinib (described later in this chapter).[12] Mean survival for adult chronic lymphocytic leukemia is 8–12 years.[13]

Lymphomas—that is, cancer of lymphocytes—are often broadly categorized into two main categories: Hodgkin's disease (HD) and non-Hodgkin's lymphoma (NHL). The presence of Reed-Stemberg cells, distinctive giant cells derived from B lymphocytes, is the hallmark abnormality associated with HD. All other types of lymphoma are considered NHL, a category that the World Health Organization has further organized into B-cell tumors, T-cell and natural-killer-cell tumors, and immunodeficiency-associated lympho-proliferative disorders.[14]

NHL is the fifth most common cancer diagnosis among both men and women in the United States,[3] and most common form of hematologic malignancy. In 2008, the American Cancer Society estimated that more than 66,000 new cases of NHL and more than 8,000 cases of HD would be diagnosed.[3] Survival rates for adults diagnosed with HD have improved dramatically over the past few decades, and now 75% of these patients can expect to achieve complete remission after receiving combination chemotherapy with or without radiation.[15] Overall 5-year survival rates for NHL are in the range of 55–65%.[3] Currently, 30–60% of aggressive forms of NHL can be cured, although survival rates are less predictable for indolent, slowly progressing forms of NHL, which are associated with higher relapse rates.[16]

Multiple myeloma is a cancer of plasma cells. The malignant plasma cells secrete proteins that stimulate the osteoclasts to break down bone, resulting in the characteristic bone lesions, bone pain, hypercalcemia, and loss of stature associated with this type of malignancy.[17] Approximately 20,000 new cases are diagnosed in the United States annually.[3] Multiple myeloma is rarely diagnosed in individuals younger than 40 years.[17] The disease responds well to treatment, but is rarely curable.[18] Current treatment modalities aim to lengthen survival time with the disease. Five-year survival rates are currently 32%.[19]

Many hematologic malignancies are now classified by cytogenetic profiling (specific genetic abnormality) or immunophenotyping (membrane surface protein expression profile) of the cancer cell. These subclassifications allow for use of more targeted treatment regimens and better estimates of patients' prognosis. An example of a genetic marker that is helpful in this regard is the Philadelphia chromosome (Ph+), the hallmark cytogenetic abnormality seen in 95% of CML cases.[20] Ph+ is a translocation of the long arms of chromosomes 9 and 22, which transfers the Abelson (*abl*) oncogene from chromosome 9 to the breakpoint cluster region (*bcr*) on chromosome 22.[21, 22] Transcription of this *bcr-abl* fusion gene produces an abnormal tyrosine kinase protein, which in turn activates a number of cytoplasmic and nuclear signal-transduction pathways, ultimately leading to the disordered myelo-proliferation seen in CML.[23]

Nutritional Interventions for Hematologic Malignancies

In general, nutrition assessment and development of a nutrition care plan for patients with any type of cancer should include consideration of two broad issues: the effects on nutritional status caused by the cancer itself and the effects on nutritional status caused by the treatment.

Impact of the Disease Process on Nutritional Status

Hematologic malignancies themselves tend not to have significant effects on an individual's nutritional status. Cancer-induced anorexia and cachexia are less common in the early phases of hematologic malignancies compared with other types of cancer, but may occur in the later stages and as side effects of certain treatments. A 1980 study by the Eastern Cooperative Oncology Group reported that weight loss in the 6 months prior to initiation of treatment occurred in only 4% of patients with AML, 10% of patients with NHL (favorable prognosis), and 15% of patients with more aggressive forms of NHL.[24] Anemias related to the cancer process, rather than nutrient deficiencies, may occur as the malignant hematopoietic cell lineage crowds out erythrocytes.

Cancer-associated hypercalcemia is most frequently described with multiple myeloma, HD and NHL, but may also occur with other hematologic malignancies. Tumor cells can disrupt the body's normally tight control of calcium homeostasis through secretion of various endocrine proteins, such as parathyroid hormone-related protein and 1,25-$(OH)_2$cholecalciferol, which in turn can lead to increased osteoclastic bone resorption and hypercalcemia.[25] Treatment for cancer-associated hypercalcemia most commonly consists of intravenous hydration to rehydrate the patient and promote renal calcium excretion, followed by bisphosphonates to inhibit bone resorption.[25] Calcium supplementation (from parenteral or oral sources) should be discontinued, and phosphorus replacement may be necessary.[26]

Impact of Treatment Regimens on Nutritional Status

Registered dietitians and other nutrition practitioners with specialized and advanced skills in oncology nutrition are able to anticipate the nutrition-related impacts of planned treatment regimens, and work with the individual to prevent or minimize these side effects.[27] Because treatment regimens are constantly evolving, the reader is referred to the National Cancer Institute's Comprehensive Cancer Database, called the Physician Data Query (PDQ; http://www.cancer.gov/cancertopics/pdq/cancerdatabase), for current recommendations by cancer type, stage, and grade.

Treatment for hematologic malignancies may include several stages of combination chemotherapy regimens: induction chemotherapy to decrease the tumor burden and assess response to chemotherapeutic agents, followed by consolidation/intensification therapy, and finally maintenance chemotherapy to keep the cancer in remission. This treatment course may extend over a lengthy period, sometimes for many months or even years.

More recently, a new class of small-molecule drugs has been developed to target the specific aberrant proteins or pathways involved in certain hematologic malignancies. These drugs, with their more specific targets, hold promise as being able to provide for better drug tolerance with improved outcomes. One of the first drugs introduced in this class, imatinib, is a tyrosine kinase inhibitor developed specifically to inhibit the abnormal tyrosine kinase that is transcribed from the Ph+ chromosome in CML. Its side effects include nausea, vomiting, diarrhea, anorexia, rash, and muscle pain, but these tend to be minor compared to the side effects observed with other chemotherapeutic agents used to treat CML.

Other chemotherapeutic classes under development for use in hematologic malignancies include biological therapies (also known as immunotherapy), such as monoclonal antibodies. Pharmacologic derivatives of vitamins A and D are also being studied for their ability to induce abnormal hematopoietic progenitor cells to differentiate normally and produce functional blood cells (known as differentiation therapy). All-*trans* retinoic acid (ATRA) and vitamin D analogs have demonstrated success at achieving remissions when combined with other chemotherapeutic agents, especially in acute promyelocytic leukemia (ATRA) and MDS (vitamin D analogs).[28] Hematopoietic cell transplantation (HCT) is also used in the treatment of hematologic malignancies; it is discussed in more detail later in this chapter.

Table 12.2 summarizes the chemotherapeutic agents commonly used in treating hematologic malignancies, as well as the potential nutritional implications of each agent.

Table 12.2 *Nutritional Implications of Chemotherapeutic Agents Commonly Used in the Treatment of Hematologic Malignancies*

Medication	Potential Side Effects with Nutritional Implications	Additional Nutrition-Related Concerns
Alkylating Agents		
Busulfan	Nausea, vomiting (<10%*), mucositis, hyperglycemia, hypomagnesemia, hypophosphatemia, weight loss	• Food may inhibit absorption of the drug.
Cyclophosphamide	Nausea, vomiting (>30%*)	• Maintain adequate hydration.
Dacarbazine	Nausea, vomiting (>90%*), anorexia	• Avoid alcohol while taking this drug.
Ifosfamide	Nausea, vomiting (30–90%*), xerostomia, abdominal pain	• Maintain adequate hydration.
Mechlorethamine	Nausea, vomiting (<90%*)	• Maintain adequate hydration.
Procarbazine	Nausea, vomiting, diarrhea, mucositis	• Avoid alcohol while taking this drug. • Avoid high-tyramine foods (such as fermented or aged foods, anchovies, caviar, liver, raisins, bananas, chocolate, avocados, fava beans, soy sauce, tofu, miso), which can cause hypertension while taking this drug.
Antimetabolites		
Cytarabine	Nausea, vomiting (10–90%*), diarrhea, mucositis, anorexia	• Maintain adequate hydration. • Avoid alcohol while taking this drug.
Fludarabine	Anorexia, nausea, vomiting (<10%*), fatigue, edema	
Hydroxyurea	Constipation	
Mercaptopurine	Diarrhea, intestinal ulcers	• Maintain adequate hydration.
Methotrexate	Nausea, vomiting (10–30%*), diarrhea, anorexia, mucositis	• Maintain adequate hydration.
Thioguanine	Nausea, vomiting, diarrhea, mucositis	• Maintain adequate hydration. • Avoid alcohol while taking this drug.

*Incidence of emesis without antiemetics for intravenous administration of the drug, according to the following source: Kris MS, Hesketh PJ, Somerfield MR, et al. American Society of Clinical Oncology guideline for antiemetics in oncology: Update 2006. *J Clin Oncol.* 2006;24:2932–2947.

(continues)

Table 12.2 *Nutritional Implications of Chemotherapeutic Agents Commonly Used in the Treatment of Hematologic Malignancies, Continued*

Medication	Potential Side Effects with Nutritional Implications	Additional Nutrition-Related Concerns
Anthracyclines		
Daunorubicin	Nausea, vomiting (30–90%*), xerostomia, dysgeusia	
Doxorubicin	Nausea, vomiting (30–90%*)	
Idarubicin	Nausea, vomiting (30–90%*), diarrhea, abdominal cramping	
Mitoxantrone	Diarrhea, nausea, vomiting (10–30%*), mucositis	
Antimitotic Drugs		
Etoposide	Nausea, vomiting (10–30%*), diarrhea, anorexia	• Avoid alcohol while taking this drug.
Vinblastine	Vomiting (<10%*), constipation, jaw pain	
Vincristine	Nausea, vomiting (<10%*), constipation, hyponatremia	
Tyrosine Kinase Inhibitors		
Dasatinib	Abdominal pain, constipation, diarrhea, anorexia, nausea, vomiting, weight gain or loss, abdominal distention, fatigue	• Do not eat grapefruit or grapefruit juice while taking this drug.
Imatinib	Nausea, vomiting, diarrhea, anorexia, weight gain, fatigue	• Take drug with meals and a large glass of water. • Do not eat grapefruit or grapefruit juice while taking this drug.
Nilotinib	Nausea, vomiting, diarrhea, constipation, hyperglycemia, hypophosphatemia	• Avoid food 2 hours before and 1 hour after taking this drug. • Do not eat grapefruit or grapefruit juice while taking this drug.

*Incidence of emesis without antiemetics for intravenous administration of the drug, according to the following source: Kris MS, Hesketh PJ, Somerfield MR, et al. American Society of Clinical Oncology guideline for antiemetics in oncology: Update 2006. *J Clin Oncol.* 2006;24:2932–2947.

(continues)

Table 12.2 *Nutritional Implications of Chemotherapeutic Agents Commonly Used in the Treatment of Hematologic Malignancies,* *Continued*

Medication	Potential Side Effects with Nutritional Implications	Additional Nutrition-Related Concerns
Monoclonal Antibodies		
Rituximab	Nausea, vomiting (<10%*)	
Miscellaneous		
Asparaginase	Nausea, vomiting, anorexia, hyperglycemia, hepatoxicity, renal insufficiency	
Bleomycin	Nausea, vomiting (<10%*), mucositis	• Avoid alcohol while taking this drug.
Bortezomib	Nausea, anorexia, diarrhea, constipation	• Maintain adequate hydration.
Cyclosporine	Renal insufficiency, hypomagnesemia, hyperlipidemia	• Maintain adequate hydration. • Magnesium supplementation is often required. Oral magnesium supplementation may cause GI upset. • Hyperlipidemia often resolves with discontinuation of medication. If duration of therapy is prolonged, the patient may benefit from modification of dietary fat intake.
Interferon	Nausea, vomiting, diarrhea, anorexia, dysgeusia, fatigue	• Maintain adequate hydration.
Prednisone	Altered body composition (increased body fat, decreased muscle stores, fluid retention), decreased bone mineralization, hyperglycemia, hyperphagia, weight gain, hypokalemia and other electrolyte disturbances, hyperlipidemia	• Encourage daily low-impact exercise. • Adequate dietary calcium, vitamins D and K intake to maximize bone density. • Diet modification and insulin may be needed to manage blood glucose levels. • Hyperlipidemia often resolves with discontinuation of medication. If duration of therapy is prolonged, the patient may benefit from modification of dietary fat intake.
Thalidomide	Nausea, constipation, hypocalcemia	• Avoid alcohol while taking this drug. • Take drug at bedtime, and at least one hour after eating.

*Incidence of emesis without antiemetics for intravenous administration of the drug, according to the following source: Kris MS, Hesketh PJ, Somerfield MR, et al. American Society of Clinical Oncology guideline for antiemetics in oncology: Update 2006. *J Clin Oncol.* 2006;24:2932–2947.

Impact of Supportive Treatments on Nutritional Status

Supportive treatments can also have nutritional implications. Transfusion iron overload can occur in patients requiring frequent red blood cell (RBC) transfusions, such as patients with myelodysplastic syndrome or patients undergoing HCT. Each unit of RBCs contains 200–250 mg iron, and with estimated daily losses of only 1–2 mg/day for the average person without blood loss,[29] iron overload can quickly become an issue for patients requiring frequent transfusions. In addition to the potential for organ damage, increased serum iron levels can increase the risk of bacterial infections.[30]

For patients with documented transfusion iron overload, or those for whom prolonged RBC support is anticipated, dietary and supplemental iron restrictions may be necessary. Multivitamin supplements without iron are increasingly available now that the major manufacturers have developed separate product lines for "seniors"—these products tend to be iron free. Dietary and supplemental vitamin C should also be limited to the Recommended Dietary Allowance for the patient's life-stage and gender, as this vitamin has been found to act as a pro-oxidant in the presence of iron.[31]

Hematopoietic Cell Transplantation

Hematopoietic cell transplantation (HCT) involves the use of chemotherapy with or without radiation, followed by infusion of donor (allogeneic) or previously stored patient (autologous) hematopoietic cells. HCT is used to treat a variety of hematologic malignancies, including leukemia and lymphoma, as well as nonmalignant conditions such as aplastic anemia, autoimmune diseases, and immune deficiency diseases. Despite significant advances in treatments over the past 40 years, HCT is associated with considerable treatment-related morbidity, prolonged hospitalizations, and long-term health problems.[32] Typical medical and nutritional issues that may arise during the myeloablative HCT process are outlined in Table 12.3.

Table 12.3 *Medical Issues and Nutritional Diagnoses That May Arise During the Myeloablative Allogeneic Hematopoietic Transplant Process**

Conditioning (Day –10 to Day 0)[†]	Neutropenia (Days 0 to 20)	Engraftment/Early Recovery (Days 20 to 100)	Long-Term Recovery (Beyond Day 100)
Possible Medical Issues with Nutritional Implications			
Tumor lysis	• Opportunistic infections • Mucositis, esophagitis, gastritis • Sinusoidal obstructive syndrome • Nausea, vomiting, diarrhea • Altered taste, smell acuity • Changes in consistency, volume of saliva	• Acute GVHD • Opportunistic infections • Altered taste acuity • Drug-induced nephrotoxicity • Transfusion-related iron overload	• Chronic GVHD • Opportunistic infections • Delayed growth and development • Relapse, secondary tumors • Cataracts • Osteopenia/osteoporosis • Transfusion-related iron overload
Possible Nutrition Diagnoses[‡]			
Increased/decreased nutrient needs: electrolytes (NI-5.1/5.4) related to tumor lysis	• Inadequate oral food/beverage intake (NI-2.1) related to mucositis, nausea, vomiting, intolerance to certain foods (especially lactose, citrus, fat) • Increased nutrient needs: fluids (NI-5.1) due to drug-induced nephrotoxicity • Increased/decreased nutrient needs: electrolytes (NI-5.1/5.4) related to drug-induced nephrotoxicity and altered electrolyte excretion or retention	• Inadequate oral food/beverage intake (NI-2.1) related to GI GVHD, altered taste acuity, transition from IV to PO medications • Increased nutrient needs: fluids (NI-5.1) related to drug-induced nephrotoxicity • Involuntary weight gain (NC-3.4) related to fluid retention • Increased/decreased nutrient needs: electrolytes (NI-5.1/5.4) related to drug-induced nephrotoxicity and altered electrolyte excretion or retention	• Impaired nutrient utilization (NC-2.1) related to malabsorption as a result of chronic GI GVHD and/or pancreatic insufficiency • Altered nutrition-related laboratory values: hyperglycemia (NC-2.2) related to chronic use of steroids • Altered nutrition-related laboratory values: hypertriglyceridemia (NC-2.2) related to chronic use of steroids, immunosuppressants

(continues)

Table 12.3 *Medical Issues and Nutritional Diagnoses That May Arise During the Myeloablative Allogeneic Hematopoietic Transplant Process, Continued*

• Altered nutrition-related laboratory values: hyperglycemia (NC-2.2) related to chronic use of steroids • Decreased nutrient needs: iron (NI-5.4) related to blood transfusions	• Increased nutrient needs: calcium, vitamin D (NI-5.1) related to chronic use of steroids • Involuntary weight gain (NC-3.4) related to chronic use of steroids • Decreased nutrient needs: iron (NI-5.4) related to blood transfusions • Chewing difficulty (NC-1.2) related to oral strictures • Swallowing difficulty (NC-1.1) related to esophageal strictures

GI = gastrointestinal, GVHD = graft-versus-host disease, IV = intravenous, PO = per os (Latin for "by mouth").

*Patients receiving autologous, syngeneic, non-myeloablative, or reduced-intensity transplants may be at lower risk of both medical and nutritional complications because of lower toxicity of conditioning and immunosuppressive regimens.

†The day of transplant is traditionally referred to as day 0.

‡Data from International Dietetics and Nutrition Terminology (IDNT) Reference Manual: *Standardized Language for the Nutrition Care Process.* American Dietetic Association, 2008. Parentheses indicate applicable nutrition diagnosis code.

Source: Adapted from Hasse JM, Robien K. Nutrition support guidelines for therapeutically immunosuppressed patients. In: Kudsk KA, Pichard C, eds. *From Nutritional Support to Pharmacologic Nutrition in the ICU.* Heidelberg, Germany: Springer-Verlag; 2000:361–383.

Disease eradication following myeloablative HCT is due not only to the chemotherapy and/or radiation given during the conditioning regimen, but also to the effect of the donor cells attacking and destroying the host malignant cells in what is known as the graft-versus-malignancy effect. Non-myeloablative and reduced-intensity treatment regimens, which utilize lower doses of radiation and chemotherapy in an attempt to utilize the graft-versus-malignancy effect to a greater degree, have made HCT feasible for patients who otherwise would not be expected to tolerate the more intense myeloablative regimens. As a result, the HCT population has expanded, to the point that older patients, patients with comorbid conditions, and patients with some premalignant diseases may receive transplants.

The current literature related to nutritional support of HCT patients relates primarily to traditional myeloablative HCT regimens. Very few studies have gathered data on non-myeloablative or reduced-intensity regimens. It is expected that these less intensive regimens will result in fewer and less intense nutritional symptoms, and will require parenteral nutrition (PN) less frequently or for shorter duration. One notable exception is that the frequency of acute and chronic graft-versus-host disease (GVHD) has been shown to be similar between myeloablative and non-myeloablative regimens, and may occur later post-transplant among patients treated with non-myeloablative regimens.[33, 34] GVHD can have severe nutritional effects, as will be discussed later in this section.

Nutritional Requirements of the HCT Patient

Because of the intensity of the treatment regimens, patients undergoing HCT—and especially allogeneic myeloablative treatment regimens—may have increased energy, protein, and fluid requirements. Whenever possible, clinicians should use indirect calorimetry to measure resting energy expenditure for patients undergoing HCT. When indirect calorimetry is not available, studies have indicated that patients receiving myeloablative treatment regimens generally require dietary intake of 30–35 kcal/kg to maintain nitrogen balance and body weight during the cytoreduction and neutropenic phases of the transplant.[35, 36] Patients receiving reduced-intensity or autologous treatment regimens may have lower energy requirements. The evidence supporting a specific protein recommendation for HCT patients is more limited, but seems to indicate that more than 2.2 g protein/kg body weight may be needed to maintain positive nitrogen balance in the early post-transplant period.[35-38]

Interest in the use of glutamine in the HCT population was stimulated by animal studies that found decreased mucosal atrophy, more rapid mucosal recovery, and decreased incidence of bacteremia following high-dose chemotherapy with oral glutamine or glutamine-supplemented PN.[39, 40] Initially, the use of glutamine in the oncology patient population had been an area of controversy owing to concerns that tumors are avid glutamine consumers. Ultimately, these concerns were allayed when studies using rat models suggested that glutamine-enhanced PN solutions did not increase tumor size compared to unsupplemented controls.[41]

Unfortunately, research into the role of glutamine supplementation in the HCT population has not lived up to the promise suggested by the earlier animal studies. While Ziegler et al[42] reported significantly improved nitrogen balance, decreased incidence of infection, and shortened length of stay among patients receiving glutamine-enhanced PN solutions compared to those who did not receive glutamine supplementation, numerous subsequent studies have failed to replicate those findings.[43-47] Therefore, the use of glutamine-enhanced PN solutions is not currently recommended because of the solutions' cost and lack of demonstrated benefit.[35] Similarly, the use of oral glutamine has failed to show a convincing benefit in improving oral intake or reducing the incidence and severity of oral mucositis or diarrhea in the HCT population[48, 49] and, therefore, is not recommended.[35]

Fluid requirements, especially in patients receiving myeloablative regimens, are also elevated because of the use of nephrotoxic conditioning regimens, immunosuppressive agents, and antimicrobial agents. Fluid requirements have been estimated to be 1,500 mL/m^2,[32] but may vary based on the individual's medical condition. Fluid restrictions may be necessary if the patient develops sinusoidal obstruction syndrome (discussed later in this chapter). Conversely, fluid requirements may increase if the patient develops renal insufficiency or has significant gastrointestinal losses from diarrhea or GVHD.

Parenteral Nutrition Support

Many HCT patients—but especially those undergoing myeloablative treatment regimens—experience significant oral mucositis, taste changes, nausea, vomiting, and diarrhea in the early post-transplant phase as a result of the conditioning regimens. These side effects can result in a significant reduction in dietary intake. PN is commonly used as the sole source of nutrition support or to supplement oral intake. However, the American Dietetic Association's evidence-based guideline on the use of PN following HCT recommends PN be used only in selected patients because of the increased risk of complications, increased cost, and lack of significant improvement in treatment outcomes.[35] Prophylactic PN is not recommended. Whenever possible, it is best to work closely with the patient and/or caregivers during this stage to find acceptable foods in an attempt to maintain oral intake and gastrointestinal integrity.

In a retrospective cohort study of 20 patients with AML undergoing HCT, Iestra et al. found that only 60% of patients required PN support based on the following criteria: (1) severe malnutrition at admission, (2) a prolonged period of minimal oral intake (7–10 days), or (3) weight loss of more than 10% of total body weight.[50] Calvo et al found that the costs associated with intensive nutritional monitoring and daily assessment of oral intake were approximately one-half of the potential cost savings achieved by avoiding inappropriate PN use and the infectious complications that could accompany unneeded PN.[51]

Concerns regarding the use of PN following HCT include the potential for intravenous lipids to contribute to an increase in infectious complications, the potential for glucose-based solutions to exacerbate efforts to maintain normal blood glucose levels and further increase infection risk, the potential for inhibiting oral intake needed to maintain gastrointestinal mucosal integrity, and the possibility of contributing to post-transplant hepatic complications as evidenced by elevated serum transaminase, alkaline phosphatase, and bilirubin levels.[52] These liver function parameters, if related to PN, often improve with discontinuation or cycling of the PN infusion.

Infectious complications, while increasingly treatable, remain a significant cause of transplant-related mortality.[53] One of the first reports suggesting PN may contribute to infectious complications following HCT came from Weisdorf et al. in 1987; in their study, these authors found that among patients receiving allogeneic HCT, bacteremias occurred in 72% of patients receiving PN and 48% of patients who did not receive PN.[54] Several studies in the late 1970s and early 1980s demonstrated that 20% intravenous lipid emulsions could inhibit phagocytosis and alter neutrophil chemotaxis in healthy volunteers,[55–57] potentially increasing the risk of infection. However, a randomized trial of 512 patients undergoing allogeneic or autologous HCT for hematologic malignancies found no significant differences in the incidence of bacterial or fungal infections between intravenous lipid emulsions (of 20% linoleic acid) at either 6–8% or 25–30% of total daily energy.[58] Similarly, a randomized trial of 66 patients receiving allogeneic HCT for hematologic malignancies comparing isocaloric glucose-based (100% glucose as nonprotein calories) and lipid-based (80% lipids and 20% glucose as nonprotein calories) PN solutions found no significant differences between the 2 groups for incidence of fever or positive blood cultures.[59]

The American Dietetic Association's evidence-based guideline on the use of lipids in PN formulations following HCT calls for providing 25–30% of energy as lipids to prevent fatty acid deficiency and improve blood glucose control.[35] The guideline also recommends monitoring triglyceride levels regularly while patients are receiving PN solutions containing lipids, and notes that the lipid infusion should be discontinued if the patient develops hyperlipidemia.[35]

Infections related to hyperglycemia in HCT patients receiving PN are also a concern. In a retrospective chart review of 208 patients undergoing HCT (including both autologous and allogeneic patients as well as those receiving myeloablative and reduced-intensity conditioning regimens), Sheean and Braunschweig found that patients who received PN were 4 times more likely to experience hyperglycemia (defined as glucose > 110 mg/dL) compared to than those who did not receive PN (OR = 3.9; 95% confidence interval: 2.7–5.5).[60] No association was observed between the dextrose administration dose (range: 1.3–3.9 mg/kg/min) and serum glucose concentrations. Sheean and colleagues also reported that the likelihood of infection was 2 times higher among patients receiving PN who had hyperglycemia compared to those who did not have hyperglycemia (OR = 2.1; 95% confidence interval: 1.3–3.5) after excluding patients on steroids.[61] Clearly, careful blood glucose monitoring and management while on PN is vital in this immunosuppressed population at increased risk of infection complications.

The potential for PN to delay resumption of oral intake is also a concern. Charuhas et al. found that providing PN once the patient has been able to transition from the hospital to the ambulatory setting (roughly corresponding to the transition from the neutropenic to the engraftment/early recovery phase) resulted in delayed resumption of oral intake.[62] In their study of 258 HCT patients, the patients who were randomized to receive intravenous hydration were able to meet more than 85% of their estimated caloric requirements an average of 6 days earlier than members of the group receiving PN.[62]

Enteral Nutrition Support

Enteral feedings are the preferred route of nutrition support in any patient population, as the presence of nutrients in the intestinal tract is thought to maintain mucosal integrity and prevent bacterial translocation. However, the use of nasoenteric feeding tubes is challenging in the early post-transplant period because of the potential for tube displacement and the risk of aspiration as a result of treatment-induced vomiting,[63, 64] increased risk of bleeding complications during tube placement, and increased risk of ulceration at contact points with the tubing.

Despite these obstacles, a small number of studies have reported successful enteral feedings in the early post-transplant period, primarily in children. In a study of 15 adult patients undergoing HCT for a variety of hematologic malignancies,[65] nasojejunal feeding tubes were placed prior to initiation of chemotherapy. Eight of the 15 patients tolerated the enteral feedings and were able to maintain their feeding tubes until the day of engraftment. One patient refused tube placement, 4 patients lost their tubes due to vomiting, and 2 patients experienced epistaxis.

Papadopoulou et al[66] reported that of 21 children undergoing HCT who elected to receive enteral feedings, only 8 patients stopped the feedings prematurely. Seven vomited the tube after an average of 10 days, and 1 stopped the enteral feeding because of diarrhea. The timing of feeding tube placement in this study is not described.

Langdana et al reported that of 49 children undergoing HCT who received nasogastric tubes during conditioning or the first week post-transplant, 42 were able to be maintained exclusively on enteral feedings.[67] Conversely, Hopman et al reported that of 12 patients who agreed to enteral feedings when they were unable to meet at least 75% of estimated caloric needs by oral intake, only 3 could be maintained exclusively by enteral feedings.[68] The researchers did note that patients who received enteral feedings for a longer time pre-transplant seemed to tolerate enteral feedings better in the post-transplant period, and that cholestasis was less common among patients who received enteral feedings compared to a group who received parenteral nutrition.

Taken collectively, these small studies suggest that enteral feedings during HCT may be possible. Clearly, though, the factors associated with successful enteral feedings require further study.

Graft-versus-Host Disease

Graft-versus-host disease (GVHD) is a common post-transplant complication.[69] Although we refer to the condition as a "disease," it actually is a normal physiologic response in which host tissue cells that were damaged during the conditioning regimen begin secreting immunostimulatory cytokines. These cytokines enhance expression of MHC antigens and adhesion molecules, thereby inducing a cascade of immune responses in the newly transplanted donor hematopoietic cells, including activation of cytotoxic T cells and natural killer cells.[69] These activated donor T cells interact with the host antigen-presenting cells, resulting in an amplification of local tissue injury and destruction.[69] The skin, liver, and intestinal tract are most often affected, as demonstrated by symptoms ranging from a mild skin rash or elevated liver function tests to fatal organ failure.

To prevent this complication, transplant patients are given immunosuppressive medications, such a cyclosporine or tacrolimus, until the donor cells are able to develop a tolerance to the host tissues. Corticosteroids are commonly used in the treatment of GVHD, and typically require a prolonged tapering schedule. Hyperglycemia and osteopenia/osteoporosis are common complications of these treatment schedules. Patients should be counseled to participate in daily weight-bearing exercise, and to consume adequate calcium and vitamin D through both diet and supplements.

Milder cases of gastrointestinal GVHD may, in part, be managed through use of diets that are low in GI stimulants or irritants, such as caffeine, lactose, acids, fats, and dietary fiber. It is especially important that patients with gastrointestinal GVHD closely follow food safety guidelines to avoid bacterial translocation across the damaged gastrointestinal mucosa. Higher grades of gastrointestinal GVHD may require PN and complete bowel rest to slow fluid losses from diarrhea and allow the gastrointestinal mucosa time to heal. The Seattle Cancer Care Alliance has developed patient education materials on its "gastrointestinal diets," which are available through the organization's website at http://www.seattlecca.org/patientsandfamilies/nutrition/nutritionDietsguidelines/.

Chronic GVHD (cGVHD), typically defined as GVHD occurring after day 100 post-transplant, is a major cause of morbidity and mortality following HCT, though the pathobiology of the disease is not well understood.[70] Nutritional concerns typically arise in conjunction with oral, hepatic, and gastrointestinal cGVHD, which can cause mouth pain, esophageal strictures, malabsorption, and weight loss.[71, 72] In particular, oral ulcerations and pain may limit oral intake.[73] Malabsorption can occur for a variety of reasons, including alterations of the intestinal mucosa, bile acid deficiency, pancreatic enzyme deficiency, or bacterial overgrowth.[72]

Low-fat diets and pancreatic enzymes may be effective in managing GI symptoms in patients with cGVHD. Patients should be evaluated for fat-soluble vitamin deficiencies, and supplements should be used as needed. Dietary intake should be monitored regularly and evaluated for nutritional adequacy.

Sinusoidal Obstruction Syndrome

Hepatic sinusoidal obstruction syndrome (SOS), previously known as veno-occlusive disease, can occur when sinusoidal epithelial cells are damaged by high-dose conditioning regimens. The damaged cells swell and eventually slough, causing congestion and obstruction of blood flow through the sinusoid.[74] SOS is characterized by hepatomegaly, fluid retention, ascites, and jaundice.[74] Fluid and sodium restrictions may be needed to limit the rapid fluid weight gain that often occurs with SOS. If hyperbilirubinemia persists for longer than a week and the patient is receiving PN, trace element solutions containing copper and manganese should be discontinued to avoid accumulation of these elements, which are normally excreted through bile.[75] Manganese toxicity can lead to neurotoxicity, whereas copper toxicity can further exacerbate hepatic damage and cause gastrointestinal side effects, such as abdominal pain, cramping, nausea, vomiting, and diarrhea.[76]

Food Safety

Because the hematopoietic system plays a significant role in the immune system, treatment for hematologic malignancies often results in neutropenia. Food-borne illnesses could easily occur, and could significantly affect a patient's recovery. Such illnesses are potentially avoidable with proper training of the patient and caregivers. Many institutions have developed neutropenic diet guidelines that are intended to exclude foods that carry a higher likelihood of bacterial contamination. These guidelines often vary from institution to institution, however, and they are rarely based on actual microbiological testing of the food items in question.

Even foods that are approved for inclusion in neutropenic diets can be a source of food-borne illness if proper food sanitation, storage, preparation, and serving procedures are not followed. In a randomized trial comparing adherence to either a neutropenic diet or the Food and Drug Administration's (FDA's) food safety guidelines among pediatric oncology patients receiving myelosuppressive chemotherapy, Moody et al. found no difference in infection rates between the two study arms.[77] The study reported a greater adherence rate with the food safety guidelines (100%) than with the neutropenic diet (94%), suggesting that the food safety guidelines, which are less restrictive regarding food choice, but more global with regard to hygiene, are more appropriate as a patient and caregiver education tool. The websites of the Centers for Disease Control and Prevention's (CDC's) Food Safety Office (http://cdc.gov/foodsafety/) and the FDA's Center for Food Safety and Applied Nutrition (http://www.cfsan.fda.gov/) offer the most current food safety guidelines and patient/client education materials.

SUMMARY

Treatment-related complications will likely have a greater impact on nutritional status than will disease-related issues for patients with hematologic malignancies. The nutritional concerns of this patient population run the gamut from fairly minor implications for patients who can be successfully treated with new small-molecule drugs such as imatinib, to some of the most challenging nutrition issues encountered in oncology among patients who receive myeloablative HCT. Food safety is a special concern for people being treated for hematologic malignancies, as these individuals are often in an immunocompromised state, either as a result of the disease or the treatment. Clinicians interested in specializing in oncology nutrition should develop their skills in anticipating nutrition-related effects of planned treatment regimens, and working with patients and caregivers to minimize the impact of treatment on nutritional status.

REFERENCES

1. Bloomfield CD, Caligiuri MA. Molecular biology of leukemias. In: DeVita VT, Hellman S, Rosenberg SA, eds. *Cancer: Principles and Practice of Oncology*. 6th ed. Philadelphia, PA: Lippincott Williams & Wilkins; 2001:2389–2404.
2. Cole P, Rodu B. Descriptive epidemiology: cancer statistics. In: DeVita VT, Hellman S, Rosenberg SA, eds. *Cancer: Principles and Practice of Oncology*. 6th ed. Philadelphia, PA: Lippincott Williams & Wilkins; 2001:228–241.
3. American Cancer Society. *Cancer Facts and Figures 2008*. Atlanta, GA: Author; 2008.
4. Scheinberg DA, Maslak P, Weiss M. Acute leukemias. In: DeVita VT, Hellman S, Rosenberg SA, eds. *Cancer: Principles and Practice of Oncology*. 6th ed. Philadelphia, PA: Lippincott Williams & Wilkins; 2001:2404–2433.
5. American Cancer Society. *Cancer Facts and Figures 2007*. Atlanta, GA: Author; 2007.
6. Kantarjian HM, Faderl S, Talpaz M. Chronic myelogenous leukemia. In: DeVita VT, Hellman S, Rosenberg SA, eds. *Cancer: Principles and Practice of Oncology*. 6th ed. Philadelphia, PA: Lippincott Williams & Wilkins; 2001:2433–2447.
7. Weinstein HJ, Tarbell NJ. Leukemias and lymphomas of childhood. In: DeVita VT, Hellman S, Rosenberg SA, eds. *Cancer: Principles and Practice of Oncology*. 6th ed. Philadelphia, PA: Lippincott Williams & Wilkins; 2001:2235–2256.
8. Pui CH, Evans WE. Treatment of acute lymphoblastic leukemia. *N Engl J Med*. 2006;354(2):166–178.
9. National Cancer Institute. *Surveillance, Epidemiology and End Results (SEER) program* (www.seer.cancer.gov): *SEER*Stat Database: Incidence-SEER 9 Regs Public Use, November 2004 sub (1973–2002)*. Washington, DC: National Cancer Institute, DCCPS, Surveillance Research Program, Cancer Statistics Branch; 2004.
10. National Cancer Institute. Adult acute myeloid leukemia treatment (PDQ): Health professional version. November 2, 2007. http://www.cancer.gov/cancertopics/pdq/treatment/adultAML/healthprofessional. Accessed December 13, 2007.
11. National Cancer Institute. Adult acute lymphoblastic leukemia treatment (PDQ): Health professional version. November 2, 2007. http://www.cancer.gov/cancertopics/pdq/treatment/childALL/healthprofessional. Accessed December 13, 2007.
12. Brenner H, Gondos A, Pulte D. Recent trends in long-term survival of patients with chronic myelocytic leukemia: Disclosing the impact of advances in therapy on the population level. *Haematologica*. 2008; 93(10):1544-9.
13. National Cancer Institute. Chronic lymphocytic leukemia treatment (PDQ): Health professional version. November 20, 2007. http://www.cancer.gov/cancertopics/pdq/treatment/CLL/healthprofessional. Accessed December 13, 2007.
14. International Agency for Research on Cancer (IARC). *World Health Organization Classification of Tumours: Pathology and Genetics of Tumours of Haematopoietic and Lymphoid Tissue*. Lyon, France: IARC Press; 2001.

15. National Cancer Institute. Adult Hodgkin lymphoma treatment (PDQ): Health professional version. November 2, 2007. http://www.cancer.gov/cancertopics/pdq/treatment/adulthodgkins/healthprofessional. Accessed December 13, 2007.

16. National Cancer Institute. Adult Non-Hodgkin lymphoma treatment (PDQ): Health professional version. November 2, 2007. http://www.cancer.gov/cancertopics/pdq/treatment/adult-non-hodgkins/healthprofessional. Accessed December 13, 2007.

17. Rajkumar SV, Kyle RA. Multiple myeloma: Diagnosis and treatment. *Mayo Clin Proc*. 2005;80(10):1371–1382.

18. National Cancer Institute. Multiple myeloma and other plasma cell neoplasms treatment (PDQ): Health professional version. December 13, 2007. http://www.cancer.gov/cancertopics/pdq/treatment/myeloma/healthprofessional. Accessed February 5, 2008.

19. *Surveillance, Epidemiology, and End Results (SEER) program* (www.seer.cancer.gov): *SEER*Stat Database: Incidence-SEER 17 Regs Limited-Use, Nov 2006 Sub (1973–2004 varying)*. Washington, DC: National Cancer Institute, DCCPS, Surveillance Research Program, Cancer Statistics Branch; April 2007, based on the November 2006 submission.

20. Rowley JD. Letter: A new consistent chromosomal abnormality in chronic myelogenous leukaemia identified by quinacrine fluorescence and Giemsa staining. *Nature*. 1973;243(5405):290–293.

21. Bartram CR, de Klein A, Hagemeijer A, et al. Translocation of *c-abl* oncogene correlates with the presence of a Philadelphia chromosome in chronic myelocytic leukaemia. *Nature*. 1983;306(5940):277–280.

22. Groffen J, Stephenson JR, Heisterkamp N, de Klein A, Bartram CR, Grosveld G. Philadelphia chromosomal breakpoints are clustered within a limited region, *bcr*, on chromosome 22. *Cell*. 1984;36(1):93–99.

23. Shteper PJ, Ben-Yehuda D. Molecular evolution of chronic myeloid leukaemia. *Semin Cancer Biol*. 2001;11(4):313–323.

24. Dewys WD, Begg C, Lavin PT, et al; Eastern Cooperative Oncology Group. Prognostic effect of weight loss prior to chemotherapy in cancer patients. *Am J Med*. 1980;69(4):491–497.

25. Clines GA, Guise TA. Hypercalcaemia of malignancy and basic research on mechanisms responsible for osteolytic and osteoblastic metastasis to bone. *Endocr Relat Cancer*. 2005;12(3):549–583.

26. Stewart AF. Clinical practice: Hypercalcemia associated with cancer. *N Engl J Med*. 2005;352(4):373–379.

27. Robien K, Levin R, Pritchett E, Otto M. American Dietetic Association: Standards of practice and standards of professional performance for registered dietitians (generalist, specialty, and advanced) in oncology nutrition care. *J Am Diet Assoc*. 2006; 106(6):946–951.

28. de vos S, Koeffler HP. Differentiation induction in leukemia and lymphoma. In: Heber D, Blackburn GL, Go VLW, Milner J, eds. *Nutritional Oncology*. 2nd ed. Burlington, MA: Academic Press; 2006:491–506.

29. Andrews NC. Disorders of iron metabolism. *N Engl J Med*. 1999;341(26): 1986–1995.

30. Bullen JJ, Rogers HJ, Spalding PB, Ward CG. Iron and infection: The heart of the matter. *FEMS Immunol Med Microbiol*. 2005;43(3):325–330.

31. Herbert V, Shaw S, Jayatilleke E. Vitamin C-driven free radical generation from iron. *J Nutr*. 1996;126(4)(suppl):1213S–1220S.

32. Lenssen P. Bone marrow and stem cell transplantation. In: Matarese L, Gottschlich MM, eds. *Contemporary Nutrition Support Practice: A Clinical Guide.* Philadelphia, PA: W.B. Saunders; 1998:561–581.

33. Antin JH. Stem cell transplantation: Harnessing of graft-versus-malignancy. *Curr Opin Hematol.* 2003;10(6):440–444.

34. Mielcarek M, Storb R. Graft-vs-host disease after non-myeloablative hematopoietic cell transplantation. *Leuk Lymphoma.* 2005;46(9):1251–1260.

35. American Dietetic Association. *Oncology Evidence-Based Nutrition Practice Guideline.* Chicago, IL: Author; September 2007.

36. Geibig CB, Owens JP, Mirtallo JM, Bowers D, Nahikian-Nelms M, Tutschka P. Parenteral nutrition for marrow transplant recipients: Evaluation of an increased nitrogen dose. *JPEN J Parenter Enteral Nutr.* 1991;15(2):184–188.

37. Cheney CL, Lenssen P, Aker SN, et al. Sex differences in nitrogen balance following marrow grafting for leukemia. *J Am Coll Nutr.* 1987;6(3):223–230.

38. Szeluga DJ, Stuart RK, Brookmeyer R, Utermohlen V, Santos GW. Energy requirements of parenterally fed bone marrow transplant recipients. *JPEN J Parenter Enteral Nutr.* 1985;9(2):139–143.

39. O'Dwyer ST, Scott T, Smith RJ, Wilmore W. 5-Fluorouracil toxicity on small intestinal mucosa but not white blood cells is decreased by glutamine [abstract]. *Clin Res.* 1987;35(3):367.

40. Fox AD, Kripke SA, De Paula J, Berman JM, Settle RG, Rombeau JL. Effect of a glutamine-supplemented enteral diet on methotrexate-induced enterocolitis. *JPEN J Parenter Enteral Nutr.* 1988;12(4):325–331.

41. Austgen TR, Dudrick PS, Sitren H, Bland KI, Copeland E, Souba WW. The effects of glutamine-enriched total parenteral nutrition on tumor growth and host tissues. *Ann Surg.* 1992;215(2):107–113.

42. Ziegler TR, Young LS, Benfell K, et al. Clinical and metabolic efficacy of glutamine-supplemented parenteral nutrition after bone marrow transplantation: A randomized, double-blind, controlled study. *Ann Intern Med.* 1992;116(10):821–828.

43. Schloerb PR, Amare M. Total parenteral nutrition with glutamine in bone marrow transplantation and other clinical applications (a randomized, double-blind study). *JPEN J Parenter Enteral Nutr.* 1993;17(5):407–413.

44. van Zaanen HC, van der Lelie H, Timmer JG, Furst P, Sauerwein HP. Parenteral glutamine dipeptide supplementation does not ameliorate chemotherapy-induced toxicity. *Cancer.* 1994;74(10):2879–2884.

45. Pytlik R, Benes P, Patorkova M, et al. Standardized parenteral alanyl-glutamine dipeptide supplementation is not beneficial in autologous transplant patients: A randomized, double-blind, placebo controlled study. *Bone Marrow Transplant.* 2002;30(12):953–961.

46. Murray SM, Pindoria S. Nutrition support for bone marrow transplant patients. *Cochrane Database Syst Rev.* 2002;2:CD002920.

47. Piccirillo N, De Matteis S, Laurenti L, et al. Glutamine-enriched parenteral nutrition after autologous peripheral blood stem cell transplantation: Effects on immune reconstitution and mucositis. *Haematologica.* 2003;88(2):192–200.

48. Jebb SA, Marcus R, Elia M. A pilot study of oral glutamine supplementation in patients receiving bone marrow transplants. *Clin Nutr.* 1995;14(3):162–165.

49. Coghlin Dickson TM, Wong RM, Offrin RS, et al. Effect of oral glutamine supplementation during bone marrow transplantation. *JPEN J Parenter Enteral Nutr.* 2000;24(2):61–66.

50. Iestra JA, Fibbe WE, Zwinderman AH, Romijn JA, Kromhout D. Parenteral nutrition following intensive cytotoxic therapy: An exploratory study on the need for parenteral nutrition after various treatment approaches for haematological malignancies. *Bone Marrow Transplant.* 1999;23(9):933–939.
51. Calvo MV, Gonzalez MP, Alaguero M, Perez-Simon JA. Intensive monitoring program for oral food intake in patients undergoing allogeneic hematopoietic cell transplantation: A cost–benefit analysis. *Nutrition.* 2002;18(9):769–771.
52. Hasse J, Robien K. Nutrition support guidelines for therapeutically immunosuppressed patients. In: Pichard C, Kudsk KA, eds. *From Nutrition Support to Pharmacologic Nutrition in the ICU.* Heidelberg, Germany: Springer-Verlag; 2000:361–383.
53. Gratwohl A, Brand R, Frassoni F, et al. Cause of death after allogeneic haematopoietic stem cell transplantation (HSCT) in early leukaemias: An EBMT analysis of lethal infectious complications and changes over calendar time. *Bone Marrow Transplant.* 2005;36(9):757–769.
54. Weisdorf SA, Lysne J, Wind D, et al. Positive effect of prophylactic total parenteral nutrition on long-term outcome of bone marrow transplantation. *Transplantation.* 1987;43(6):833–838.
55. Fraser I, Neoptolemos J, Darby H, Bell PR. The effects of intralipid and heparin on human monocyte and lymphocyte function. *JPEN J Parenter Enteral Nutr.* 1984;8 (4):381–384.
56. Wiernik A, Jarstrand C, Julander I. The effect of intralipid on mononuclear and polymorphonuclear phagocytes. *Am J Clin Nutr.* 1983;37(2):256–261.
57. Nordenstrom J, Jarstrand C, Wiernik A. Decreased chemotactic and random migration of leukocytes during intralipid infusion. *Am J Clin Nutr.* 1979;32(12):2416–2422.
58. Lenssen P, Bruemmer BA, Bowden RA, Gooley T, Aker SN, Mattson D. Intravenous lipid dose and incidence of bacteremia and fungemia in patients undergoing bone marrow transplantation. *Am J Clin Nutr.* 1998;67(5):927–933.
59. Muscaritoli M, Conversano L, Torelli GF, et al. Clinical and metabolic effects of different parenteral nutrition regimens in patients undergoing allogeneic bone marrow transplantation. *Transplantation.* 1998;66(5):610–616.
60. Sheean P, Braunschweig C. The incidence and impact of dextrose dose on hyperglycemia from parenteral nutrition (PN) exposure in hematopoietic stem cell transplant (HSCT) recipients. *JPEN J Parenter Enteral Nutr.* 2006;30(4):345–350.
61. Sheean PM, Freels SA, Helton WS, Braunschweig CA. Adverse clinical consequences of hyperglycemia from total parenteral nutrition exposure during hematopoietic stem cell transplantation. *Biol Blood Marrow Transplant.* 2006;12 (6):656–664.
62. Charuhas PM, Fosberg KL, Bruemmer B, et al. A double-blind randomized trial comparing outpatient parenteral nutrition with intravenous hydration: Effect on resumption of oral intake after marrow transplantation. *JPEN J Parenter Enteral Nutr.* 1997;21(3):157–161.
63. Szeluga DJ, Stuart RK, Brookmeyer R, Utermohlen V, Santos GW. Nutritional support of bone marrow transplant recipients: A prospective, randomized clinical trial comparing total parenteral nutrition to an enteral feeding program. *Cancer Res.* 1987;47(12):3309–3316.
64. Lenssen P, Bruemmer B, Aker SN, McDonald GB. Nutrient support in hematopoietic cell transplantation. *JPEN J Parenter Enteral Nutr.* 2001;25(4):219–228.

65. Sefcick A, Anderton D, Byrne JL, Teahon K, Russell NH. Naso-jejunal feeding in allogeneic bone marrow transplant recipients: Results of a pilot study. *Bone Marrow Transplant.* 2001;28(12):1135–1139.

66. Papadopoulou A, MacDonald A, Williams MD, Darbyshire PJ, Booth IW. Enteral nutrition after bone marrow transplantation. *Arch Dis Child.* 1997;77(2):131–136.

67. Langdana A, Tully N, Molloy E, Bourke B, O'Meara A. Intensive enteral nutrition support in paediatric bone marrow transplantation. *Bone Marrow Transplant.* 2001; 27(7):741–746.

68. Hopman GD, Pena EG, Le Cessie S, Van Weel MH, Vossen JM, Mearin ML. Tube feeding and bone marrow transplantation. *Med Pediatr Oncol.* 2003;40(6):375–379.

69. Reddy P, Ferrara JL. Immunobiology of acute graft-versus-host disease. *Blood Rev.* 2003;17(4):187–194.

70. Shlomchik WD, Lee SJ, Couriel D, Pavletic SZ. Transplantation's greatest challenges: Advances in chronic graft-versus-host disease. *Biol Blood Marrow Transplant.* 2007;13(1)(suppl 1):2–10.

71. Bhushan V, Collins RH Jr. Chronic graft-vs-host disease. *JAMA.* 2003;290(19): 2599–2603.

72. Stern JM. Nutritional assessment and management of malabsorption in the hematopoietic stem cell transplant patient. *J Am Diet Assoc.* 2002;102(12): 1812–1815; discussion 1815–1816.

73. Treister NS, Cook EF Jr, Antin J, Lee SJ, Soiffer R, Woo SB. Clinical evaluation of oral chronic graft-versus-host disease. *Biol Blood Marrow Transplant.* 2008;14 (1):110–115.

74. Wingard JR, Nichols WG, McDonald GB. Supportive care. *Hematology Am Soc Hematol Educ Program.* 2004:372–389.

75. Lenssen P, Aker SN. Nutritional support of patients with hematologic malignancies. In: Hoffman R, Benz E, Shattil S, Furie B, Cohen H, eds. *Hematology: Basic Principles and Practice.* 4th ed: Philadelphia, PA: Churchill Livingstone; 2005: 1591–1609.

76. Institute of Medicine. *Dietary Reference Intakes for Vitamin A, Vitamin K, Arsenic, Boron, Chromium, Copper, Iodine, Iron, Manganese, Molybdenum, Nickel, Silicon, Vanadium and Zinc.* Washington, DC: Institute of Medicine, Standing Committee on the Scientific Evaluation of Dietary Reference Intakes; 2001.

77. Moody K, Finlay J, Mancuso C, Charlson M. Feasibility and safety of a pilot randomized trial of infection rate: Neutropenic diet versus standard food safety guidelines. *J Pediatr Hematol Oncol.* 2006;28(3):126–133.

Chapter 13

Brain Tumors

Cathy Scanlon, MS, RD, LD

INTRODUCTION

Brain tumors are made of cells that demonstrate unrestrained growth in the brain.[1] A primary brain tumor originates in the brain and does not spread outside the brain. A secondary brain tumor travels, or *metastasizes*, to the brain by cancer cells. from another place in the body—most commonly, tumors in the lungs, breast, or kidney, or melanomas in the skin. A primary brain tumor can be either malignant or benign. Whether malignant or benign, primary brain tumors do not spread outside the brain to other locations in the body. Rarely, a malignant primary brain tumor will shed cancer cells to other parts of the brain or spinal cord. Benign primary brain tumors can be just as dangerous and deadly as malignant tumors if they exert pressure on vital areas of the brain, causing interference with brain function, or if they increase the intracranial pressure (ICP). Usually, however, benign primary brain tumors can be treated successfully.[1]

Because no two brain tumors or patients are alike, treating a brain tumor is quite challenging. Many factors influence the type of treatment approach, prognosis, and survival, including the genetic composition and location of the tumor, and the age, cognition, and overall health of the person with the tumor. The approach to treating a primary brain tumor can be often multimodal in nature, including chemotherapy, surgery, and radiation as well as hormonal drugs such as steroids, immunologicals, antiangiogenics, and antivirals.[2] These treatment approaches and their nutrition-related side effects are addressed later in this chapter.

Interpreting Reports of Statistical Data

Using statistical information related to brain cancer can be quite challenging because statistics simply provide a "slice" of information that may not reflect an individual person's prognosis.[3] This statement is not intended to imply that there is no role for statistical data in cancer treatment, but rather suggest that statistics should be viewed objectively and with a full understanding of what they represent.[3] For example, incidence rates from various reporting agencies or registries often cannot be compared because of the organizations' use of different case definitions, study populations, data collection methods, or statistical calculation methods. This issue is exemplified by the two brain tumor databases in the United States.

The Central Brain Tumor Registry of the United States (CBTRUS) and the Surveillance, Epidemiology, and End Results (SEER) Program are the two centralized brain tumor databases in the United States. CBTRUS is a non-profit corporation "committed to providing a resource for gathering and dis-seminating current epidemiologic data on all primary brain tumors, malignant and non-malignant, for the purposes of accurately describing their incidence and survival patterns, evaluating diagnosis and treatment, facili-tating etiologic studies, establishing awareness of the disease, and ulti-mately, for the prevention of all brain tumors."[4] The SEER program was established in response to the 1971 congressional legislation known as the National Cancer Act, which mandated the National Cancer Institute (NCI) to "collect, analyze, and disseminate data useful to prevent, diagnose, and treat cancer."[5]

The current CBTRUS statistical report for 2005–2006 is compiled from data collected over the period 1998–2002. CBTRUS incidence rates include all primary malignant and nonmalignant tumors of the brain, central nervous system (CNS), pituitary and pineal glands, and olfactory tumors of the nasal cavity. The 1973–2002 SEER report includes incidence rates for all primary malignant tumors of the brain, CNS, pituitary and pineal glands, and olfac-tory tumors of the nasal cavity, as well as lymphomas and leukemias. The 1975–2002 SEER report includes primary malignant tumors of the brain and CNS, but excludes lymphomas, leukemias, and tumors of the pituitary and pineal glands.[4] Many other details also differentiate the two registries. Even with the few differences described here, however, it is obvious these differ-ences must be considered when reviewing and drawing conclusions from the statistical reports.

One commonality between CBTRUS and SEER is that both report rates in terms of "person-years," usually "per 100,000 person-years," which means 1 person over 1 year of time. Other agencies, such as the National Program of Cancer Registries (NPCR) and the Centers for Disease Control and Preven-tion (CDC), report rates in terms of "per 100,000 persons." Table 13.1 con-tains cancer surveillance data for adult primary brain and CNS cancer from several reporting entities.

Table 13.1   *Brain Cancer Surveillance Data*

Database	Incidence	Mortality	Lifetime Risk	Prevalence
CBTRUS	Total: 7.4 per 100,000 person-years Males: 14.5 Females: 15.1	—	—	130.8 per 100,000 people
SEER	Total: 6.4 per 100,000 person-years Males: 7.6 Females: 5.3	Males: 0.49% Females: 0.39%	Males: 0.65% Females: 0.50%	—
ACS	—	12,760 primary brain and CNS cancers in United States in 2005	—	—
IARC	Worldwide per 100,000 person-years: Males: 3.7 Females: 2.6	—	—	—

CBTRUS = Central Brain Tumor Registry in the United States.
SEER = Surveillance, Epidemiology, and End Results program.
ACS = American Cancer Society.
CNS = Central nervous system.
IARC: International Agency for Research on Cancer.

Incidence in Primary Malignant Brain and CNS Tumors

The current CBTRUS report indicates that the "incidence rate of all primary non-malignant and malignant brain and central nervous system tumors is 14.8 per 100,000 person-years." Interestingly, half of these cases (7.4 per 100,000 person-years) are malignant; the other half are considered either benign or "borderline" tumors. Females have a higher incidence (15.1 per 100,000 person-years) than do males (14.5 per 100,000 person-years). CBTRUS estimated there would be 43,800 new cases of malignant and non-malignant primary brain and CNS cancer diagnosed in 2005.[4]

SEER reports the incidence rate of primary malignant brain and CNS tumors as 6.4 cases per 100,000 person-years. The rate is higher in males (7.6 per 100,000 person-years) than in females (5.3 per 100,000 person-years).

According to the American Cancer Society (ACS), an estimated 18,500 new cases of primary malignant brain and CNS tumors were expected to be diagnosed in the United States in 2005 (10,620 male cases and 7,880 female cases). These figures represent 1.35% of all primary malignant cancers diagnosed in the United States in 2005.

The International Agency for Research on Cancers (IARC) reports the worldwide incidence of primary malignant brain and CNS tumors is 3.7 per 100,000 person-years in males and 2.6 per 100,000 person-years in females. Incidence rates per 100,000 person-years are higher in more developed countries (5.8 in males and 4.1 in females) than in less developed countries (3.0 in males and 2.1 in females).[4]

Lifetime Risk and Mortality in Primary Malignant Brain and CNS Tumors

The lifetime risk of receiving a diagnosis of a primary malignant brain or CNS tumor is 0.65% for men and 0.50% for women. The chance of dying from these tumors is 0.49% for men and 0.30% for women. These statistics do not include the diagnoses of lymphoma, leukemia, tumors of the pineal or pituitary glands, or olfactory tumors of the nasal cavity.[4] CBTRUS's first annual report in 1995 estimated that approximately 12,760 deaths in the United States in 2005 would be attributed to primary malignant brain and CNS tumors.[4]

Prognostic Factors in Primary Brain Tumors

"Pretreatment variables affect survival more than does the treatment itself."[6] Most experts agree the top three prognostic factors for survival of a primary brain tumor in an adult are young age, performance status, and the histology of the tumor.[6, 7]

Adult Malignant Primary Brain Tumors

Each year more than 200,000 people in the United States are diagnosed with a primary or secondary brain tumor. Primary brain tumors account for approximately 40,000 of these cases.[3, 4] As mentioned previously in this chapter, primary brain tumors do not generally metastasize to other parts of the body.[3, 8] More than 120 different types of brain tumors exist, making diagnosis and treatment difficult. As described earlier, a nonmalignant brain tumor can cause just as much damage and danger of death as a malignant tumor.[1, 3] Consequently, there is an enormous—even overwhelming—amount of information available on both malignant and nonmalignant brain and CNS tumors, which cannot be adequately described in one chapter. Therefore, this chapter will limit its scope to adult malignant primary brain tumors.

Incidence and Mortality Rates

For the last decade, the incidence and mortality rates for primary brain cancers have remained relatively unchanged. For Caucasians, the incidence and mortality rates are much higher than for members of any other ethnic or racial group, and regardless of race or ethnicity there are much higher incidence and mortality rates among men than among women.[9]

In a descriptive study, Deorah and co-workers at the University of Iowa employed statistical analyses of population-based data from the SEER program and found the incidence of brain cancer increased to 1.68% of the population in 1987, only to then decline to the present 0.44%. The researchers concluded that, despite the hypothesis that increased levels of environmental toxins might lead to a rise in brain cancer rates, the incidence of brain cancer is not actually increasing. They also found an increased risk associated with being male, elderly, white, and residing in a metropolitan county.[10]

Etiology

The cause of most primary brain tumors is not known. Exposure to ionizing radiation, such as x-rays and nuclear energy, is the only known risk factor for a primary brain cancer.[6, 11] Ionizing radiation is very high in energy, which enables it to break chemical bonds, thereby damaging deoxyribonucleic acid (DNA) and leading to cancer. Indeed, one definition of *ionize* is "to dissociate atoms or molecules into electrically charged atoms or radicals."[12] Ionizing radiation is made of neutrons, electrons, or gamma (electromagnetic) radiation.[12]

Gliomas have been linked to irradiation of the skull, with many persons experiencing a 10- to 20-year latency period after exposure.[6, 11] Other proposed causes of brain tumors include usage of cell phones and hair dyes, head trauma, exposure to high-tension wires, and dietary factors including fat, cholesterol, and dietary exposure to nitrates used in food processing. These areas of investigation have yet to yield any convincing evidence for a relationship to an increased risk of brain cancer.[6, 9, 13–15]

Defective oncogenes and defective tumor suppressor genes are thought to be responsible for the process of cancer growth or the failure to suppress tumor growth, respectively.[1] Glioblastomas, anaplastic astrocytomas, and medulloblastomas have been linked to either the defective gene *MMAC1* (mutated multiple advanced cancers) or the "Patched 2" gene. These acquired genetic defects are not to be confused with inherited genetic defects, which are acquired as part of one's family DNA.[1]

Clinical Signs and Symptoms

Signs and symptoms of brain tumors are categorized as either focal or generalized.[1, 9, 16, 17] Focal signs and symptoms include nausea, vomiting, dysphagia, hemiparesis, aphasia, seizures, and various levels of cognitive dysfunction; these phenomena are related to the actual location of the tumor in the brain. Generalized signs and symptoms include headache, nausea, vomiting, seizures, drowsiness, and visual changes; they reflect an increase in ICP as a result of the tumor's presence in the brain. Headache is the most common initial symptom of a brain tumor and can be distinguished from a non-tumor-related headache by the following features:

- Worse in the morning and is gone within a few hours
- Onset while sleeping and occurs in conjunction with at least one other symptom such as vomiting or mental confusion
- Accompanied by weakness, numbness, or double vision

Cognitive and mental changes may present as memory loss, problems with concentration, speech, ability to reason, and increased sleepiness. Persons with brain stem tumors always experience gastrointestinal symptoms of nausea and vomiting. Other signs and symptoms may be an unsteady gait, double vision or loss of vision, a gradual loss of movement or sensation in an arm or leg, and loss of hearing. The loss of vision, dilated pupils, a fixed gaze, and any feelings of paralysis on one or both sides of the body are considered a sign of a life-threatening emergency. Experiencing any one or more of these events requires prompt intervention in the nearest emergency room. Depending on the location of the tumor in the brain, seizures may occur, and do in 15–95% of persons with a brain tumor.[1]

Diagnosis of Brain Tumors

Magnetic resonance imaging (MRI) of the cranium is all that is required to diagnose a brain tumor. Using "normal contrast-enhanced MRI can essentially rule-out the possibility of a brain tumor"; however, if a brain tumor is suspected, the test of choice is an MRI using the contrast medium gadolinium.[9] Computerized tomography (CT) scan is not recommended as it is not sensitive enough to detect certain tumors. Indeed, even when administered with contrast, a CT may not detect certain low-grade non-enhancing tumors.[9]

Once the presence of a tumor is confirmed, the subsequent steps are to obtain tumor cells through lumbar puncture or tissue biopsy, so as to determine the type of tumor and select the optimal therapy. Lumbar puncture, also known as a spinal tap, is a procedure in which a sample of cerebrospinal fluid (CSF) is obtained to ascertain if it contains tumor cells. A tissue biopsy is a procedure in which a piece of tumor is obtained and examined to identify which cell types are present and whether those cells are malignant or benign.

Oftentimes, it is considered too dangerous to obtain a tissue biopsy, such as in the case of a brain stem glioma, when an attempt to obtain a biopsy may result in the removal of healthy tissue vital to normal functioning. In these cases, stereotactic techniques, called stereotaxy, are used to obtain a tissue biopsy. Sterotaxy involves the use of computers to create a three-dimensional image of the area, which allows for a precise biopsy without injury to healthy tissue. Stereotaxy can also be used to deliver treatment to the tumor site. Sometimes, the neurosurgeon must decide if a stereotactic biopsy is too risky for the patient, just as conventional surgery or radiosurgery can be too risky.[1] Refer to Tables 13.2 and 13.3 for more information related to treatment using radiation.

Table 13.2 *Types of Radiation Treatments*

External-beam radiation	Conventional method of radiation in which beams are aimed directly at the tumor
Conformal radiation	Highly targeted technique in which beams of radiation are formed in the shape of the tumor
Hyperfractionated radiation	Many small doses of radiation are given and the sum total is a very high radiation dose
Stereotactic radiosurgery	Delivers very high doses directly to the tumor in an attempt to avoid surrounding healthy tissue
Balloon catheter or "glia site"	Gives radiation directly to the tumor bed after surgery has removed the tumor bulk
Brachytherapy or interstitial radiation	Radioactive "seeds" are placed directly at the tumor site

Source: Brain tumors: Primary. Available at www.mdconsult.com/das/patient/body/81670263-3/643425000/10041/9428.html. Accessed November 13, 2007.

Table 13.3 *Methods of Delivery of Radiation Beams*

Gamma knife	Many gamma rays converge into a single point delivered to the tumor to provide a synergistic effect when all the rays converge. Used for small tumors.
Linear accelerator	Produces photons (atomic particles with positive charges) formed to the shape of the tumor and treatment can be fractionated. Used for larger tumors.
Cyclotron	Produces photons directed at the tumor. Some research involves the intravenous injection of boron neutron-capture therapy (BNCT), which is more readily taken up by tumor cells than healthy cells. With BNCT, a single dose of radiation is rendered more powerful because the boron releases high-energy particles that kill the tumor cells.

Source: Brain tumors: Primary. Available at www.mdconsult.com/das/patient/body/81670263-3/643425000/10041/9428.html. Accessed November 13, 2007.

Malignant Gliomas, Neuromas, and Meningiomas

Adult primary brain cancer tumors are classified according to the cells from which they originate—either glial, neuronal, or meningial.[2, 3, 18] Glial cells provide physical support to neurons via the myelin sheath, as well as physiologic support for the many processes of the neurons in the brain. Neurons are cells that make up the nerves, which themselves transmit impulses and give rise to neuromas.[2, 6] Meningiomas arise from the meningothelial cells, which form the membranous lining that covers the outside of the brain. Although technically meningothelial cells are outside the brain, meningiomas are still classified as brain tumors because the outer lining of the brain is located within the intracranial cavity and their presentation involves neurologic signs and symptoms.[9] Angiomas, another type of brain tumor, are composed of abnormal blood vessels and found either on the surface of the brain or inside the brain itself.[6]

Primary CNS lymphoma traditionally represented approximately 1% or less of all primary brain tumors. In the past 20 years, however, its incidence has tripled in the United States. The risk for primary CNS lymphoma is significantly increased in persons with congenital immune deficiency or an acquired immune deficiency, such as acquired immune deficiency syndrome (AIDS). No behavioral or environmental risk factors for this relationship have been identified.[9]

Gliomas

Glial tumors are called gliomas[2, 3, 19]; they arise from the many types of glial cells, necessitating creation of several subcategories—astrocytomas, ependymomas, and oligodendrogliomas—to distinguish them.[2, 6] Gliomas are the most common brain cancer.

Astrocytomas, the most common type of glioma, arise from star-shaped glial cells, whose shape inspires their name, astrocytes. Astrocytomas are graded according to their aggressiveness, with grade I being the least aggressive and grade IV being the most aggressive and usually requiring more aggressive treatment. Most astrocytomas seen in children are low-grade, whereas adults typically have high-grade astrocytomas. These tumors can occur in any area in the brain, including the brain stem. Astrocytomas spread by invading brain connective tissue, making it very difficult to completely remove them without causing significant damage to vital structures in the brain.[6]

Grade I astrocytomas, called pilocytic astrocytomas or juvenile pilocytic astrocytomas, are not only low-grade in their behavior initially but remain low-grade even if they recur.[19] These tumors have the highest 5-year survival rate, at greater than 70%; conversely, if they are located in an inaccessible area, they are life-threatening.[1] Pilocytic astrocytomas very rarely undergo malignant transformation.[16] If the pilocytic astrocytoma is located in the cerebellum, it can often be completely removed with surgery. In cases where the tumor is unresectable and is leading to progressive problems for the patient, radiotherapy and possibly carboplatin-based chemotherapy can be attempted. Carboplatin-based chemotherapy has been shown to be useful in children, although its effectiveness in adults has not been evaluated.[16] A recurrence can be treated with additional surgery, as well as radiation or chemotherapy, according to the individual circumstances. If needed, investigational drugs may be used. The prognosis for pilocytic astrocytoma includes a 10-year survival of 90% if the tumor is surgically accessible.[1]

Grade II astrocytomas not otherwise specified (NOS), include three subtypes:

- Fibrillary—fibrous and derived from fibrillary astrocytes
- Gemistocytic or gemistocytoma—possesses a round or oval shape and is derived from gemistocytin-type astrocytes
- Protoplasmic astrocytic—resembles a protoplasm

Grade II astrocytomas are usually seen in young adults, with the peak ages of onset being from the thirties to the forties.[1] A complete surgical resection is impossible to achieve in such cases.[19] The average postoperative survival in astrocytoma NOS is 5 years.[1] Chemotherapeutic treatment options include cisplatin (Platinol) or carboplatin (Paraplatin), etoposide (VePesid), and paclitaxel (Taxol).[19]

Grade III astrocytoma is also called anaplastic astrocytoma (AA). The mean age of persons with AA is 45 years, and the tumors are associated with a median overall survival of 3–4 years.[17] Approximately 40% of these astrocytomas are found in the frontal lobes.[20] The chief symptoms seen in persons with an AA are headaches and convulsions.[19] Average survival is 2–3 years after diagnosis, though this span decreases with increasing patient age. Evidence of any tumor necrosis would change the diagnosis to a glioblastoma multiforme (GBM).[6, 18, 20] Treatment of AA usually consists of surgical resection followed by cranial radiation.[6] Chemotherapy can be associated with a small yet significant improvement in remission and survival.[18, 21]

Grade IV astrocytoma, also called GBM, accounts for almost two-thirds of all astrocytomas and is the most malignant of all gliomas.[6, 18, 20] It is also the most common malignant brain tumor that occurs in persons from 45 to more than 85 years of age.[4] The mean age of the person with GBM is 54 years, in whom median survival is 10–12 months.[20] GBM is the only astrocytoma that includes the presence of necrosis, a feature necessary for its diagnosis.[6] A GBM can develop from a grade II or III astrocytoma or from normal astrocytes, bypassing the lower grades.[22] The main symptoms seen in persons with GBM are personality changes and focal neurological deficits. The average prognosis for survival is 18–24 months. Neither chemotherapy nor radiation therapy is curative, although these measures do lead to increased survival.[18]

Treatment of Astrocytomas

Because malignant astrocytomas are considered incurable, the treatment goals are directed toward improving neurological problems, such as poor mental functioning, and maintaining optimal quality of life.[19] According to Lefranc and colleagues, current treatment recommendations for GBM are maximum surgical resection followed by concurrent chemoradiation.[23] The chemotherapy used concurrently with radiation consists of the novel alkylating drug temozolomide (TMZ). After the concurrent chemoradiation is complete, the patient should then receive adjuvant therapy using the same chemotherapy drug, TMZ, for up to 6 months.[23]

Mortality, Survival, and Prognosis of Astrocytomas

The prognosis of an astrocytoma varies between grades. Grades I and II are considered low-grade gliomas, and grades III and IV are considered high-grade gliomas.[5, 6] There is a significant difference in prognoses among grades I/II, III, and IV, but not between grades I and II. The median survival for the low grades is 8 years after diagnosis, that for grade III is 2–3 years, and that for grade IV (GBM) is approximately 1 year.[6]

Ependymomas arise from the ependymal cells, which line the ventricles and spinal cord. In adults, ependymomas most often occur in the fourth ventricle or spinal cord.[3, 18] As with astrocytomas, ependymomas are graded from I to IV, from least to most aggressive. The fourth ventricle is located at the back of the brain stem, making total tumor resection difficult or even impossible in patients with ependymomas. The goal of surgery is to ensure maximum resection without damaging the brain stem.[6]

Two types of grade I ependymomas exist: myxopapillary, which is usually found in the spine, and subendymoma, which is typically located in the fourth ventricle. Both types are benign. The standard treatment for grade I ependymoma is surgical resection, which is usually curative.[1]

The three types of grade II ependymomas are papillary cellular (found in the fourth ventricle and midline area), clear cell (also located in the fourth ventricle and midline area), and papillary (rare; found in the cerebellopontine angle). The grade II ependymomas usually affect adults,[1] and their treatment consists of surgery followed by radiation. If these measures are not successful, nitrosourea-based chemotherapies or investigational drugs are used.[1]

Grade III anaplastic ependymomas are commonly located in the cerebral hemispheres, and these tumors can often spread to the spinal fluid. The usual treatment is surgery followed by radiation to the brain or spinal cord.[1]

Grade IV ependymoblastomas are found along the CSF pathway, are very rare, and are more common in children than in adults. They are usually found in the cerebellum. Other names for these tumors include primitive neuroecto-dermal tumors (PNET) and neuroblastomas. The usual treatment is surgery followed by radiation to the brain and spinal cord.[1]

Oligodendrogliomas arise from glial cells called oligodendroglia. Oligodendroglia cells make up the myelin sheath, which insulates and protects nerve endings inside the brain. "Pure" oligodendrogliomas are rare; instead, most of these tumors contain a mix of astrocytes, mineral deposits, and oligodendroglia. For this reason, they are often called "mixed" gliomas or oligodendrocytoma. Under a microscope, oligodendrocytomas look like fried eggs.[6, 18] Oligodendrogliomas account for approximately 10–20% of all gliomas, typically occur in middle age, and often present with seizures.[1, 6] They are graded according to prognosis: I and II are considered low grades with a better prognosis, and III and IV considered high grades with a less favorable prognosis. Most cases are low grade (II), with prognoses that are more favorable than for astrocytomas. Median survival is 2–7 years, with the extremes corresponding to high-grade tumors and low-grade tumors, respectively. Survival is improved with more aggressive surgical resection. Although radiation therapy has not been shown to lengthen survival, many oligodendrogliomas respond to PCV [procarbazine, lomustine (CCNU), vincristine] chemotherapy.[6]

Treatment of low-grade oligodendroglioma is not usually undertaken until the disease's progression causes symptoms. Once symptoms are present, surgery to remove the entire tumor is the first step. Surgery is usually followed by radiation when the entire tumor cannot be removed and in those patients older than age 40, but this pattern is controversial because strong evidence of its benefits has not been shown.[1] The role of chemotherapy following radiation is under investigation and shows promise: Two-thirds of patients who receive PCV have a tumor response to this regimen.[1] Sustained remissions averaging 16 years have been seen with PCV therapy.[1] A "pure" oligodendroglioma tends to demonstrate a better response to TMZ than does a mixed glioma, with TMZ showing promise as a second-line treatment in mixed gliomas.[1]

High-grade (III and IV) oligodendrogliomas are also known as anaplastic oligodendrogliomas. They are treated with immediate surgery, with a goal of complete tumor removal. Radiation usually follows surgery; chemotherapy can be given before or concurrently with radiation. Recommended chemotherapeutic agents include TMZ, retinoic acid, melphalan, thiotepa, carboplatin, cisplatin, and etoposide.[1] The nutrition-related side effects of these chemotherapy agents are discussed later in this chapter.

Neuromas

Vestibular schwannoma, also called acoustic neuromas, grow in the vestibulocochlear nerve (cranial nerve VIII). The most common symptoms are progressive hearing loss, ringing in the ears (tinnitus), and difficulty with balance. A large tumor can lead to compression of the brain stem or obstructive hydrocephalus.[2] Treatment may include microsurgical resection or stereotactic radiosurgery using devices such as a gamma knife or linear accelerator. Gamma knife radiosurgery has been shown to be safe and effective for a variety of intracranial disorders, but it may have higher toxicity than fractionated radiation, and no evidence exists to prove its long-term efficacy.[18] The main complication of treatment is damage to and dysfunction of the facial nerve (cranial nerve VII).[2] The remission rate of acoustic neuroma after radiosurgery is 91% at 5 years.[21]

Meningiomas

Approximately 20% of all primary brain tumors are meningiomas, which have an annual incidence rate of 7.8 per 100,000. The incidence is higher in females than males (3:2 female-to-male ratio). According the World Heath Organization (WHO), the ratio is as high as 2:1 in some reports.[9]

Most meningiomas are benign and asymptomatic. Indeed, meningiomas are often discovered incidentally at autopsy.[6, 9] Benign meningiomas rarely invade nearby tissue, and their long-term prognosis is favorable. Most meningiomas grow very slowly and occur at the base of the skull. Whether malignant or benign, a tumor located near the base of the skull may at best be difficult, if not impossible, to remove. The incidence of symptomatic cases is 2 per 100,000.[9] Manifestations will depend on the location of the tumor, and symptoms are due to the compression of tissue from the tumor mass itself and not actual invasion of surrounding brain tissue.[6]

Two percent of meningiomas are frankly malignant.[9] The malignant forms, which are called anaplastic meningioma and hemangiopericytoma, are rare and difficult to remove with surgery. Malignant tumor attributes consist of invasion into brain, tumor necrosis, and numerous mitoses. A meningioma can invade bone, the dura mater, and the venous sinus. Signs and symptoms include headache, seizure, increased ICP, and focal neurological signs. The standard treatment consists of surgery that provides for complete tumor removal if possible, although the chance of complete removal may be limited by the tumor's location.[6, 9] Gamma knife radiosurgery and fractionated external-beam radiation have also shown promising results in the treatment of malignant meningioma.[1, 21]

Categories of Brain Tumors by Location

Brain tumors are also named for their location in the brain (see Figures 13.1 and 13.2). This is one of the reasons why understanding the various names used for the same brain tumor can be confusing. This section briefly describes the categorization of brain tumors by their anatomical location.[1]

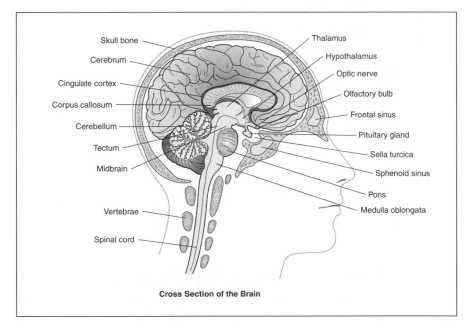

Cross Section of the Brain

Figure 13.1   *Cross Section of the Brain*

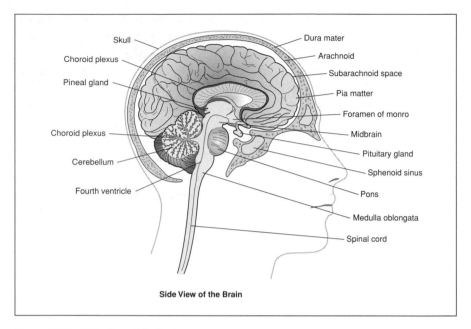

Figure 13.2 *Side View of the Brain*

Meningioma—a usually benign tumor that is found in the membrane covering the brain and spinal cord, called the meninges

Cerebral astrocytoma—a glioma in the cerebrum

Cerebellar astrocytoma—a glioma in the cerebellum

Brain stem glioma—may be found in any of the following three sections of the brain stem:

- **Medulla**—regulates breathing, swallowing, blood pressure, and heart rate
- **Pons**—the area linking the cerebrum to the cerebellum
- **Midbrain**—the area that controls vision and hearing

Medulloblastoma—a tumor found in the cerebellum

Pituitary tumor—usually benign, slow-growing tumor in the pituitary gland

Treating Malignant Primary Brain Tumors

The most common treatment modalities used in brain cancer are surgery, radiation, and chemotherapy. However, treatment can also involve the use of biotherapy, antiangiogenics, genetics, diet therapy, and various drugs to treat the side effects of the tumor and its treatments. These treatments are used alone as well as in various combinations to obtain optimal results.

Surgery

Surgery is usually the first approach to treating a primary brain tumor. Such procedures are performed by a neurosurgeon, whose objective is to remove as much tumor as possible. Reducing the size of the tumor can make other therapies, such as radiation, more effective. Some sources suggest that extensive surgery for a high-grade glioma may not improve survival and that radiation is the best approach for these patients.[1]

Craniotomy is a surgical procedure that involves the removal of a piece of the cranium (skull) in an effort to locate and remove the tumor. During a craniotomy, options for tumor removal include laser microsurgery (vaporizing the tumor using heat) and ultrasonic aspiration (breaking the tumor into small pieces to allow the tumor to be suctioned out of the brain).[1]

Because the brain stem is the area that controls life-sustaining processes, surgery may pose too much danger when tumors are located on the brain stem. In these cases, radiation is the usual therapy of choice. If the tumor is located in the cerebellum, which is more accessible, gross total resection is easier to accomplish and is usually curative. Grade I gliomas can be treated with surgery only. Whether surgery is appropriate or useful for treating low-grade astrocytomas remains debatable, and there is little research evidence to demonstrate survival benefit from this course of action. Most malignant tumors will require additional treatments after surgery, as well as repeat surgeries.[1]

Removing a solid tumor from an area outside the brain usually entails removing some healthy tissue along with the tumor. This prospect may be just as problematic for the patient as the effects of the tumor itself. Depending on the function of the healthy brain tissue removed, the losses for the patient may outweigh the benefits of surgery. Therefore, additional radiosurgery procedures have been developed to aid the surgeon in removing as little healthy brain tissue as possible. In cortical localization or stimulation, a small electrical current is used to stimulate an area of the brain to allow for observation of the part of the body the area controls, enabling the surgeon to identify areas of the brain to avoid during surgery. In image-guided surgery, a three-dimensional (3-D) picture of the patient's brain is obtained from a CT or MRI scan. The 3-D picture is placed in view of the surgeon. As the surgical instruments touch a part of the brain, a camera sends an image to the 3-D picture, allowing the surgeon to see where the instrument is located in the patient's brain and, therefore, which areas to avoid during surgery. Stereotactic surgery is an adjunctive treatment to traditional surgery in which a dose of radiation is directed precisely at the tumor while avoiding healthy tissue nearby.[1]

Radiation

A variety of radiation therapies exist for brain tumors (Tables 13.2 and 13.3 on pages 327 and 328), and those treatments are used for a variety of purposes. This chapter highlights only the most common types of radiation therapy.

As mentioned earlier, surgery is the preferred first step in brain tumor treatment. Many times, radiation is used to treat the tumor tissue left behind when the entire tumor was unable to be removed, or to treat any microscopic cancer cells left behind after an entire tumor is removed. Radiation can be used when the tumor is unreachable by traditional surgery or when a particular type of tumor is known to respond well to radiation. Radiochemotherapy, in which radiation is combined with chemotherapy, is a technique commonly used to treat high-grade gliomas.[1]

Chemotherapy

The effective use of chemotherapy to treat brain tumors is not always possible due to limitations associated with the blood–brain barrier. The most common chemotherapy agents used to treat brain cancer are carmustine, PCV [procarbazine, N-(2-chloroethyl)-N-cyclohexyl-N-nitrosurea (CCNU), and vincristine], and TMZ.[1, 24]

Carmustine (BCNU), which is used to treat gliomas, is either given intravenously or delivered directly to the tumor site by way of a biodegradable wafer called a Gliadel Wafer. Intravenous BCNU has been used for more than 30 years as the standard treatment for GBM; even though it carries significant risk of toxicity, it has been more successful than other chemotherapy drugs in treating this type of brain cancer. The use of the Gliadel Wafer limits the toxicity associated with this drug, because the wafer is exposed only to the tumor bed, thereby avoiding systemic toxicity.[25] Unfortunately, use of carmustine has not led to any increase in survival rates because most patients develop a resistance to this drug.[1]

Temodar®—the brand name for temozolomide (TMZ)—entered the market in 1999 and was the first drug to be approved in 20 years for treatment of brain tumors. At the time of its launch, it was specifically indicated for adults with anaplastic astrocytoma who did not respond to other treatments.[1] It subsequently won approval for use in GBM, but only to be used several months after patients received radiation and their tumors returned. In 2005, TMZ was approved for use immediately after diagnosis and concurrent with radiation rather than after the tumor recurs.[26, 27]

Table 13.4 lists the nutrition-related side effects of carmustine, PCV, and TMZ.

Investigative and Novel Therapies

Until recently, GBM, a "rapidly fatal" form of malignant brain cancer, had a survival time of approximately 6–12 months; patients almost never lived longer than 24 months after diagnosis. Treatment consisted of radiation therapy alone.[28] Phase III trial data published by Stupp in 2005 demonstrated the 6- to 12-month survival time could be increased to 2 years by using concurrent radiation and TMZ compared to treatment with radiation only.[29] This study enrolled 573 adult subjects who were newly diagnosed with histologically proven GBM, had good performance status, had no history of chemotherapy or radiation, and were no more than 6 weeks from biopsy or surgical resection. The 573 subjects were randomized (1) to receive TMZ during and after radiation or (2) to receive only radiation.[29] The patients who received the TMZ survived 2 years after diagnosis, whereas the patients who received radiation alone did not experience a change in the usual survival time of 6–12 months.[29] The patients with better survival were younger than 50 years of age and otherwise healthy with no major medical conditions prior to their GBM diagnosis. Based on this trial report, TMZ immediately became the standard treatment around the world.[28]

Due to these promising results, the study was extended to determine if the 2-year survival benefit could be lengthened even further. The treatment

Table 13.4   *Nutrition-Related Side Effects of the Chemotherapy Agents Commonly Used to Treat Brain Cancer*

Drug	Potential Nutrition-Related Side Effects
Carmustine	Diarrhea, kidney and lung damage, dysphagia, mucositis, anemia
PCV agents	Anorexia, weight loss, nausea and vomiting, diarrhea, constipation, abdominal pain and cramps, dysphagia, xerostomia, jaw pain, weakness*
Temozolomide	Anorexia, diarrhea, nausea, vomiting, constipation, stomach pain and cramps, fever, weakness,* numbness,* tiredness,* difficulty walking,* back pain,* fatigue,* confusion,* anxiety*

PCV = Procarbazine + CCNU [*N*-(2-chloroethyl)-*N*-cyclohexyl-*N*-nitrosurea] + vincristine.
*These side effects can indirectly lead to poor nutrition.
Source: Radiation plus chemo quadruples survival time for fatal brain cancer. http://virtualtrials.com/news3.cfm?item=4021. Accessed December 25, 2007.

group received TMZ before and after radiation, while the control group received radiation only.[28] The treatment group demonstrated survival of more than 4 years after a diagnosis of GBM. The study enrolled 573 adult subjects who were newly diagnosed with histologically proven GBM, had good performance status, had no history of chemotherapy or radiation, and were no more than 6 weeks from biopsy or surgical resection. Survival was improved in patients younger than 50 years of age and otherwise healthy with no major medical conditions prior to their GBM diagnosis.[28] The trial's lead author, Rene-Olivier Mirimanoff, states, "Considering how quickly this type of cancer grows, patients who live 4 or 5 years after diagnosis are indeed considered long-term cancer survivors."[28]

Bionanocapsules (BNCs), a novel drug delivery system, are hollow nanoparticles that can be filled with various substances and used in many different industries, including the drug industry. Nanoparticles are so small that they are measured in micrometers (mcm); a micrometer is one-millionth of a meter and was formerly called a micron. Bionanocapsules are composed of L protein, the same protein of which the hepatitis B virus surface antigen is made; as a consequence, they have an affinity for liver cells. A hybrid bionanocapsule was developed that has an affinity for abnormal glioma cells and avoids healthy cells.[30] Research thus far has been carried out in vivo in mice brain cancer tumors and in vitro in rat astrocyte and human glioma cell cultures.[30] These experiments have successfully provided cancer therapeutic drug delivery to mice with brain cancer tumors in vivo while preserving healthy tissue, and hold much promise for future use in human brain cancer treatment.[30]

Photodynamic Radiation Therapy

Currently under research for use in recurrent GBM, photodynamic therapy uses a light-sensitive drug called photofrin that is administered intravenously and concentrates itself in the tumor.[1,3] Photofrin causes the tumor to become fluorescent so that during surgery the surgeon can focus a laser light on the tumor. The laser light, in turn, activates the photofrin to kill the cancer cells.[1,3]

Magnetic-Tipped Catheters

Magnetic-tipped catheters are flexible devices that neurosurgeons can guide to the tumor site by using magnetic fields located outside the skull. This technique allows the surgeon to direct the catheter in such a way as to avoid areas of the brain where damage would cause harm to the patient.[1]

Therapies on the Horizon

Although concurrent TMZ and radiation with adjuvant TMZ appears to quadruple survival times in persons with GBM, more research into this combination of therapies is under way. Currently, two areas are being investigated: increasing the dose of TMZ and adding targeted agents to the concurrent TMZ/radiation therapy.[31]

Complementary Treatment Used in Brain Cancer: Melatonin

Melatonin is a hormone that is synthesized from the amino acid tryptophan and is produced by the pineal gland located in the brain. Melatonin is involved in the body's sleep/wake cycle, also known as the circadian rhythm. The release of melatonin by the pineal gland is stimulated by light and suppressed by darkness, so that blood levels of melatonin are highest just before bedtime.[24] Synthetic melatonin is sold as a dietary supplement and marketed as a therapy for a variety of conditions, most commonly sleep problems or disorders. Melatonin also has potent antioxidant properties and has been studied to evaluate its action in reducing chemotherapy-related side effects.[24] The Natural Standard evidence-based validated grading rationale assigned an evidence grade of "C" to the results of this research, which means the evidence is "unclear or conflicting" for the use of melatonin for sleep disorders and amelioration of chemotherapy side effects.[24]

Nutritional Issues in Malignant Brain Cancer

Diet and Brain Cancer Prevention

According to the ACS, "there are no known nutritional risk factors for brain cancer."[32] Several factors have led to the lack of conclusive scientific evidence for dietary links to brain cancer development. Some proposed explanations for the lack of evidence point to problems inherent to the research design and the heterogenic nature of the studies, which prevent analyses of cumulative data.[33] However, many population studies show a reduction in cancer incidence in persons who consume fruits, vegetables, and grains on a regular basis.[34, 35]

The cancer-preventive effect of plant foods is attributed to phytochemicals present in plants.[35] To date, several hundred phytochemicals have been identified, and researchers believe there are hundreds, possibly thousands, more awaiting discovery. Phytochemicals protect plants from disease and damage to keep it alive. When consumed as part of foods, phytochemicals can also provide protective effects at the cellular level in humans and animals. Plant foods are thought to be "cancer-fighting" foods because of phytochemicals' protective functions.

The intake of certain phytochemicals has been shown to have an inverse association in the development of gliomas in adults.[36] In a study by Tedeschi-Blok and colleagues, statistical comparisons were made comparing the consumption of specific antioxidants and phytochemicals among 802 adult glioma cases and 846 control cases from the San Francisco Bay Area Adult Glioma Study, 1991–2000.[36] The results revealed a statistical significance for the inverse relationship between the intake of certain phytochemicals, including alpha- and beta-carotene, daidzein and coumestrol, and the occurrence of a glioma.[36]

Phytochemicals are promoted to help "fight cancer" at the cellular level and as cancer preventive agents. In contrast, research demonstrating the benefits of phytochemicals once cancer has been diagnosed is limited. In fact, depending on the type of cancer, a high intake of fruits and vegetables may be contraindicated during treatment. Advice for nutrition during cancer treatment should come from a registered dietitian (RD) to ensure that evidence-based recommendations are provided.

Nutrition Status at Diagnosis

Unlike patients with some types of cancer, who experience significant weight loss and nutrient deficits as part of their disease, persons diagnosed with malignant primary brain cancers do not necessarily present with obvious weight loss. Nutrient deficits are usually subclinical and related to the focal effects of the tumor rather than being systemic effects of chemicals produced by the brain tumor. Varying degrees of nutritional status are seen in persons with newly diagnosed brain cancer, which is considered a low nutrition-risk cancer.[37] Pretreatment factors, such as a normal nutrition status and a high Karnofsky Performance Score (KPS), can enable a person to handle treatment of a brain tumor more successfully.[34] The KPS plays an even more important role in patients who are older than 50 years. In this age group, patients with a KPS $\geq$ 70 survive a median of 10.3 months, whereas those with a KPS < 70 survive a median of 5.3 months.[35]

Nutritional Assessment and Therapy During Brain Cancer Treatment

Nutritional intervention and therapy for patients with brain cancer are best provided by a RD who possesses specialized training, education, and experience as well as access to a network of other nutrition professionals and evidence-based information that no other discipline can provide. Because nutrition is an art and a science, the skills of a RD are optimal to assess all aspects of a patient's life that may be interfering with appropriate nutrition. The RD can help the patient or caregiver with problem solving or referral to other clinicians for areas out of the RD's scope of practice.

Nutrition therapy involves designing a customized, realistic plan based on the patient's individual nutritional, medical, and social history and current clinical and personal issues. If the patient has cognitive and memory issues preventing him or her from fully benefiting from individual counseling, the caregiver should be included to assist with accomplishing the nutritional goals at home or during any subsequent admissions. Standard nutrition care involves both verbal and written information, and includes a plan for follow-up. Additionally, it is helpful to provide the patient and caregiver parameters for when to contact the RD (e.g., significant or ongoing weight changes or difficult blood glucose management) or when to call the physician (e.g., uncontrolled pain).

Brain cancer is considered a low-nutrition-risk (LR) cancer.[38] Persons with brain cancer do not often experience undernutrition as opposed to those persons receiving treatment for a high-nutrition-risk (HR) cancer. HR cancers typically include the head and neck cancers and those in the gastrointestinal system; LR cancers include those affecting the prostate, breast, lung, brain, gallbladder, and uterus.[38]

A study done by Ravasco and colleagues[37] compared 125 patients who were diagnosed with either a HR or LR cancer. The purpose of the study was threefold: (1) to determine quality of life (QOL), nutrition status, and nutrition intake at the onset of radiation therapy; (2) to determine whether individual nutrition counseling would enhance nutrient intake over time and whether nutrition status influenced QOL; and (3) to determine which symptoms may be predictive of a poor QOL and/or a reduction in nutrient intake. Prior to and following radiation each patient was assessed on these parameters. Results revealed a significant difference in malnutrition prior to treatment between the HR and LR groups ($p = 0.02$). Nutrient intake was associated with nutritional status ($p = 0.007$), and there was no significant change in nutritional status during treatment. At baseline, the LR patients not only had a higher calorie intake than their personal recommended energy requirements ($p = 0.001$), but also consumed more calories compared to the HR group ($p = 0.002$). QOL was higher in the LR group both before and after treatment compared to the HR group ($p = 0.01$). At the end of treatment, QOL had improved for the HR group—an outcome that was directly correlated with improved nutrient intake ($p = 0.001$). For the LR group, QOL and nutrient intake were stable before and after treatment.

If surgery such as a craniotomy is performed, then wound healing and bone knitting will require adequate diet and controlled blood sugar to support healing. If the patient has preexisting diabetes or is receiving steroids, then blood glucose should be tightly controlled to promote immune function not only for healing purposes, but also for optimizing any planned cancer treatments. When making appropriate calorie, protein, and fat recommendations for any patient receiving steroids, it is important to consider a therapeutic diet to promote the control of blood glucose if hyperglycemia has been a problem. If it has not, the patient should be informed that drug-induced hyperglycemia may become a problem in the future.

After brain surgery, patients may require mechanical ventilation. In such cases, attention must be paid to avoid both overfeeding and underfeeding related to issues of ventilator dependence and to prevent increased intracranial pressure in those patients in which this issue is a problem. The etiology of nausea and vomiting should be identified so it can be properly treated to prevent nutritional deficits.

Food–Drug Interactions

The chemotherapy drug procarbazine is a monoamine oxidase (MAO) inhibitor, and its use requires dietary modifications to avoid severe drug–nutrient interactions. The patient must follow a low-tyramine diet, which involves the avoidance of tea, coffee, cola drinks, cheese, yogurt, bananas, cigarettes, and alcoholic beverages including wine and beer.[24] According to one source, a tyramine-restricted diet should not include cheese, pickled or smoked fish, nonfresh meats and livers, dry sausage, sauerkraut, meat extracts, broad beans, banana peels, brewer's yeast and yeast extracts, Chianti and vermouth wines, or beer and ale. Foods to consume with caution include avocados, raspberries, soy sauce, chocolate, peanuts, unpasteurized yogurt or cream, distilled spirits, red and white wines, and port wines.[39] Drinking alcohol while taking procarbazine can cause severe nausea and vomiting.[24, 39] It may also cause a decrease in serum potassium, phosphorus, and calcium.[39]

Management of Nutrition-Related Side Effects of Treatment

Surgery

Besides the need for appropriate nutrition and blood glucose control following surgery, other surgery-related nutritional issues include pain, constipation due to pain medication, and diarrhea from antibiotic use. Uncontrolled pain is known to place additional stress on the patient as well as affect vital signs. Prolonged pain can lead to depression and loss of appetite. "Patients with . . . pain are rarely interested in eating."[40] Pain control experts advise that on the 0–10 pain scale, controlled postsurgical pain is considered to be in the range of 3–4. The RD, as a member of the healthcare team, should be cognizant of the patient's pain as a nutritional risk factor. If necessary, the RD should speak to appropriate healthcare team members about a patient's uncontrolled pain, especially if the patient is not communicating this information on his or her own behalf.

Consistent use of opioid pain medicine usually leads to constipation, and the best approach for managing this side effect is prevention, not treatment after the constipation has developed. If opioid-induced constipation does occur, the best treatment approach is a combination of a stool softener and laxative, rather than use of enemas or suppositories. Fortunately, long-term use of pain medication is not generally an ongoing issue in patients with brain cancer. Current research is promising in regard to use of two opioid-receptor antagonists, methylnaltrexone and alvimopan, in reducing the occurrence of ileus and reduction in hospital length of stay, while preserving analgesic effects of the opioids given for pain.[41]

Radiation

The nutrition-related side effects of radiation to the brain include nausea, vomiting, and fatigue.[1, 20] According to the American Society of Clinical Oncology (ASCO), the risk for vomiting with radiation to the brain is minimal (less than 30%) and the recommended treatment for this level of risk is on an "as-needed basis only" with the use of dopamine or serotonin-receptor antagonists. If vomiting occurs, a prophylactic antiemetic should be used for each remaining radiation treatment day.[42]

Radiation has been known to worsen dysphagia, a common focal effect of a tumor in the brainstem.[1, 20] Dysphagia will require involvement of a speech pathologist for proper diagnosis, and recommendations should be made for the appropriate texture modifications of food and fluid and swallowing therapy.

The synergistic tumor and radiation side effects are usually temporary and are commonly treated with steroids; steroids, of course, posses their own nutrition-related side effects, such as hyperglycemia and water and fat weight gain. Radiation commonly causes changes in mental functions, such as thinking and concentration, and these symptoms along with fatigue can significantly hamper a person's ability to plan, purchase, and prepare adequate meals.[1, 20]

Chemotherapy

An intermittent chemotherapy administration schedule is one technique used to minimize chemotherapy toxicity. Toxicity occurs when chemotherapeutic agents cause damage or death to normal healthy cells and is relative to the degree of damage. By giving chemotherapy intermittently, the damaged normal cells have a chance to recover and replenish their numbers. Common nutrition-related chemotherapy side effects include nausea, vomiting, fatigue, and infection.[1]

Nausea and Vomiting

ASCO has developed guidelines for the prevention of nausea and vomiting, with the guidelines being categorized by the risk of nausea or vomiting associated with each chemotherapy agent. Chemotherapy drugs that very frequently cause nausea and vomiting are labeled "high risk." Carmustine (BCNU), for example, is a high-risk chemotherapy drug commonly used to treat brain cancer. Patients receiving high-risk chemotherapeutics should also receive an antiemetic regimen.[42] The recommended antiemetic regimen combination is a 5-HT_3 serotonin-receptor antagonist (dolasetron, granisetron, ondansetron, or palonosetron), dexamethasone for 1–3 days, and aprepitant for 3 days.[42]

Fatigue

Fatigue can be experienced with all cancer treatment modalities and is considered a secondary nutrition risk factor because it interferes with the ability to plan, purchase, and prepare an adequate diet.[43] Ideally, a person experiencing the level of fatigue that interferes with adequate nutrition will have access to the resources needed to overcome this obstacle, such as friends, family, community groups, food delivery services, or social services. Persons with extreme fatigue and compromised ability to care for themselves may benefit from the services of an oncology social worker. Ideas for maintaining adequate intake during times of fatigue involve the use of easy-to-prepare convenience and prepackaged foods, such as pudding, snack foods, cheese, peanut butter, microwave foods, caloric beverages for hydration, and nutrient-dense, high-calorie, high-protein commercial nutritional supplements.

Seizures

Seizures are a common side effect of chemotherapy, radiation to the brain, or changes deriving from the tumor itself. In many patients, antiseizure and antiepileptic medications are required to control these seizures. Medications used to treat seizures include carbamazepine, phenytoin, and phenobarbital. These drugs require monitoring by the medical oncologist because they interact with some chemotherapy drugs, such as paclitaxel, irinotecan, interferon, and retinoic acid. Because medications used to treat seizures have numerous other drug–drug interactions, collaboration with a pharmacist who specializes in oncology is beneficial when such medications are prescribed.

Carbamazepine

The main nutrition-related side effect of carbamazepine relates to its concurrent use while consuming grapefruit juice or grapefruit products. Four levels of recommendations are made regarding the consumption of grapefruit while taking certain medications: "avoid grapefruit juice," "use with caution," "no significant interaction," and "safe." Carbamazepine falls under the category of "use with caution" because of the need for monitoring the serum plasma levels of the drug if it is taken with grapefruit products; carbamazepine levels may become too high in this setting.[43]

Additionally, if carbamazepine is used for more than six months, a supplemental or dietary increase in vitamin D and calcium is indicated because of the effects that this drug has on the metabolism of these nutrients. Carbamazepine may cause nausea, vomiting, or diarrhea. Alcohol should be avoided while taking this drug, and may increase CNS depression. Patients receiving enteral feedings should use the suspension form of this medication and mix it with equal parts of a diluting agent before administration into the feeding tube.[43] Administering the medication with adequate water will help reduce any risk of gastrointestinal (GI) irritation.

Phenytoin

Phenytoin is subject to many of the same food–drug interactions as carbamazepine. It should be taken with food and/or milk consistently to help reduce its potential for GI irritation.

Phenytoin increases the metabolism of folate and vitamins D and K, which can lead to bone disorders or osteoporosis; for this reason, supplementation with these nutrients may be needed. The patient should take 1 mg folate per day, as well as calcium, vitamin D, and thiamine supplements. However, taking supplements requires consideration of interactions that can reduce phenytoin's bioavailability when it is taken with certain substances. For example, supplementation with calcium, magnesium, or antacids requires a 2-hour separation before or after taking phenytoin.[43] If the patient is receiving an enteral feeding, the usual course of action is to stop the feeding 1 hour before and 1 hour after the administration of phenytoin. Depending on the facility where the patient is admitted, varying degrees of time may be used, such as 30 minutes to 2 hours before and after the enteral feeding. Attention to adequate fluid flushes is needed when administering this medication to help reduce GI irritation.[39]

Phenobarbital

Phenobarbital increases the rate of metabolism of vitamins D and K and folate, and it can lead to an increase in cholesterol, low-density lipoprotein (LDL), high-density lipoprotein (HDL), and lipoprotein α. Intake of dietary vitamin D and calcium should be increased, or supplemented if increased dietary intake is not possible.[39, 43]

Corticosteroids

Persons receiving chemotherapy and/or radiation for brain cancer often receive steroids to help control treatment-induced nausea and vomiting and to reduce cerebral edema, which can be life-threatening. Dexamethasone is often the treatment of choice and is very effective in reducing cerebral edema.[39, 44]

Steroids can cause increased gastric and intestinal irritation when combined with alcohol, aspirin, and certain arthritis medications, leading to an increased risk of GI ulcers. Steroids should be consumed with food and/or milk to reduce the chance of GI irritation and discomfort.[24]

The metabolic effects of high doses or long-term steroid use include increased fat and water stores and alterations in calcium and protein metabolism. Dietary modifications (low sodium, increased potassium and calcium, high-quality protein) are often needed to counteract the side effects of the steroids. Compared with other steroid medications, dexamethasone is associated with less sodium retention, edema, and potassium losses. Liver enzymes can become elevated due to steroid use, however, and should be monitored by a physician.[38, 39]

Hyperglycemia is a major complication associated with steroid therapy that can make glucose control in a patient with preexisting diabetes quite challenging. Additionally, it can lead to drug-induced hyperglycemia in persons with no history of diabetes.[38, 39] A patient without a history of diabetes and a chromium deficiency who receives steroid therapy is at increased risk for the development of drug-induced diabetes.[38] Diet therapy in the presence of hyperglycemia includes limiting concentrated sweets, such as non-diet carbonated beverages, cakes, candies, pies, pastries, and ice cream. The addition of or adjustment to oral hypoglycemic agents and insulin may be necessary.[38]

The Ketogenic Diet

The ketogenic diet is a high-fat, very-low-carbohydrate, adequate-protein diet designed to increase the body's dependence on fat rather than glucose for energy. The goal of the ketogenic diet is to produce ketones, which are the products of rapid incomplete fat breakdown and include β-hydroxybutyrate, acetoacetate, and acetone.[45] This diet is currently used to treat intractable seizures in adults and children, weight loss, and certain metabolic disorders that involve abnormal utilization of glucose.

Normally brain cells prefer glucose as their main energy source. If glucose is not available, however, normal brain tissue can easily switch to use of ketones as a fuel source. Normal brain cells are considered metabolically flexible. In contrast, brain tumor cells are not flexible and depend on glucose for their growth and survival.[46] One reason for this inflexibility is that tumor cells possess dysfunctional mitochondria in abnormal amounts. Mitochondria, which serve as the "powerhouse" of the cell, generate most of the energy for the cell and control cellular growth. Under normal circumstances, mitochondria are key to the utilization of ketones for energy. Theoretically, if mitochondria are lacking in number and function, limited or no access to glucose could cause brain cancer cells to die.[46]

In 1995, Nebeling and colleagues published a landmark clinical study involving utilization of the ketogenic diet to interfere with tumor metabolism without affecting the subject's nutritional status.[47] The study, which is the only human study of the diet ever conducted, consisted of two subjects, both female children with nonresectable high-grade gliomas. After experiencing "severe life-threatening adverse effects" after treatment with extensive radiation and chemotherapy, both girls had "measurable" tumor remaining. Both children responded well to the ketogenic diet and experienced long-term tumor management without further chemotherapy or radiation. Glucose uptake by the tumor cells was measured using positron emission tomography with fluoro-deoxy-glucose and demonstrated a 21.8% reduction of glucose uptake at the tumor site in both patients. As of 2005, one girl was still alive.[44]

SUMMARY

Brain cancers are complex for a number of reasons, including the various types of brain tumors, the numerous treatment options, questions about the optimal treatment plan, and side effects associated with therapies. In general, individuals with brain cancer are not at high risk for malnutrition when compared to their counterparts with other types of cancers. However, because of the inherent nutritional risk associated with cancer therapies, persons with a brain cancer diagnosis should undergo nutrition screening and be referred to a registered dietitian if risk factors, such as unintentional weight loss and poor appetite, are identified. Attention to potential nutrition-related problems deriving from specific treatment modalities, drug–nutrient interactions, and medication side effects is necessary. Additionally, a multi-disciplinary approach is essential to ensure the most positive outcome for the patient.

REFERENCES

1. Brain tumors: Primary. Available at http://www.mdconsult.com/das/patient/body/81670263-3/643425000/10041/9428.html. Accessed November 13, 2007.
2. Smith ML, Grady MS. Neurosurgery. In: Brunicardi FC, Anderson DK, Billiar TR, et al, eds. *Schwartz's Principles of Surgery*. 8th ed. New York: McGraw Hill; 2005. http://www.accessmedicine.com/content.aspx?aID=82106. Accessed September 6, 2006.
3. Black P. Brain Tumor Society. Brain tumor facts and statistics 2006. Available at http://www.tbts.org. Accessed July 18, 2006.
4. Central Brain Tumor Registry of the United States (CBTRUS). *Statistical Report: Primary Brain Tumors in the United States, 1998–2002.* CBTRUS; 2005.
5. The National Cancer Act of 1971, Public Law No. 92-218, S 1828, 92nd Congress (December 23, 1971). http://www.cancer.gov/aboutnci/national-cancer-act-1971. Accessed February 1, 2009.
6. Brain tumor. Available at http://www.DynamicMedical.com. Accessed September 25, 2007.
7. Bauman G, Lote K, Larson D, et al. Pretreatment factors predict overall survival for patients with low-grade glioma: A recursive partitioning analysis. *Intl J Radiation Oncol Biol Physics.* 1999;45(4):923–929.
8. Hinkle JL. In: Kors E, ed. *Brunner and Suddarth's Textbook of Medical–Surgical Nursing*. 10th ed. Philadelphia, PA: Lippincott Williams & Wilkins; 2004: 1856–1860, 1969–1977.
9. National Cancer Institute. A snapshot of brain and central nervous system cancers. http://planning.cancer.gov/brain-snapshots.pdf.shtml. Accessed November 18, 2007.
10. Deorah S, Lynch CF, Sibenaller ZA, Ryken TC. Trends in brain cancer incidence and survival in the United States: Surveillance, Epidemiology, and End Results program, 1973 to 2001. *Neurosurg Focus.* 2006;20(4):1–7. Available at www.aans.org. Accessed October 10, 2008.
11. DeAngelis LM. Brain tumors. *New Engl J Med.* 2001;344(2):114–123.
12. MediLexicon. http://www.medilexicon.com/. Accessed December 10, 2007.
13. Hepworth SJ, Schoemaker MJ, Muir KR, Swerdlow AJ, van Tongeren MJ, McKinney PA. Mobile phone use and risk of glioma in adults: Case-control study. *Br Med J.* 2006;332(7546):883–887.
14. Maier M. Brains and mobile phones. *Br Med J.* 2006;332:864–865.
15. Lahkola A, Tokola K, Auvinen A. Meta-analysis of mobile phone use and intracranial tumors. *Scand J Work Environ Health.* 2006;32(3);171–177.
16. Behin A, Hoang-Xuan K, Carpentier AF, Delattre JY. Primary brain tumours in adults. *Lancet.* 2003;361(9354):323–331.

17. *Cancer Medicine.* 6th ed. Lewiston, NY: BC Decker; 2003. Available at www.ncbi .nlm.nih.gov/books/. Accessed November 12, 2007.

18. Kelly PJ, Daumas-Duport C, Kispert DB, et al. Imaging-based stereotaxic serial biopsies in untreated intracranial glial neoplasms. *J Neurosurg* 1987;66: 865–874.

19. Pollock BE, Gorman DA, Schomberg PJ, Kline RW. The Mayo Clinic gamma knife experience: Indications and initial results. *Mayo Clinic Proc.* 1999;74:5–13.

20. Enam SA, Rock JP, Rosenblum ML. Malignant gliomas. In: Berger MS, Bernstein M, eds. *Neuro-oncology: The Essentials.* New York: Thieme; 2000:309–318.

21. Brada M. Radiosurgery for brain tumours: Triumph of marketing over evidence based medicine. *Br Med J.* 1999;318(7181):411–412.

22. Dolinsky C. Development of glioblastoma multiforme. Available at http://cancer.med .upenn.edu/custom_tags/print_article.cfm?Page=2444&Section. Accessed November 20, 2007.

23. Lefranc F, Sadeghi N, Camby I, Metens, T, Dewitte O, Kiss R. Present and potential future issues in glioblastoma treatment. *Expert Rev Anticancer Ther.* 2006;6 (5):719–732.

24. MedlinePlus. Available at http://www.nlm.nih.gov/medlineplus/druginfo/drug_Aa .html. Accessed December 29, 2007.

25. Aoke T, Hashimoto N, Matsutani M. Management of glioblastoma. *Expert Opin Pharmacother.* 2007;8(18):3133–3146.

26. Pierson R. Schering-Plough brain cancer drug wins expanded OK. Available at http://virtualtrials.com/news3.cfm?item=3052. Accessed December 25, 2007.

27. Spiegel BM, Esrailian E, Laine L, Chamberlain MC. Clinical impact of adjuvant chemotherapy in glioblastoma multiforme: A meta-analysis. *CNS Drugs.* 2007;21 (9):775–787.

28. Radiation plus chemo quadruples survival time for fatal brain cancer. Available at http://virtualtrials.com/news3.cfm?item=4021. Accessed December 25, 2007.

29. Stupp R, Mason WP, van den Bent MJ, et al. Radiotherapy plus concomitant and adjuvant temozolomide for glioblastoma. *N Engl J Med.* 2005;352:987–996.

30. Tsutsui Y, Tomizawa K, Nagita M, et al. Development of bionanocapsules targeting brain tumors. *J Controlled Release.* 2007;122:159–164.

31. London S. Radiation/temozolomide raises possibility of cure in glioblastoma. *Oncol News Intl.* 2007;16(12):1–3.

32. Ressel GW. American Cancer Society releases guidelines on nutrition and physical activity for cancer prevention. Available at www.mdconsult.com. Accessed November 13, 2007.

33. Wardlaw GM, Smith AM. *Contemporary Nutrition.* 6th ed. New York, NY: McGraw Hill; 2006:36.

34. Bauer JD, Capra S. Nutrition intervention improves outcomes in patients with cancer cachexia receiving chemotherapy: A pilot study. *Support Care Cancer.* 2005;13 (4):270–274.

35. Curran WJ Jr, Scott CB, Horton J, et al. Recursive partitioning analysis of prognostic factors in three Radiation Therapy Oncology Group malignant glioma trials. *J Natl Cancer Inst.* 1993;85:704–710.

36. Tedeschi-Blok N, Lee M, Sison JD, Miike, R, Wrensch M. Inverse association of antioxidant and phytoestrogen nutrient intake with glioma in the San Francisco Bay Area: A case-control study. *BMC Cancer.* 2006,6:148. Available at http://www .biomedcentral.com/147-2407/6/148. Accessed December 25, 2007.

37. Ravasco P, Monteiro-Grillo I, Camilo ME. Does nutrition influence quality of life in cancer patients undergoing radiotherapy? *Radiother Oncol.* 2003;67(2):213–220.

38. Grant B, Byron J. Nutritional implications in chemotherapy. In: Elliott L, Molseed L, McCallum PD, eds., with Grant B, technical ed. *Medical Nutrition Therapy in Oncology.* 2nd ed. Chicago, IL: American Dietetic Association; 2006:72–87.

39. Haken V. Interactions between drugs and nutrients. In: Mahan LK, Escott-Stump S, eds. *Krause's Food, Nutrition, and Diet Therapy.* Philadelphia, PA: W.B. Saunders; 2000:399–414.

40. Wilkes G. Nutrition: The forgotten nutrient in cancer care. *Am J Nurs.* 2004:100 (4):46–51.

41. Kurz A, Sessler DI. Opioid-induced bowel dysfunction: Pathophysiology and potential new therapies. *Drugs.* 2003;63(7):650–671.

42. Mark KG, Hesketh PJ, Somerfield MR, et al. American Society of Clinical Oncology guidelines for antiemetics in oncology: Update 2006. Available at www.asco.org. Accessed January 1, 2007.

43. Pronsky ZM. *Food–Medication Interactions.* 13th ed. Birchrunville, PA: Food–Medication Interactions; 2004:96, 251, 254.

44. Seyfried TN, Mukherjee P. Targeting energy metabolism in brain cancer: Review and hypothesis. *Nutr Metabol.* 2005;21(2):30.

45. National Cancer Institute. Nausea and Vomiting. http://www.cancerweb.ncl.ac.uk/cancernet/304466.html. Accessed January 3, 2007.

46. Zhou W, Mukherjee P, Kiebish MA, Markis WT, Mantis JG, Seyfried TN. The calorically restricted ketogenic diet, an effective alternative therapy for malignant brain cancer. *Nutr Metabol.* 2007;22(4):5.

47. Nebeling LC, Miraldi F, Shurin SB, Lerner E. Effects of a ketogenic diet on tumor metabolism and nutritional status in pediatric oncology patients: Two case reports. *J Am Coll Nutr.* 1995;14:202-208.

Chapter 14

Palliative Care

Kelay Trentham, MS, RD, CD

WHAT IS PALLIATIVE CARE?

Palliative treatment is defined as treatment that is designed to ease the symptoms of a disease rather than attempting to cure it.[1] The term "palliative care" refers to both a care philosophy and a comprehensive, organized, and highly structured interdisciplinary care system provided to persons with debilitating or life-threatening illness for the purpose of physical, spiritual, and psychological comfort.[2, 3] It is suggested that palliative care begins at the time of such diagnosis and continue through cure or until death, and into the family's bereavement period.[4] Palliation may be either the primary focus of care, or it may be provided concurrently with life-prolonging treatment.[3]

Key components of palliative care include a family-centered approach; a focus on effective pain and symptom management; presence of spiritual, psychosocial and bereavement support; and provision of individualized care plans and coordinated services in any setting used by the patient.[2, 3] Hospice is well-established as the means for delivering palliative care at the end of life.[4] Other organizational delivery models include the following approaches:

- Consultation service team (hospital, nursing home, office practice, or home settings)
- Dedicated inpatient unit (acute or rehabilitation hospital, nursing home) or as part of freestanding inpatient hospice
- Combined consultative service and inpatient unit (hospital, nursing home)
- Combined hospice and palliative care program (hospital, nursing home, freestanding inpatient hospice)
- Hospital- or private-practice-based outpatient care clinic
- Hospice-based home care or outpatient consultation[4]

In settings without direct access to a palliative care specialist, it is advised that consultation be sought via telemedicine or other remote means.[4]

It is well documented that communication issues among these care settings may result in discontinuity of care and, therefore, cause distress for the patient and family.[4] Thus a core value of palliative care is to facilitate continuity of care to avoid needless suffering and errors, eliminate the perception of abandonment, and ensure respect of the patient's choices.[4]

General goals of palliative care include prevention and relief of suffering, enhancement of quality of life, optimization of function, assistance with decision making, and provision of personal growth opportunities for patients and families.[4, 5] More specifically, the World Health Organization (WHO) states that palliative care performs the following functions:

- Provides relief from pain and other distressing symptoms
- Affirms life and regards dying as a normal process
- Intends neither to hasten nor to postpone death
- Integrates psychological and spiritual aspects of patient care
- Offers a support system to help patients live as actively as possible until death
- Offers a support system to help the family cope during the patient's illness and in their own bereavement
- Uses a team approach to address the needs of patients and their families, including bereavement counseling, if indicated
- Enhances quality of life and will possibly influence the outcome of illness
- Is applicable early in the course of illness, in conjunction with other therapies that are intended to prolong life, including chemotherapy and radiation therapy, and includes those investigations needed to better understand and manage distressing complications[5]

Comprehensive evaluation and treatment should be patient-centered and focused on the role of the family unit in decision making while honoring their values, beliefs, and cultures. This approach may require the expertise of a wide variety of healthcare team members, including physicians, nurses, social workers, chaplains, pharmacists, psychologists, rehabilitation specialists, child life specialists, bereavement coordinators, trained volunteers, and dietitians.[4] Effective integration of these disciplines and services requires excellence in communication, leadership, collaboration, and coordination.[4]

The Dietitian's Role in Palliative Care

An integral part of the healthcare team, the dietetics professional is an important advocate for the advanced cancer patient receiving palliative care.

The registered dietitian (RD), who has a distinctive education encompassing nutrition, medical, behavioral, and psychosocial sciences as well as ethics, can provide a balanced perspective regarding the appropriateness of various nutrition interventions, including artificial nutrition and hydration.[6] The RD serves as educator and advisor for the patient and family, as well as for other healthcare clinicians. Throughout a patient's course of care, it is the RD's responsibility to assess the patient's nutritional status, identify his or her nutrition care needs, and implement a nutrition care plan based on current evidence of best practice. Development of a nutrition care plan entails involving the patient, the patient's family, and the healthcare team. The resulting plan should be consistent with the patient's goals and focused on quality of life, with an objective both to prevent and relieve any suffering associated with the symptoms and complications of advanced cancer.[7]

Caring for the Patient with Advanced Cancer

Ideally, supportive nutrition care should begin at the time of cancer diagnosis.[8] Although aggressive nutrition care may be warranted for the patient undergoing curative treatment, the goals of medical nutritional therapy will change when it is determined that the disease is incurable.[9] As the treatment mode shifts away from curative therapy and toward end-of-life care, there is greater focus on well-being and quality of life (QoL).[10] For the patient with advanced cancer, early palliative care is described as the period when disease is incurable and life-threatening, but death is not necessarily imminent. In contrast, late palliative care is delivered when the disease is in the terminal phase, life expectancy is less than one month, and maintaining QoL is considerably more difficult.[8, 9] During early palliative care, nutritional interventions should be a priority to aid in the healing process, to ensure that nutrition therapy options can be proactively identified and discussed, and to improve the patient's sense of well-being.[9] In the terminal phase of disease, patients and their families may require guidance regarding artificial nutrition and hydration in addition to less invasive measures to address nutritional status.

Prevalence of Nutritional Impact Symptoms

Along with the late stage of cancer disease, deteriorating nutritional status (weight loss) and declining nutritional intake (loss of appetite) have been shown to be major determinants of patients' QoL.[11–13] Severe chemosensory dysfunction has been correlated with significantly decreased food enjoyment and QoL as well.[14] Table 14.1 illustrates the prevalence of nutrition-related symptoms of patients with advanced cancer in four studies.[15–18]

Additionally, symptoms of fatigue and diminished sense of well-being have been noted to be among the most distressing symptoms reported by cancer patients.[19] Given that significant decreases in energy intake have been seen in patients with late-stage cancer,[20] and that symptoms such as anorexia and chemosensory dysfunction are known to result in significantly reduced calorie intake, nutrition-related symptoms that impair adequate intake are likely to be partly responsible for fatigue.[14] Clearly, the declines seen in patients' nutritional

Table 14.1   *Nutrition-Related Symptoms in Patients with Advanced Cancer (Prevalence as a Percentage of Total Cases)*

Symptom	Inpatient and Outpatient[1] (N = 352)	Outpatient[2] (N = 200)	Inpatient[3] (N = 50)	Inpatient and Outpatient[4] (N = 1,000)
Weight loss*	85%	54%	76%	50%
Anorexia	81%	59%	56%	66%
Early satiety	69%	49%	71%	51%
Xerostomia	69%	67%	84%	57%
Constipation	59%	39%	58%	52%
Nausea	49%	26%	48%	36%
Bloating	43%	50%	50%	18%
Vomiting	38%	11%	34%	23%
Diarrhea	24%	10%	16%	8%
Taste changes	16%	32%	60%	28%

Other symptoms observed include belching (18–35%), indigestion (19–35%), hiccups (9–25%), sore mouth/throat (5–22%), dysphagia (18–32%), and odynophagia (15%).

*Defined as more than >10% body weight lost.
Data Sources
[1]Sarhill N, Mahmoud F, Walsh D, et al. Evaluation of nutritional status in advanced metastatic cancer. *Support Care Cancer.* 2003;11:652–659.
[2]Homsi J, Walsh D, Rivera N, et al. Symptom evaluation in palliative medicine: Patient report vs systematic assessment. *Support Care Cancer.* 2006;14:444–453.
[3]Komurcu S, Nelson KA, Walsh D, Ford RB, Rybicki L. Gastrointestinal symptoms among inpatients with advanced cancer. *Am J Hosp Palliat Care.* 2002;19:351–355.
[4]Walsh D, Donelly S, Rybicki L. The symptoms of advanced cancer: relationship to age, gender and performance status in 1000 patients. *Support Care Cancer.* 2000;8:175–179.

status are multifactorial, with any one symptom or a combination thereof potentially contributing to significant distress for patients with advanced cancer.

Cancer cachexia, a wasting syndrome of nutritional deterioration, is characterized by severe weight loss and, unlike starvation, includes loss of both lean body mass and adipose tissue.[21, 22] Cachexia is present in more than 80% of patients with gastric and pancreatic cancers, and in more than 50% of patients with lung, prostate, and colon cancers.[23] Overall, approximately 50% of cancer patients suffer from cachexia,[24] which is typically accompanied by anorexia, fatigue, anemia, and edema.[23] In addition, one study showed that 52% of patients surveyed indicated concern about either eating less or weight loss[25] ultimately contributing to decreased QoL.

Symptom Etiology and Management

Anorexia, Cachexia, and Weight Loss

Etiology

Cancer cachexia syndrome is thought to be the result of multiple factors that can be categorized as follows: anorexia leading to inadequate nutrient intake, metabolic disturbances, and the presence of inflammatory and other humoral factors.[26] Anorexia in cachexia may be primarily caused by cytokine-induced *hypothalamic resistance*—the inability of the hypothalamus to respond appropriately to signals that indicate an energy deficit.[22] Additional contributing factors to cachexia–anorexia include depression, anxiety, taste alterations, intestinal obstruction, chemotherapy and radiotherapy, previously mentioned nutrition-related symptoms, and pain.[23, 26, 27] Compared to controls, cancer patients have been found to have normal, reduced, or increased metabolic rates.[24] Glucose turnover and gluconeogenesis (glucose production from body tissues) are increased in the presence of insulin resistance, elevated peripheral fat mobilization, and excessive fatty acid oxidation, leading to depletion of lipid stores[26]; whole-body protein turnover is increased while muscle protein synthesis is reduced, resulting in loss of lean body mass.[24, 26] In addition to affecting appetite regulation, cytokines are thought to play a role in inducing the catabolic state.[22, 26] However, the specific mechanism of their involvement remains unclear and continues to be studied.

Management

Although anorexia is only one of several factors resulting in cachexia, anorexia is considered a primary contributing factor to this wasting syndrome.[28] For this reason, most nutritional interventions are geared toward improving appetite and maximizing nutrition intake.[22, 28] Studies have indicated that nutritional counseling positively affects patient outcomes—and particularly QoL—in patients undergoing curative treatment.[29-32] In these studies, counseling was individualized, based on regular food, and given in the form of written dietary guidelines with detailed explanation.[32]

The use of oral supplements containing bioactive substances has also been extensively studied in patients undergoing curative treatment. One review evaluating the use of fish-oil–enriched nutrition supplements providing 2–6 g/day of eicosapentaenoic acid (EPA) indicated that the supplementation led to weight stabilization, gains in lean body mass, reversal of negative nitrogen balance, prolonged survival, and improved or stabilized QoL.[33] Conversely, another study showed no positive benefits related to ingestion of EPA supplementation in terms of weight, appetite, or well-being.[34] Researchers speculate that the benefits obtained related to EPA ingestion are associated with the doses consumed, as Fearon et al. found a dose-response relationship between n-3 fatty acid intake and weight gain, increase in lean tissue, and improvements in QoL.[35]

Recent reviews investigating the effects of n-3 fatty acid supplementation have yielded conflicting results.[36, 37] In their review of 17 studies, Colomer and colleagues concluded that oral supplements providing at least 1.5 g/day of n-3 fatty acids were beneficial in increasing weight and appetite, improving QoL, and reducing postsurgical morbidity, particularly in patients with upper digestive tract and pancreatic cancers.[36] Another review of 5 trials that enrolled a total of 587 patients, however, found insufficient evidence to conclude that EPA supplementation improves symptoms of cachexia syndrome.[37] Further studies including patients with curable or terminal disease will be helpful in determining whether there is sufficient cause to routinely recommend EPA supplementation.

Pharmacological approaches are also considered an important part of integrative therapy for cachexia.[22] The primary drugs that have been used to improve appetite include progestins (megestrol acetate [MA], medroxyprogesterone acetate [MPA]), cannabinoids (dronabinol), corticosteroids (dexamethasone),[22] and prokinetics (metoclopramide).[28] Other agents studied include hydrazine sulfate, cyproheptadine, pentoxifylline, melatonin, erythropoietin, androgenic steroids, ghrelin, interferon, and nonsteroidal anti-inflammatory drugs (NSAIDs; indomethacin).[28] In a review of 55 studies, only 2 medications garnered sufficient evidence to support their use in cancer cachexia: corticosteroids and progestins.[28] The most commonly studied progestins, MA and MPA, have been found to increase weight and exhibit a dose response up to a dosage of 800 mg/day.[28] Whether corticosteroids are associated with significant benefits is difficult to evaluate, because the studies investigating their use have used varied dosages and different types, making it difficult to determine the optimal dose and duration of use.[28] Short courses of use are generally recommended for corticosteroids, as their benefits typically diminish after 4 weeks.[28]

Dry mouth, early satiety, and taste changes have been identified as an additional symptom cluster that occurs together with fatigue/anorexia, which supports the concept that anorexia–cachexia syndrome is multifactorial in origin.[38] Other symptoms that may affect anorexia, and thereby promote weight loss, include pain, depression, and other nutrition-related symptoms such as nausea, vomiting, malabsorption, and constipation.[23]

Table 14.2 summarizes the therapeutic strategies used for treating the anorexic–cachectic patient. Specific recommendations for addressing individual nutrition-related symptoms are discussed later in this chapter, as well as indications and contraindications for use of artificial nutrition and hydration.

Early Satiety

Etiology

As previously discussed, early satiety is common in advanced cancer, occurring in 49% to 71% of patients,[15–18] and is likely to be a significant contributing factor in reduced intake. Despite this fact, early satiety is a symptom that

Table 14.2 *Palliative Nutrition and Medical Therapy Approaches for Anorexia–Cachexia*

Provide individualized dietary counseling.	• Provide one-on-one instruction including written information. • Recommendations: small, frequent meals; energy-dense foods; eat at regular times; pleasant surroundings at mealtime; avoid unpleasant odors; exercise as tolerated and with doctor's permission; avoid extremes in taste and temperature; take liquids between meals; oral supplements to aid calorie intake
Address nutrition-related symptoms.	Nausea, vomiting, dry mouth, early satiety, taste changes, constipation, malabsorption
Address non-nutrition-related symptoms.	Pain, depression
Provide drug therapy.	• Progestins (MA, MPA) • Corticosteroids

Sources: Laviano A, Meguid MM, Inui A, et al. Therapy insight: Cancer anorexia–cachexia syndrome: When all you can eat is yourself. *Nat Clin Pract.* 2005;2:158–165; Stewart G, Skipworth RJE, Fearon KCH. Cancer cachexia and fatigue. *Clin Med.* 2006;6:140–143; Finley J. Management of cancer cachexia. *AACN Clin Issues Ad Pract Acute Crit Care.* 2000;11:590–603.

is rarely discovered unless the healthcare provider specifically inquires about it.[39] Early satiety may be attributed to a number of things, but is most commonly thought to be related to decreased gastric motility due to paraneoplastic syndrome or chemotherapy.[39] Other causes include impaired gastric motility and decreased gastric capacity related to dysfunction of the autonomic nervous system, medications (opioids, chemotherapy), gastric surgery, fibrosis, or gastritis.[39]

Management

Nutrition intervention for early satiety should address known causes. If impaired gastric motility is a known or suspected cause, prokinetic agents may be beneficial.[23] Patients may also be advised to eat small, frequent, and nutrient-dense meals or snacks; focus on eating earlier in the day; avoid consumption of foods that have very high fat content (which may increase gastric transit time); drink liquids between meals; limit intake of gas-forming foods; and, if appropriate, consider light activity to help stimulate digestion.[39, 40]

Nausea and Vomiting

Etiology

Nausea and vomiting are considered two of the more distressing symptoms experienced by patients with advanced cancer[41] and appear to be more prominent than prevalence statistics might suggest (see Table 14.1 on page 354). Vomiting is less prevalent than nausea and seems to be less bothersome as well.[42] In advanced cancer, nausea and vomiting are more likely seen in patients diagnosed with stomach or breast malignancies, and may be of moderate to great severity.[42] The most common causes of these symptoms include mechanical issues (impaired gastric emptying, GI obstructions), chemical sources (cytotoxic agents, opioids, NSAIDs), therapeutic side effects (as in palliative radiation therapy), and metabolic factors (infections, comorbidities, renal or hepatic failure).[39, 43] Other contributing factors include pain, fear and anxiety, and unpleasant odors or tastes.[39]

Management

Etiology-based management of nausea and vomiting is recommended for promoting a systematic approach to patient care, identifying all possible causes, and providing specific and appropriate therapy in a population already at risk for overmedication.[41] Mechanical issues, such as impaired gastric emptying or bowel obstruction, may require either pharmacological or nonpharmacological management techniques.[41] Impaired gastric emptying can be treated with prokinetics, as previously described.[23] Appropriate treatment of bowel obstruction requires careful consideration of the tumor location and burden, patient's prognosis, patient's performance status, and presence of concurrent complications.[44] Options for treatment include surgery, nasogastric suction, pharmacological treatment, self-expanding metallic stents, venting gastrostomy, and bowel rest with total parenteral nutrition (TPN) or hydration.[44] Clinical practice recommendations for managing bowel obstruction from an expert panel endorsed by the European Association for Palliative Care are summarized in Table 14.3.

Table 14.3 *Palliative Therapy Recommendations for Management of Bowel Obstruction*

Surgery	• Not recommended for patients with poor prognostic criteria: intra-abdominal carcinomatosis, poor performance status, massive ascites. • Successful palliation is associated with absence of palpable abdominal or pelvic masses, ascites volume < 3 L, unifocal obstruction, and preoperative weight loss < 9 kg.
Nasogastric tube (NGT) for suction	Temporary use only recommended if inoperable obstruction not manageable by drugs alone
Drugs: antisecretory, analgesics, antiemetics	Recommended alone or in combination; efficacy supported by literature
Self-expanding metallic stents	May be useful in advanced metastatic disease, poor surgical risk; not without complications; further studies warranted to determine who may best benefit
Venting gastrostomy	Consider if drugs unsuccessful; preferred for long term decompression over NGT; percutaneous endoscopic gastrostomy (PEG) tube is superior to surgical gastrostomy tube; 90% effectiveness in controlling nausea and vomiting
Total parenteral nutrition (TPN)	Controversial; indicated for patients who may die of starvation rather than tumor spread; consider in young patients with Karnofsky Performance Score (KPS) > 50
Hydration	May be indicated to correct nausea; may be difficult, uncomfortable for some patients; regular mouth care is preferred treatment for correcting dry mouth

Source: Ripamonti C, Twycross R, Baines M, et al. Clinical-practice recommendations for the management of bowel obstruction in patients with end-stage cancer. *Support Care Cancer.* 2001;9:223–233.

Drug-induced nausea and vomiting are typically treated with antiemetics, rotation (in the case of opioids), steroids, mucosal protectants (in the use of NSAIDs), and changing, reducing dosage of, or discontinuing use of the causal agent.[45] Nausea and vomiting related to radiation therapy is prophylactically treated with serotonin-receptor antagonists, dopamine-receptor agonists, or dexamethasone.[42] Metabolic causes may be adequately treated with hydration (uremia) or appropriate medications (such as bisphosphonates for hypercalcemia), or by otherwise addressing the cause (such as correcting electrolyte imbalances).[42]

Individualized dietary intervention for the management of nausea and vomiting has been found to be useful.[39, 42] Basic recommendations include those previously described for early satiety. Also recommended are the following measures: avoidance of strong odors; keeping foods cold or at room temperature; eating dry, starchy, or salty foods; taking sips of ginger ale; eating candied ginger or peppermint candies; avoiding liquids on an empty stomach; and avoiding lying down for at least one hour after eating.[40] If vomiting occurs secondary to gagging on secretions, the following measures may help: increasing fluid intake to thin secretions; frequent rinsing and gargling with a baking soda solution (1 tablespoon baking soda in 1 quart of water); eating fresh pineapple to thin oral and pharyngeal secretions; use of a cool mist humidifier; and avoiding alcohol-based mouthwashes, which can further dry the mouth.[40]

Xerostomia

Etiology

Xerostomia, or dry mouth, is very common in patients with advanced cancer, and particularly if they undergo radiation to the head and neck areas.[45] In addition to being distressing, dry mouth impairs swallowing, lessens taste and enjoyment of food, and can lead to infections, denture problems, bad breath, and difficulty communicating.[45, 46] Opioids are thought to be the most common cause of dry mouth.[39] Other medications that can cause dry mouth include antibiotics, antiemetics, tricyclic antidepressants, anticholinergics, antihistamines, beta blockers, cytotoxics, and diuretics, all of which reduce saliva flow.[39, 45, 46] Other causes include dehydration, mouth breathing, anxiety, advanced age (age > 65 years), smoking, and poor fluid intake.[45] Exposure to alcohol, either by drinking or from oral rinses, also contributes to oral dryness.[46]

Management

Effective management of xerostomia can prove challenging for patients with advanced cancers. Adequate oral hydration is an essential element of care, but may be a difficult goal for the patient who is struggling with other symptoms such as nausea, vomiting, dysgeusia, and anorexia.[46] For this reason, both fluid intake and good oral hygiene should be encouraged. Toothbrushing with a soft brush and fluoride toothpaste is recommended on a twice daily basis.[39, 47, 48] Denture cleaning is recommended after each meal and after removal of the dentures in the evenings, and gums/soft tissue should be brushed with a soft brush.[47]

Several types of mouth rinses have been suggested to alleviate xerostomia, including chlorhexidine (antibacterial), sodium bicarbonate, dilute hydrogen peroxide, and salt water or saline.[49] In an extensive review, however, only saline rinses were found to have no apparent detrimental effects.[49] Chlorhexidine causes burning and stinging, and patients complain that it has an unpleasant taste.[49] Sodium bicarbonate promotes an alkaline environment, which allows for bacterial growth, and some patients find that it has an unpleasant taste.[49] Hydrogen peroxide, even diluted, is highly astringent and is noted to cause stinging, pain, nausea, exacerbation of dryness; it may also lead to fungal overgrowth.[49] In patients with oral lesions, peroxide inhibits mucosal tissue granulation.[49] Water-based mouthwashes, such as Biotene and Oral Balance, should be used in place of alcohol-containing ones.[50] Saline solution (0.9% sodium chloride) is non-irritating and may promote granulation and healing.[49] Patients may also rinse the mouth with a meat tenderizer solution ($1/2$ teaspoon unseasoned tenderizer mixed into $1/2$ cup water) to help manage sticky saliva.[51] It is recommended that lemon and glycerin be avoided, as the former quickly exhausts salivary production while the latter may further dry the mouth.[48, 49]

Pharmacological symptom management consists primarily of either salivary stimulation or use of salivary substitutes.[52] For patients who may still have some salivary activity, pharmacological treatment options include pilocarpine, cevimeline, citric acid, sodium fluoride, chlorhexidine, and nicotinamide.[39, 46, 52] Salivary substitutes may also help relieve the discomforts associated with dry mouth. These solutions mimic the physical and chemical characteristics of saliva, but do not contain the protein, digestive, and antibacterial enzymes found in actual saliva.[46] Carboxymethyl cellulose- and mucin-based lubricants are thought to be the most useful.[17, 52]

Additional recommendations for managing xerostomia include avoiding tobacco and using a cool mist humidifier.[40] Table 14.4 lists dietary interventions useful in the management of xerostomia. Food and fluid should be provided via the oral route only if this practice is comfortable for the patient. In addition, the reasoning behind the dietary restrictions should be explained so that patients may make informed decisions regarding avoidance of foods that may exacerbate symptoms.

Table 14.4 *Palliative Nutrition Therapy for Management of Xerostomia*

Sip cool, smooth liquids or suck on ice chips, popsicles throughout the day.
Encourage water over highly acidic fruit juices; fruit nectars may also be better tolerated.
Try very soft, moist foods with added sauces, gravies, dressings, oil, or butter.
Avoid alcohol, caffeine, tobacco, and hard or spicy foods.
Try tart foods for stimulating saliva flow unless they cause discomfort.
Chew sugar-free gum.

Sources: Appendix A: Tips for managing nutrition impact symptoms. In: Elliott L, Molseed L, McCallum PD, Grant B, eds. *The Clinical Guide to Oncology Nutrition.* 2nd ed. Chicago, IL: American Dietetic Association; 2006:241–245; Amerongen AVN, Veerman ECI. Current therapies for xerostomia and salivary gland hypofunction associated with cancer therapies. *Support Care Cancer.* 2003;11: 226–231; Grant B, Hamilton KK. *Management of Nutrition Impact Symptoms in Cancer and Educational Handouts.* Chicago, IL: American Dietetic Association; 2004.

Constipation

Etiology

Constipation is another symptom that is multifactorial in origin. It is most commonly attributed to medications—in particular opioids, but also antiemetics, antidepressants, anticholinergics, phenothiazine, 5-hydroxytryptamine-3 antagonists, iron, calcium, antacids, barium, anticonvulsants, and vinca alkaloids.[39, 45] Metabolic abnormalities such as dehydration, hypokalemia, and hypercalcemia (the last of which slows gastric motility) may also result in constipation.[53] Other causes are neurogenic (spinal cord compression, neurotoxicity) or physiologic (debility, diet, poor intake, age) in nature.[39] Constipation may be the cause of other symptoms such as anorexia, early satiety, nausea, vomiting, bloating, and abdominal pain.[39, 53] It may also be a first sign of bowel obstruction.[45]

Management

A bowel management program is indicated for any patient who requires opioids, with the best results usually achieved by combining a stool softener and a bowel stimulant.[45] If impaired motility is suspected, prokinetic agents may prove useful.[39] Consumption of a high-fiber diet and use of bulking agents (methylcellulose, psyllium) should be recommended with caution. If the patient does not have adequate fluid intake (minimum 2–3 L/day), these measures may cause impaction; consequently, they are not indicated for persons at risk for bowel obstruction.[40, 53] Table 14.5 lists dietary interventions to treat or prevent constipation, including guidelines for using fiber.

Table 14.5 **Palliative Nutrition Therapy for Management of Constipation**

Encourage adequate fluid intake.
Recommend prunes or prune juice if tolerated.
Use of Fiber
Encourage increased fiber intake only if it does not cause the patient distress.
Do not encourage fiber intake for persons at risk for or with known bowel obstruction.
Encourage fiber intake only if adequate fluid intake is possible.
Increase fiber intake gradually to improve tolerance.
If adding wheat germ, bran, or flaxseed to foods, begin with 2 tsp and build up to 2 tbsp per day.
Advise limiting gas-forming foods (which may cause discomfort) or using Beano with them.

Sources: Appendix A: Tips for managing nutrition impact symptoms. In: Elliott L, Molseed L, McCallum PD, Grant B, eds. *The Clinical Guide to Oncology Nutrition.* 2nd ed. Chicago, IL: American Dietetic Association; 2006:241–245; Grant B, Hamilton KK. *Management of Nutrition Impact Symptoms in Cancer and Educational Handouts.* Chicago, IL: American Dietetic Association; 2004.

Taste Changes

Etiology

Altered taste sensation, also known as dysgeusia, is a significant nutrition-related symptom in the cancer setting. It has been reported to affect 50% to 90% of patients with advanced cancer.[54] The presence of chemosensory complaints (including alterations in taste and smell) is significantly correlated with reduced food enjoyment, poor nutrient intake, and decreased quality of life.[14] That this issue is so prevalent in patients who are not undergoing active treatment suggests that its more significant causes are factors other than cancer therapy.[54] Common causes of taste changes include smoking; dentures; dry mouth; thick saliva; poor dental hygiene; stomatitis; oral infections; micronutrient deficiencies (e.g., vitamin A, zinc, niacin); medications; nerve damage; radiation to head, neck, or cerebral areas; and advanced age.[39, 54] Surgeries such as partial glossectomy, laryngectomy, thyroidectomy, hypophysectomy, and adrenalectomy are also known to cause reduced or altered taste sensation.[39] Patients may experience either decreases or increases in taste sensitivity, particularly in response to bitter or sour stimuli,[14] and often complain that foods taste metallic, distorted, or bland.[54]

Management

Suggestions for managing dysgeusia include good oral hygiene, which is recommended to prevent infections, manage stomatitis, and maintain good oral health.[39, 51] Encourage regular toothbrushing or cleansing of dentures as well as use of mouth rinses.[51] Use of non-mint flavored or unflavored toothpastes and rinses is suggested for oral care done prior to eating.[51] Rinsing with a baking soda and salt water solution may prove beneficial in between meals to lessen bad tastes in the mouth.[51] Patients should also be monitored for the presence of candidiasis, with the appropriate treatment being prescribed to lessen issues related to dysgeusia.[51] Suggestions for obtaining relief from dry mouth or thick saliva should also be provided. If nutrient deficiencies are a suspected cause of the dysgeusia, supplementation may be of benefit if not otherwise contraindicated (such as for the imminently terminal patient, or if adverse nutrient–drug interactions would occur).[54] It has been suggested that cannabinoids (such as in Marinol®) may enhance taste sensation in addition to stimulating appetite, and their use warrants further study for a role in treating dysgeusia.[54] Table 14.6 summarizes dietary interventions to address altered taste sensation.

Other Symptoms

Less prevalent symptoms that warrant discussion include diarrhea, difficult or painful swallowing (dysphagia, odynophagia), and hiccups.[45]

Diarrhea may result from drugs, palliative chemotherapy or radiotherapy, bowel obstruction, malabsorption, or islet cell tumors.[45] Its medical management includes opioids, particularly loperamide, or octreotide for refractory

Table 14.6   *Palliative Nutrition Therapy for Management of Dysgeusia*[39, 51]

When not eating, lemon drops, gum, or mints may help mask a bad taste in the mouth.
Suggest use of marinades, spices, and herbs, particularly with meats.
Suggest that poultry, fish, eggs, cheese, or other protein sources be substituted for red meats, the taste of which may be significantly altered.
Counteract heightened tastes with other flavors. For example, use lemon juice or salt for sensitivity to sweet taste, or sweeteners for sensitivity to bitter tastes.
Use moist cooking methods, gravies, and sauces, and encourage sips of liquid with meals (especially for dry mouth).
Sources: Komucru S, Nelson K, Walsh D. The gastrointestinal symptoms of advanced cancer. *Support Care Cancer.* 2000;9:32–39; Grant B, Hamilton KK. *Management of Nutrition Impact Symptoms in Cancer and Educational Handouts.* Chicago, IL: American Dietetic Association; 2004.

chemotherapy-induced diarrhea; nutrition care should focus on rehydration and replacement of electrolytes.[45]

Dysphagia is often the result of mechanical obstruction caused by tumors of the mouth or esophagus, or by esophageal stricture.[45] Other causes include fibrosis, nerve damage, extrinsic compression, and mucosal inflammation.[45, 51] Consultation with a speech therapist may help identify appropriate food and liquid textures or swallowing techniques.[51] For patients with esophageal tumors, treatment options include dilatation, brachytherapy, endoscopic stenting, endoscopic laser, or photodynamic therapy (PDT).[45] In treating smaller tumors, laser therapy appears to offer better palliation than stent placement.[45] However, studies comparing laser therapy with PDT suggest that PDT is safer and more effective.[45] Topical anesthetics, sprays, and lozenges may help ease painful swallowing.[51]

Hiccups, which may be caused by diaphragmatic irritation, uremia, or medications (corticosteroids) and less commonly by hyponatremia, hypocalcemia, or myocardial infarction, are frequently seen in patients with cancer.[45] Hiccups may be managed by pharyngeal stimulation techniques such as nebulized saline, palatal massage with a cotton ball, or more traditional means such as drinking from the wrong side of a cup or swallowing two teaspoons of granulated sugar.[45] Baclofen is the most effective pharmacological therapy for hiccups, but may not be appropriate for patients with renal insufficiency.[55]

Artificial Nutrition and Hydration in Palliative Care

Whether to use artificial nutrition or hydration (ANH) has long been a difficult and sometimes controversial question facing patients with terminal cancer, as well as their physicians, families, and caregivers. American society clearly supports a person's right to self-determination such that individuals who possess decision-making capacity have the right to make decisions regarding medical interventions according to their own reasoning and values system.[56, 57] The legal consensus is that all medical interventions can be refused by patients with decision-making capacity, and that ANH, as a medical treatment, is no exception—even if refusing it results in death.[57] An individual's approach to medical decision making may involve many different religious, philosophical, and personal values, all of which deserve and require respect from the healthcare team.[56]

The American Dietetic Association's position paper regarding nutrition, hydration, and feeding underscores the importance of the patient's informed choice regarding the degree of nutrition intervention, and suggests that the palliative care plan need not exclude nutrition support while acknowledging that nutrition support may also be futile care for the terminally ill.[56] In addition, it is suggested that the concept of "when in doubt, feed" applies to all patients, with the decision to stop feeding being based on the patient's wishes, medical contraindications, or diagnosis of persistent unconsciousness with evidence of the patient's wish to stop nutrition and hydration in that circumstance.[56]

Clinicians have a responsibility to educate patients, families, and healthcare team members regarding the benefits and burdens of artificial nutrition and hydration while giving due consideration to each individual's circumstances. It has been suggested that nutrition support be considered a separate issue from hydration.[58] As such, the benefits and burdens of artificial nutrition and artificial hydration are presented separately here.

Use of Artificial Nutrition

When considering whether to utilize artificial nutrition, it must be determined whether this therapy aligns with the primary goals of palliation: relief of suffering and improvement of quality of life. Healthcare providers may find it challenging to offer this therapy; likewise, patients and families find it difficult to decide whether to initiate or discontinue it. For all involved, an understanding of current relevant research is critical to evaluating, for each individual case, whether the benefit of artificial nutrition outweighs the burden.

Benefits

In a review of nonrandomized, controlled clinical trials, enteral versus routine nutrition therapy in patients receiving palliative care resulted in no significant impact on body weight, while in patients undergoing chemotherapy or radiotherapy there was no effect on mortality (esophageal cancer patients) or infectious complications (leukemia patients).[59] A meta-analysis of randomized clinical trials of nutrition support (NS) enrolling surgical patients found that NS had no significant effect on mortality, mixed effects on body weight, and minimal effects on biochemical outcomes.[59] An observational study of patients in a palliative care unit in Taiwan noted that there was no significant impact of artificial nutrition and hydration on survival.[60]

In contrast, enteral nutrition has been found to reduce length of stay and infections versus parenteral nutrition in patients undergoing surgical procedures for various stages of gastrointestinal cancer.[59] Another review demonstrated that home parenteral nutrition when initiated in cancer patients with intestinal obstruction at a time when they had good life expectancy, significantly improved quality of life up until several weeks before death.[59] In other studies, enteral or parenteral nutrition has been shown to increase body weight and performance status, although in one study this effect was limited to patients with a survival time of greater than three months.[59] In patients surviving more than three months, approximately two-thirds were assessed as having improved quality of life. In another study of patients who received either supplemental oral or parenteral nutrition (when intake decreased below specified amounts) along with other treatments, the as-treated analysis showed improvement in survival and other outcomes.[61] In a qualitative study evaluating the experiences of patients with advanced cancer receiving home parenteral nutrition (HPN), patients and family members reported physical, social, and psychological benefits from the HPN, including relief that nutritional needs were met, and increased energy, strength, activity, and quality of life.[62] It is noteworthy that these patients were able to eat orally and received HPN as a supplemental measure.

Burdens and Risks

A large study of patients with head and neck cancer who underwent gastrostomies, and most of whom had advanced disease, showed a complication rate of 42% with 3 fatalities following use of artificial nutrition.[63] Wound infections were the most common severe complication reported; other complications included abdominal pain and leakage of gastric acids. As noted in Dy's review,[59] several other studies reported similar results. When a percutaneous endoscopic-placed gastrostomy (PEG) could not be placed, an open gastrostomy was sometimes required. Additional adverse effects associated with HPN reported by Dy included catheter-related issues, such as bacteremia, occlusions, and dislocations, as well as an estimation that at least 1% of deaths may be attributable to HPN.[59]

In another review reflective of the general population using HPN, burdens included disruption of common activities (work, travel, going to the bathroom, sleeping, and maintaining employment), fatigue, fear of complications or hospitalizations, loss of sexual interest, and concern about the burden on caregivers.[64] As reported by Orrevall et al. in another qualitative study, similar burdens were noted; patients reported that HPN negatively affected sleep, increased urinary frequency, and restricted participation in social and family activities.[62]

Recommendations Regarding Use of Artificial Nutrition

As discussed, enteral or parenteral nutrition may be beneficial in limited circumstances, but is not without significant risks or burdens. Based on clinical practice guidelines and position papers as reviewed by Dy, enteral or parenteral nutrition may be of benefit only in those patients with gastrointestinal obstruction or other conditions precluding oral intake.[59] Published guidelines regarding palliative or terminal nutrition for patients with progressive cancer suggest that the use of enteral or parenteral nutrition is not recommended in patients with a prognosis of less than 3 months or a Karnofsky score of less than 50%.[10] Suggested criteria for the use of parenteral nutrition in advanced cancer, when enteral nutrition is not an option, are the potential survival benefit, expected duration of more than 6 weeks, Karnofsky score of more than 50%, and the presence of a supportive home environment.[65] Psychological support and counseling are recommended for patients not meeting these criteria, as they are unlikely to survive long enough to benefit from the provision of artificial nutrition.[59]

Artificial Hydration

Although it has been discussed in the literature for more than 20 years, the decision of whether to provide artificial hydration (AH) to terminally ill patients remains a controversial and much-debated topic.[66] A review of the literature regarding the attitudes and actions of medical professionals indicates considerable differences in both understanding and practice across care settings. A 1994 review, which included studies evaluating the use of AH for patients with terminal conditions from the United States, United Kingdom, Canada, and Switzerland, found that 27% to 73% of physicians would prescribe AH to terminal cancer patients; with as many as 88% reporting that if the IV infiltrated, AH would be restarted for palliative care patients; and as many as 40% being willing to replace or relocate IV access if needed to continue AH.[67] It was also noted that terminally ill patients dying from malignancies in hospitals were more likely to receive AH than those dying in hospice or at home.[67]

In 2001, McAulay indicated that hospital nurses are more likely to believe that dehydration causes unpleasant symptoms; this author suggests that the use of AH in hospital settings may be related to the negative perception of "giving up" should fluids be discontinued or not offered.[68] Conversely, Zerwekh noted that hospice, oncology, and gerontology specialists support her assertion that AH should not routinely be given to dying patients based on the following observations: (1) terminal patients remained comfortable during prolonged periods of dehydration, and (2) those hospitalized for symptom relief who were receiving AH developed many signs of fluid overload.[69]

More recently, a study assessed knowledge, attitudes, and behavioral intentions of hospital nurses toward providing ANH for terminal cancer patients in Taiwan.[70] While the nurses surveyed viewed ANH as having more burden than benefit, their behavioral intentions still favored provision of ANH.[70] In an informal survey of U.S. nurses designed to elicit beliefs regarding benefits of ANH in terminal care, home health nurses were divided in their beliefs, while the hospice nurses unanimously believed that ANH leads to further discomfort.[71] Van der Riet et al. found that Australian palliative care physicians and nurses believe dehydration to be a normal component of the dying process that does not result in thirst or suffering, with these health-care providers suggesting that AH may contribute to suffering rather than relieve it.[72]

As with AN, it is important that the benefits versus burdens of AH therapy be carefully considered before it is employed. A clear understanding of the potential beneficial and detrimental effects of dehydration and rehydration in terminal illness is of key importance to this evaluation.

Dehydration

Dehydration is defined as a fall in the body's water content often accompanied by a loss of sodium and other electrolytes.[1] General features of dehydration include reduced skin turgor, altered renal function, electrolyte abnormalities, dry mouth, headaches, nausea, vomiting, cramps, lethargy, hypotension, and impaired cognitive function (ranging from confusion to coma).[67, 68, 73] Thirst occurs as a result of increased plasma osmolality (hypernatremia) or decreased intravascular volume.[74] The core of the debate about AH therapy is whether the experience of dehydration in the terminally ill patient differs from that in the patient who is not terminal, if it is distressing, or if it tenders any benefit.

Potential Benefits

Although the findings do not come from randomly controlled trials, many observed possible benefits of dehydration have been reported in the literature. Dehydration may result in reduced urine output, gastrointestinal fluids, and pulmonary secretions, which may in turn reduce incontinence, need for catheterization, vomiting, coughing, choking, use of tracheal suction, and sensation of drowning.[75, 76] Reduction in edema, and therefore pressure on internal organs, may decrease pain.[77] It has also been suggested that analgesia or anesthesia may result from metabolic imbalances (acidosis, hypernatremia, and hypercalcemia), hypovolemia, or the production of opioid peptides and ketones that occurs with both dehydration and malnutrition.[67] In contrast, other studies have found no differences in either electrolyte balance or comfort level in hydrated versus dehydrated patients.[78]

Thus, while some suggest that decreased awareness and therefore decreased suffering can be attributed to electrolyte imbalances, others suggest that normal electrolyte balance is the reason that a dehydrated state promotes comfort in the terminally ill.[67, 69] Decreases in the need for analgesia, incidence of distressing symptoms (vomiting, choking) and pain as well as increased mental acuity have also been observed by those working with dehydrated, terminally ill patients.[68, 78] Other postulated advantages of dehydration are somnolence and peaceful death.[67]

Potential Detrimental Effects

Although many researchers have reported beneficial effects of terminal dehydration, some contend that this condition produces detrimental effects that warrant consideration when contemplating whether to employ AH. Physiological changes attributed to dehydration include postural hypotension, altered blood viscosity and electrolyte imbalances, and decreased skin perfusion, urine output, and fluid volume.[67] Proposed negative effects of these changes include increased risk of pulmonary emboli or deep vein thrombosis, increased risk of pressure sores, and increased risk of urinary tract infection, constipation, and gastrointestinal tract pain.[67, 79] Apathy, depressive states (ranging from lethargy to coma), and neuromuscular irritability and twitching are said to result from electrolyte imbalances; postural hypotension may increase the risk of falls.[67] Nevertheless, several studies have reported that electrolyte levels remain normal in dying patients, and that even those patients whose levels are abnormal remain comfortable.[73] Dehydration is also noted to cause restlessness, confusion, and potentially myoclonus and seizures in patients receiving opioid therapy without fluid intake,[79] although van der Riet et al. note that the occurrence of seizures is rare.[80]

Dry mouth and thirst—terms that are often used interchangeably in the literature[81]—along with nausea, vomiting, and fatigue, are thought to be the most commonly experienced symptoms of terminal dehydration.[82] Dry mouth, which is the most consistently reported symptom, has also been attributed to medications (opioids, phenothiazines, antihistamines, and antidepressants), history of local radiation therapy, mouth breathing, food debris or dried sputum coating the oral mucosa, and oral infection.[69, 77, 83] McCann et al. found that in 63% of patients studied who were dying of cancer or stroke, thirst was not reported or was reported only on initial assessment, and that it was easily relieved with good oral care and ice chips.[81] Phillips et al. demonstrated a reduced perception of thirst in dehydrated, healthy, elderly men, suggesting that reduced thirst perception may be related more to age or cognitive function.[84]

Dehydration may be physiologically different in terminal illness than in nonterminal illness, which may partially account for the disparity between thought and observation. Billings described dehydration as being hypernatremic (loss of more water than salt), hyponatremic (loss of more salt than water), or eunatremic (proportionate loss of salt and water).[85] While hypernatremic and hyponatremic dehydration may result in profound or mild thirst, respectively,[77] Billings suggests that eunatremic dehydration, which occurs over a long period of time, is common in end-stage illness and leads to a negligible amount of thirst.[85]

Rehydration

Potential Benefits

Patients may be artificially rehydrated by intravenous, subcutaneous (hypo-dermatoclysis), and rectal routes as well as through continued use of a feeding tube.[66] Often, the perceived benefits of hydration are ideological in nature. Physicians and family may feel that hydration is a way to demonstrate caring and to honor the sanctity of life.[78] Clinicians or family may wish to provide hydration to avoid feeling as though they have abandoned the patient, and they may see this therapy as a standard of care to help prevent distress.[78]

Suggested clinical benefits of AH are that it may provide comfort by preventing confusion, restlessness, and neuromuscular irritability; may improve myoclonus and sedation; may decrease thirst and dry mouth; may decrease cognitive impairment; and may prolong survival.[77, 82] Smith and Andrews assert that there is a role for low-volume AH in patients with cancer by increasing comfort through alleviation of symptoms of opioid toxicity.[73] It is implied by reviewing the potential detriments of dehydration that AH may also prevent risks associated with reduced blood viscosity, urine output, and skin perfusion as well as postural hypotension, with secondary benefits including relief of constipation and reduced risk of falls.

It is worthy to note that many reported benefits are considered to be observational, rather than research-based.[77, 82] A significant quantity of data exists indicating that AH does not prolong life. For example, Smith reviewed several studies that found no difference in survival of patients receiving such treatments as nasogastric tube feedings, TPN, or IV therapy versus patients receiving less aggressive treatment and no ANH.[78] In fact, in some of these studies, patients who did not receive AH survived longer than those who did. More recent studies suggested that symptoms of myoclonus, sedation, dry mouth, thirst, and nausea may be relieved in certain patients, and that further study of the effect of AH on these conditions is warranted.[77, 86]

Potential Detrimental Effects

In Bavin's review, suggested possible negative clinical effects of rehydration include increased pulmonary and gastric secretions leading to increased congestion, rattle, nausea, and vomiting; increased peritumor, cerebral, and peripheral edema; catheter site infection; and increased urine output.[77] Other negative effects include repeated needle punctures, congestive heart failure, increased intracranial pressure, tumor swelling, and exacerbation of ascites.[82] In a 2004 study, physicians and nurses in oncology and palliative care settings frequently reported increased symptoms of fluid retention (edema, pleural effusions/ascites, bronchial secretion) in patients with lung and gastric cancer who received AH.[87] Another study evaluating the use of AH in acute versus palliative care settings found a significantly higher use of diuretics in the acute care group, which also had the highest mean hydration volumes, suggesting the potential for overhydration symptoms in these patients.[88] Nonclinical negative effects include invasiveness of intravenous access, diversion from holistic care, and the potential for AH to be a barrier to physical affection and closeness with the patients' loved ones.[77]

Because of associated ethical and other difficulties, few well-designed studies exist to help clarify the benefits and burdens of AH. As a result, most claims as to its benefits and burdens are anecdotally supported.[77, 82]

Recommendations Regarding Use of Artificial Hydration

Artificial hydration remains controversial, with no clear evidence for or against its use for palliation. Indeed, consensus-based standards or guidelines for AH are lacking. Several authors propose that key factors be considered when AH is being deliberated. Dalal and Bruera[89] proposed the following as useful questions to consider:

1. Is the patient dehydrated?
2. What are the symptoms caused and/or aggravated by dehydration?
3. What are the expected advantages of rehydration?
4. What are the disadvantages of hydration?
5. What are the views of the patient and family?
6. What are the individualized goals of care?

Some practitioners have stressed a holistic approach to caring for patients with advanced cancers, and have suggested that the interdisciplinary team, including a social worker, chaplain, and dietitian, participate in assessing the anticipated effects of any intervention on spiritual, social, and psychological care.[77] Initiating or continuing hydration, as well as nutrition, may be an important means of honoring beliefs and values of some cultural or religious groups.[90] Assessment of survival is also important, as a longer prognosis (weeks or months versus days) may significantly influence the decision, especially if patients need a little more time to express their end-of-life needs and wishes.[77]

Ethics and Decision Making

Ethics is a key component of decision making when either artificial nutrition or hydration is being considered. The American Dietetic Association (ADA) describes the skill of ethical decision making as focusing on the patient's best interests while allowing all stakeholders to participate in the decision-making process, and balancing rules, goals, and virtues to achieve a morally justified decision.[56] Key principles are that of autonomy (honoring the patient's wishes), nonmaleficence (doing no harm), beneficence (doing what is in the patient's best interests), justice (doing what is fair), informed consent (providing succinct explanation of pros and cons), and capacity (ensuring the patient understands the information needed to give informed consent).[56, 77]

According to the ADA's position paper, the dietitian has a duty to facilitate collaborative ethical deliberation.[56] First, the dietitian needs sound technical judgment on how and whether, in the given situation, ANH can achieve desired goals. Second, the dietitian should, as a primary contact for patient and family regarding nutrition and feeding, assess the patient's wishes, ensure that feeding and hydration issues are discussed, and ensure that all appropriate options are considered. Finally, the dietitian has a duty to understand and explain the position of the ADA, whether or not that position conflicts with the dietitian's own personal professional opinion.

SUMMARY

The primary focus of palliative care is prevention of suffering and enhanced quality of life. Although it is commonly considered to be synonymous with terminal care, palliative care is not limited to persons forgoing curative therapy; indeed, it may be provided concurrently with aggressive measures. While it may be initiated at any stage of disease, its use should be considered upon diagnosis and at regular intervals throughout the course of care. Palliative care may be delivered through a variety of systems: inpatient, outpatient, nursing home, private-practice consultation, and home care. In particular, hospice services are widely recognized for providing palliative care at the end of life.

Provision of palliative care is an interdisciplinary process involving a wide variety of professionals. Regardless of the setting where care is delivered, the dietitian fills an important role on the team. Given that as many as 80% of palliative care patients experience anorexia, weight loss, and a broad range of gastrointestinal symptoms, the dietitian has the training and skills required to assist with symptom management, help improve function, and enhance quality of life for these individuals. The dietitian is responsible for assessing the patient's needs and wishes at regular intervals and as care goals change, and for designing and implementing a nutrition care plan accordingly. Additionally, the dietitian should take an active role in educating and advising patients, families, and members of the healthcare team.

The decision of whether to use artificial nutrition and hydration in the setting of advanced cancer remains a difficult and controversial topic not only for patients and families, but often among healthcare professionals. Available evidence suggests that artificial nutrition may have palliative benefit in specific circumstances. However, evidence to support a consensus on the palliative use of artificial hydration is lacking. Assisting with decision making requires educating those involved regarding the benefits and burdens, both known and perceived, of initiating, abstaining from, or withdrawing these therapies. The dietitian can help all parties involved in patient care by providing a balanced perspective regarding ANH, and by facilitating collaborative deliberation regarding the overall nutrition care plan.

REFERENCES

1. In: Marcovitch H, ed. *Black's Medical Dictionary*. 41st ed. Lanham, MD: Scarecrow Press; 2006: 185–186, 529.
2. Billings A. Recent advances in palliative care. *BMJ.* 2000;321:555–558.
3. National Comprehensive Cancer Network (NCCN). NCCN clinical practice guidelines in oncology: Palliative care. V.1.2007. 2007. Available at http://www.nccn.org/professionals/physician_gls/PDF/palliative.pdf. Accessed January 5, 2008.
4. National Consensus Project for Quality Palliative Care. Clinical practice guidelines for quality palliative care. 2004. http://www.nationalconsensusproject.org/Guideline.pdf. Accessed January 5, 2008.
5. World Health Organization (WHO). Palliative care definition. 2008. http://www.who.int/cancer/palliative/definition/en/. Accessed January 5, 2008.
6. Posthauer ME. The role of nutritional therapy in palliative care. *Adv Skin Wound Care.* 2007;20:32–33.
7. MacDonald N. Nutrition as an integral component of supportive care. *Oncology*. Available at http://cancernetwork.com/article/showArticle.jhtml?articleId=177105541. Accessed December 1, 2007.
8. Caro MMC, Laviano A, Pichard C. Nutritional intervention and quality of life in oncology patients. *Clin Nutr.* 2007;26:289–301.
9. Eberhardie C. Nutrition support in palliative care. *Nurs Stand.* 2002;25:47–52.
10. Bachmann P, Marti-Massoud M, Blanc-Vincent MP, et al. Summary version of the standards, options, and recommendations for palliative or terminal nutrition in adults with progressive cancer. *Br J Cancer.* 2003;89(suppl 1):S107–S110.
11. Ravasco P, Monteiro-Grillo I, Vidal PM, Camilo ME. Cancer: Disease and nutrition are key determinants of patients' quality of life. *Support Care Cancer.* 2004; 12:246–252.
12. Labori K, Hjermstad MJ, Wester T, Buanes T, Loge JH. Symptom profiles and palliative care in advanced pancreatic cancer: A prospective study. *Support Care Cancer.* 2006;14:1126–1133.
13. Persson C, Glimelius B. The relevance of weight loss for survival and quality of life in patients with advanced gastrointestinal cancer treated with palliative chemotherapy. *Anticancer Res.* 2002;22:3661–3668.

14. Hutton JL, Baracos VE, Wismer WV. Chemosensory dysfunction is a primary factor in the evolution of declining nutritional status and quality of life in patients with advanced cancer. *J Pain Symptom Manage.* 2007;33:156–165.
15. Sarhill N, Mahmoud F, Walsh D, et al. Evaluation of nutritional status in advanced metastatic cancer. *Support Care Cancer.* 2003;11:652–659.
16. Homsi J, Walsh D, Rivera N, et al. Symptom evaluation in palliative medicine: Patient report vs systematic assessment. *Support Care Cancer.* 2006;14:444–453.
17. Komurcu S, Nelson KA, Walsh D, Ford RB, Rybicki, L. Gastrointestinal symptoms among inpatients with advanced cancer. *Am J Hosp Palliat Care.* 2002;19: 351–355.
18. Walsh D, Donelly S, Rybicki L. The symptoms of advanced cancer: Relationship to age, gender and performance status in 1000 patients. *Support Care Cancer.* 2000;8: 175–179.
19. Braiteh F, Osta BE, Palmer JL, Reddy SK, Bruera, E. Characteristics, findings, and outcomes of palliative care inpatient consultations at a comprehensive cancer center. *J Palliat Med.* 2007;10:948–955.
20. Ravasco P, Monteiro-Grillo I, Vidal PM, Camillo ME. Nutritional deterioration in cancer: The role of disease and diet. *Clin Oncol.* 2003;15:443–450.
21. Skipworth RJE, Stewart GD, Dejong CHC, Preston T, Fearon KCH. Pathophysiology of cancer cachexia: Much more than host–tumour interaction? *Clin Nutr.* 2007; 26:667–676.
22. Laviano A, Meguid MM, Inui A, et al. Therapy insight: Cancer anorexia–cachexia syndrome: When all you can eat is yourself. *Nat Clin Pract.* 2005;2:158–165.
23. Stewart G, Skipworth RJE, Fearon KCH. Cancer cachexia and fatigue. *Clin Med.* 2006;6:140–143.
24. Tisdale M. Biology of cachexia. *J Natl Cancer Inst.* 1997;89:1763–73.
25. Hopkinson J, Wright DNM, McDonald JW, Corner JL. The prevalence of concern about weight loss and change in eating habits in people with advanced cancer. *J Pain Symptom Manage.* 2006;32:322–331.
26. Nitenberg G. Nutritional support of the cancer patient: issues and dilemmas. *Crit Rev Hem Oncol.* 2000;34:137–168.
27. Finley J. Management of cancer cachexia. *AACN Clin Issues Ad Pract Acute Crit Care.* 2000;11:590–603.
28. Yavuzsen T, Davis MP, Walsh D, LeGrand S, Lagman R. Systematic review of the treatment of cancer-associated anorexia and weight loss. *J Clin Oncol.* 2005;23: 8500–8511.
29. Isenring EA, Capra S, Bauer JD. Nutrition intervention is beneficial in oncology patients receiving radiotherapy to the gastrointestinal or head and neck area. *Br J Cancer.* 2004;91:447–452.
30. Ravasco P, Monteiro-Grillo I, Vidal PM, Camilo ME. Dietary counseling improves patient outcomes: A prospective, randomized, controlled trial in colorectal patients undergoing radiotherapy. *J Clin Oncol.* 2005;23:1431–1438.
31. Ravasco P, Monteiro-Grillo I, Vidal PM, Camilo ME. Impact of nutrition on outcome: A prospective randomized controlled trial in patients with head and neck cancer undergoing radiotherapy. *Head Neck.* 2005;27:659–668.
32. Ravasco P, Monteiro-Grillo I, Camilo ME. Cancer wasting and quality of life react to early, individualized nutritional counseling! *Clin Nutr.* 2007;26:7–15.

33. Barber M. Cancer cachexia and its treatment with fish-oil–enriched nutritional supplementation. *Nutr.* 2001;17:751–755.
34. Bruera E, Strasser F, Palmer JL, et al. Effect of fish oil on appetite and other symptoms in patients with advanced cancer and anorexia/cachexia: A double-blind, placebo-controlled study. *J Clin Oncol.* 2003;21:129–134.
35. Fearon K, von Meyenfeldt MF, Moses AGW, et al. Effect of a protein and energy dense *n*-3 fatty acid enriched oral supplement on loss of weight and lean tissue in cancer cachexia: A randomized double blind trial. *Gut.* 2003;52:1479–1489.
36. Colomer R, Moreno-Nogueira JM, Garcia-Luna PP, et al. *n*-3 fatty acids, cancer and cachexia: A systematic review of the literature. *Br J Nutr.* 2007;97:823–831.
37. Dewey A, Baughan C, Dean T, Higgins B, Johnson I. Eicosapentaenoic acid (EPA, an omega-3 fatty acid from fish oils) for the treatment of cancer cachexia (review). *Cochrane Database of Systematic Reviews.* 2007; 1. Art. No: CD004597. DOI: 10.1002/14651858.CD004597.pub2.
38. Walsh D, Rybicki L. Symptom clustering in advanced cancer. *Support Care Cancer.* 2006;14:831–836.
39. Komucru S, Nelson K, Walsh D. The gastrointestinal symptoms of advanced cancer. *Support Care Cancer.* 2000;9:32–39.
40. Appendix A: Tips for managing nutrition impact symptoms. In: Elliott L, Molseed L, McCallum PD, Grant B, eds. *The Clinical Guide to Oncology Nutrition.* 2nd ed. Chicago, IL: American Dietetic Association; 2006: 241-245.
41. Wood GJ, Shega JW, Lunch B, Von Roenn JH. Management of intractable nausea and vomiting in patients at the end of life. *JAMA.* 2007;298:1196–1207.
42. Wickham R. Nausea and vomiting. In: Yarbro CH, Frogge MH, Goodman M, eds. *Cancer Symptom Management.* Sudbury, MA: Jones and Bartlett; 2004:187–214.
43. Stephenson J, Davies A. An assessment of aetiology-based guidelines for the management of nausea and vomiting in patients with advanced cancer. *Support Care Cancer.* 2006;14:348–353.
44. Ripamonti C, Twycross R, Baines M, et al. Clinical-practice recommendations for the management of bowel obstruction in patients with end-stage cancer. *Support Care Cancer.* 2001;9:223–233.
45. Cherny NI. Taking care of the terminally ill cancer patient: Management of gastrointestinal symptoms in patients with advanced cancer. *Ann Oncol.* 2004;15 (suppl 4):iv205–iv213.
46. Maher K. Xerostomia. In: Yarbro CH, Frogge MH, Goodman M, eds. *Cancer Symptom Management.* Sudbury, MA: Jones and Bartlett; 2004:215–229.
47. Kinley J, Brennan S. Changing practice: Use of audit to change oral care practice. *Intl J Palliat Nurs.* 2004;10:581–587.
48. Regnard C, Allport S, Stephenson L. ABC of palliative care: Mouth care, skin care, and lymphoedema. *BMJ.* 1997;315:1002–1005.
49. Miller M, Kearney N. Oral care for patients with cancer: A review of the literature. *Cancer Nurs.* 2001;24:241–254.
50. Amerongen AVN, Veerman ECI. Current therapies for xerostomia and salivary gland hypofunction associated with cancer therapies. *Support Care Cancer.* 2003; 11:226–231.
51. Grant B, Hamilton KK. *Management of Nutrition Impact Symptoms in Cancer and Educational Handouts.* Chicago, IL: American Dietetic Association; 2004.
52. Sweeney MP, Bagg J. The mouth and palliative care. *Am J Hosp Palliat Med.* 2000;17:118–124.

53. Massey RM, Haylock PJ, Curtiss C. Constipation. In: Yarbro CH, Frogge MH, Goodman M, eds. *Cancer Symptom Management.* Sudbury, MA: Jones and Bartlett; 2004: 512–527.

54. Brisbois T, Hutton J, Baracos V, Wismer W. Taste and smell abnormalities as independent cause of failure of food intake in patients with advanced cancer: An argument for the application of sensory science. *J Palliat Care.* 2006;22:111–114.

55. Smith HS, Busracamwongs A. Management of hiccups in the palliative care population. *Am J Hosp Palliat Care.* 2003;20:149–154.

56. Maillet JO, Potter RL, Heller L. Position of the American Dietetic Association: Ethical and legal issues in nutrition, hydration, and feeding. *J Am Diet Assoc.* 2002;102:716–726.

57. Ganzini L. Artificial nutrition and hydration at the end of life: Ethics and evidence. *Palliat Supp Care.* 2006;4:135–143.

58. Dunlop RJ, Ellershaw JE, Baines JM, Sykes N, Saunders CM. On withholding nutrition and hydration in the terminally ill: Has palliative medicine gone too far? A reply. *J Med Ethics.* 1995;21:141–143.

59. Dy SM. Enteral and parenteral nutrition in terminally ill cancer patients. *Am J Hosp Palliat Med.* 2006;23:369–377.

60. Chiu TY, Hu WY, Chuang RB, Chen CY. Nutrition and hydration for terminal cancer patients in Taiwan. *Support Care Cancer.* 2002;10:630–636.

61. Lundholm K, Daneryd P, Bosaeus I, Korner U, Lindholm E. Palliative nutritional intervention in addition to cyclooxygenase and erythropoietin treatment for patients with malignant disease: Effects on survival, metabolism, and function. *Cancer.* 2004;100:1967–1977.

62. Orrevall Y, Tishelman C, Permert J. Home parenteral nutrition: A qualitative interview study of the experiences of advanced cancer patients and their families. *Clin Nutr.* 2005;24:961–970.

63. Ehrsson YT, Langius-Eklof A, Bark T, Laurell G. Percutaneous endoscopic gastrostomy (PEG): A long-term follow-up study in head and neck cancer patients. *Clin Otolaryngol Allied Sci.* 2004;29:740–746.

64. Winkler M. Quality of life in adult home parenteral nutrition patients. *J Parenter Enteral Nutr.* 2005;29:162–170.

65. Mirhosseini N, Fainsinger RL, Baracos V. Parenteral nutrition in advanced cancer: Indications and clinical practice guidelines. *J Palliat Med.* 2005;8:914–918.

66. Fainsinger RL, Bruera E. When to treat dehydration in a terminally ill patient? *Support Care Cancer.* 1997;5:205–211.

67. Sutcliffe J, Holmes S. Dehydration: Burden or benefit to the dying patient? *J Adv Nurs.* 1994;19:71–76.

68. McAulay D. Dehydration in the terminally ill patient. *Nurs Standard.* 2001;16: 33–37.

69. Zerwekh JV. Do dying patients really need IV fluids? *Am J Nurs.* 1997;97:26–30.

70. Ke LS, Chiu TY, Lo SS, Hu WY. Knowledge, attitudes, and behavioral intentions of nurses toward providing artificial nutrition and hydration for terminal cancer patients in Taiwan. *Cancer Nurs.* 2008; 31:67–76.

71. Suter P, Rogers J, Strack C. Artificial nutrition and hydration for the terminally ill: A reasoned approach. *Home Healthcare Nurs.* 2008;26:23–29.

72. van der Riet P, Good P, Higgins I, Sneesby L. Palliative care professionals' perceptions of nutrition and hydration at the end of life. *Intl J Palliat Nurs.* 2008;14: 145–151.

73. Smith SA, Andrews M. Artificial nutrition and hydration at the end of life. *Medsurg Nurs.* 2000;9:233–47.

74. Whitmire SJ. Water, electrolytes, and acid–base balance. In: Mahan K, Escott-Stumpf S, eds. *Krause's Food, Nutrition, and Diet Therapy.* 11th ed. Philadelphia, PA: Saunders; 2004: 164-179.

75. Zerwekh JV. The dehydration question. *Nursing.* 1983;13:47–51.

76. Dolan MB. Another hospice nurse says. *Nursing.* 1983;13:51.

77. Bavin L. Artificial rehydration in the last days of life: Is it beneficial? *Intl J Palliat Nurs.* 2007;13:445–449.

78. Smith SA. Controversies in hydrating the terminally ill patient. *J Intraven Nurs.* 1997;20:193–200.

79. Welk TA. Clinical and ethical considerations of fluid and electrolyte management in the terminally ill client. *J IV Nurs.* 1999;22:43–47.

80. van der Riet P, Brooks D, Ashby M. Nutrition and hydration at the end of life: Pilot study of a palliative care experience. *JLM.* 2006;14:182–198.

81. McCann RM, Hall WJ, Groth-Juncker A. Comfort care for terminally ill patients: The appropriate use of nutrition and hydration. *JAMA.* 1994;272:1263–1266.

82. Burge F. Dehydration and provision of fluids in palliative care: What is the evidence? *Can Fam Physician.* 1996;42:2383–2388.

83. Lawlor PG. Delirium and dehydration: Some fluid for thought? *Support Care Cancer.* 2002; 10:445–454.

84. Phillips P, Rolls B, Ledingham J, et al. Reduced thirst after water deprivation in healthy elderly men. *N Engl J Med.* 1984;311:753–759.

85. Billings A. Comfort measures for the terminally ill: Is dehydration painful? *J Am Geri Soc.* 1985;33:808–810.

86. Bruera E, Sala R, Rico MA, et al. Effects of parenteral hydration in terminally ill cancer patients: A preliminary study. *J Clin Oncol.* 2005;10:2366–2371.

87. Morita T, Shima Y, Miyashita M, Kimura R, Adachi I. Physician- and nurse-reported effects of intravenous hydration therapy on symptoms of terminally ill patients with cancer. *J Palliat Med.* 2004;7:683–693.

88. Lanuke K, Fainsinger RL, DeMoissac D. Hydration management at the end of life. *J Palliat Med.* 2004;7:257–261.

89. Dalal S, Bruera E. Dehydration in cancer patients: To treat or not to treat. *Support Oncol.* 2004;2:467–479.

90. HPNA Board of Directors. Artificial nutrition and hydration in end-of-life care: HPNA position paper. *Home Healthcare Nurse.* 2004;22:341–345.

Chapter 15

Pharmacologic Management of Cancer Cachexia–Anorexia and Other Gastrointestinal Toxicities Associated with Cancer Treatments

Todd W. Mattox, PharmD, BCNSP

Dawn E. Goetz, PharmD, BCOP

Recent data demonstrate a clear trend toward increased survival and declining incidence of cancer in the United States.[1] However, data that characterize occurrence and severity of adverse events associated with the malignancy or its treatment are limited.[2,3] Cancer and the related treatments often result in a wide variety of metabolic abnormalities that are associated with increased morbidity and mortality.[2-4] In general, gastrointestinal (GI) toxicities associated with cancer treatments have the potential to cause life-threatening medical complications, contribute to development of malnutrition, and worsen quality of life.

The gastrointestinal tract (GIT) is a common target for end-organ toxicity from localized effect of the tumor or treatments such as surgery, radiation, and chemotherapy (Table 15.1).[4] Adverse effects associated with surgery depend on many factors, including the site of the tumor and the extent of the surgical resection. The potential degree of GI toxicity caused by radiation therapy generally depends on the site of the tumor, the dose fractionization, the field of radiation, and the total radiation dose. The impact of chemotherapy on the GIT depends on the agent, dose, administration route, and length of therapy. Combinations of these therapies generally produce greater numbers of adverse effects that are usually more serious.

Toxicities may occur early in the course of treatment, usually during treatment or within a few weeks after completing treatment. Later toxicities may occur months or even years after treatment.[2, 4] Many of these problems are reversible, but some may progress to become persistent, chronic disorders. Although the type and severity of adverse events is generally dependent upon the treatment, toxicities may vary widely among patients receiving the same therapy.[2]

GI toxicities may also contribute to weight loss and malnutrition by hindering adequate nutrient intake or disrupting normal digestive processes (Table 15.1).[4] Approximately 50% of the most frequently reported and most

Table 15.1 *Gastrointestinal Abnormalities Associated with Cancer or Antitumor Therapies*

Cancer-Induced Abnormalities	Obstruction/perforation
	Fistula
	Intestinal secretory abnormalities
	Malabsorption
	Intestinal dysmotility
	Fluid/electrolyte abnormalities
Treatment-Induced Abnormalities	
Chemotherapy	Anorexia
	Altered taste
	Nausea, vomiting
	Mucositis, enteritis
	Intestinal dysmotility
Surgery	Malabsorption, diarrhea
	Adhesion-induced obstruction
	Ileus
	Fluid/electrolyte abnormalities
	Vitamin/mineral abnormalities
Radiation	Anorexia
	Altered taste
	Nausea/vomiting
	Mucositis, enteritis
	Xerostomia, dysphagia
	Obstruction
	Perforation, fistula
	Stricture
	Intestinal dysmotility
Infection-Induced Abnormalities	Malabsorption, diarrhea
	Intestinal dysmotility

Source: Schattner M, Shike M. Nutrition support of the patient with cancer. In: Shils ME, Shike M, Ross AC, Caballero B, Cousins RJ, eds. *Modern Nutrition in Health and Disease.* 10th ed. Baltimore, MD: Lippincott Williams & Wilkins; 2006:1290–1313.

distressing symptoms for patients with advanced cancer are related to GI abnormalities.[5] Dry mouth, weight loss, early satiety, and anorexia are among the most frequently reported symptoms. The etiology of continued nutritional wasting in patients without apparent GI toxicities is likely to be tumor-induced abnormalities in appetite regulation and nutrient utilization.[6] Frequently, pharmacological intervention is used to treat adverse effects associated with cancer treatments that negatively affect GI function and contribute to malnutrition. This chapter reviews supportive care treatments for common GI toxicities associated with antitumor treatments and unintentional weight loss associated with cancer cachexia–anorexia.

Unintentional Weight Loss and Cancer Cachexia

Weight loss occurs in cancer patients as a result of inadequate nutrient intake, abnormal metabolism, or the combined effects of both. It tends to occur more frequently in patients with GIT malignancies and lung cancer compared to those with hematological malignancies.[7] Nevertheless, no consistent relationship has been found between the degree of weight loss and tumor types, extent of tumor burden, performance status, and effect on survival.[6, 7]

Tumor-induced alterations in GI function may cause altered nutrient metabolism or preclude adequate nutrient intake (Table 15.1, page 380). Patients with a functional GIT, however, may develop progressive wasting associated with anorexia or cancer cachexia (CC).[6, 8, 9] Both anorexia and CC are clinical diagnoses.

Anorexia is the abnormal loss of appetite that is frequently associated with a lack of interest in foods that were previously satisfying, which results in the reduced oral nutrient intake and weight loss seen with CC. Anorexia may occur secondary to learned food aversion, altered taste or smell, or other psychological factors such as depression and fear of disease.[10] Other proposed mechanisms based on experimental animal data suggest altered hypothalamic function caused by cytokine-induced abnormalities in peripheral and central neurohormonal appetite regulators such as ghrelin, leptin, and serotonin.[6, 8, 9]

Cancer cachexia is a syndrome characterized by unintentional weight loss, anorexia, early satiety, progressive asthenia, and malnutrition that results in a greater risk of organ dysfunction and death.[6, 8] Decreased nutrient intake caused by anorexia may contribute to CC. However, the characteristic progressive loss of body fat mass and skeletal protein seen with CC is thought to be caused by a complex interaction between host neuroendocrine and cytokine systems that promote systemic inflammation and tumor-derived products such as lipid-mobilizing factor and proteolysis-inducing factor that promote direct tissue catabolism.[6, 8]

The approach to treatment of unintentional weight loss varies according to the underlying cause and the patient's goals and clinical condition.[10, 11] For example, weight loss due to GI dysfunction requires correction of the underlying abnormality. Treatment options for anorexia and weight loss in patients with a functional GIT are less clear. Further complicating clinical decisions is the potentially distressing reaction to poor appetite and weight loss by patients and their families and the limited success in enhancing appetite and weight achieved with use of currently available agents.

Several single nutrients or pharmacologic agents have been used to alter appetite favorably or counter abnormalities in nutrient metabolism associated with CC with varying degrees of success (Table 15.2). Numerous investigations of oral nutrients or pharmacologic agents have reported statistically significant improvement with weight gain in the CC treatment group compared to the control group.[12, 13] Despite these results, a large percentage of those patients who receive CC treatment demonstrate very little or no weight gain.[14] In addition, the number of patients who continue to lose weight has not been clearly reported in many investigations. Indeed, improved appetite and weight gain have been reported in patients who received placebo treatments in randomized controlled trials.[8, 13, 15] When body composition was reported, patients who gained weight increased their fat stores instead of improving their lean body mass. However, prevention of further weight loss and improved appetite or sense of well-being may be desirable and achievable goals for many patients who want increased enjoyment of food with appropriate use of currently available pharmacologic treatments of CC.[10, 11]

The most effective therapies used for treating CC appear to have the best effect on anorexia, an inconsistent effect on weight, and no positive effect on lean tissue mass or survival.[6, 8] Multiple investigations have reported appetite stimulant properties with use of the progestational agents megestrol acetate (MA) and medroxyprogesterone (MPG), although MA has been investigated more frequently in cancer patients.[11–14] MA is approved by the U.S. Food and Drug Administration (FDA) for the treatment of anorexia, cachexia, or unexplained, significant weight loss in patients with a diagnosis of acquired immune deficiency syndrome (AIDS).[16] However, it has been widely investigated in randomized controlled trials of cancer patients.[11–14, 17–20]

A recent meta-analysis reported improved appetite and weight gain with MA compared to placebo.[12] However, the effect on health-related quality of life was not clear. The pooled analysis of comparison studies of MA and other drugs on appetite and weight gain included trials of patients with AIDS. The analysis reported no difference in appetite improvement, and inconclusive results for weight gain, although comparison trials of MA and dronabinol, and of MA and an eicosapentaenoic acid (EPA)-containing supplement, were not included in the analysis.[17, 18] These individual investigations reported

Table 15.2   *Pharmacologic Treatments for Cancer Anorexia–Cachexia*

Pharmacologic Category	Agent
Cytokine Antagonists	Omega-3 fatty acids Melatonin Pentoxiphylline Thalidomide
Anabolic Agents	Testosterone derivatives Fluoxymesterone Oxandrolone Nandrolone decanoate
Metabolic Inhibitors	Hydrazine sulfate
Appetite Stimulants	
Atypical antipsychotic	Olanzapine
Antidepressant	Mirtazapine
Cannabinoids	Dronabinol
Antihistamine	Cyproheptadine
Glucocorticoids	Dexamethasone Methylprednisolone Prednisolone
Progestational agents	Megestrol acetate Medroxyprogesterone

Sources: Palesty JA, Dudrick SJ. What we have learned about cachexia in gastrointestinal cancer. *Dig Dis.* 2003;21:198–213; Laviano A, Meguid MM, Rossi-Fanelli F. Cancer anorexia: Clinical implications, pathogenesis, and therapeutic strategies. *Lancet Oncol.* 2003;4:686–694; Mattox TW. Treatment of unintentional weight loss in patients with cancer. *Nutr Clin Pract.* 2005;20:400–410; Yavuzsen T, Davis MP, Walsh D, et al. Systematic review of the treatment of cancer-associated anorexia and weight loss. *J Clin Oncol.* 2005;23:8500–8511.

improved appetite and weight gain in patients who received MA compared to patients who received dronabinol, and improved weight with no difference in appetite with MA compared to patients who received an EPA-containing supplement. MA use has no positive effect on survival and the effect on quality of life is inconclusive.[11–14, 20]

The most appropriate MA dose to maximize response and minimize toxicities is not known.[12–14, 19] Initiating therapy at lower doses of 160 mg/day and titrating the dose based on patient response or to a maximum of 480–800 mg/day has

Table 15.9 *National Cancer Institute's Toxicity Criteria for Constipation*

Grade	1	2	3	4	5
Constipation	Occasional or intermittent symptom, occasional use of stool softeners, laxatives, or dietary modification or enema	Persistent symptoms with regular use of laxatives or enema indication	Symptoms interfering with ADL; constipation with manual evacuation indicated	Life-threatening consequences (obstruction or toxic megacolon)	Death
Ileus	Asymptomatic, radiographic findings only	Symptomatic altered GI function; IV fluids; tube feeding or TPN indicated < 24 hours	Symptomatic and severe altered GI function; IV fluids; tube feeding or TPN indicated ≥ 24 hours	Life-threatening consequences	Death

ADL = Activities of daily living; GI = gastrointestinal; IV = intravenous; TPN = total parenteral nutrition.

Source: Gibson RJ, Keefe DMK. Cancer chemotherapy-induced diarrhea and constipation: Mechanisms of damage and prevention strategies. *Support Care Cancer.* 2006;14:890–900.

been recommended to alleviate cost concerns and improve patient compliance.[11–14, 19] Most of the adverse effects associated with MA use as an appetite stimulant have been reported with short-term use, usually less than 12 weeks. The risk of adverse effects with longer-duration use is not known.

Increased risk of thromboembolism is a concern with MA use, especially in patients with a history of thrombophlebitis or deep vein thromboembolism (DVT), although no statistically significant differences in thrombolic events between treatment and placebo groups were reported in two recent meta-analyses.[12, 20] Cautious use of MA in patients with a history of thromboembolic disease is recommended by the drug's manufacturer, whereas other sources have recommended not using any progestational agents in these patients.[11, 16]

Other adverse effects associated with the glucocorticoid properties of MA have been reported, such as biochemical evidence of adrenal insufficiency with abrupt discontinuation after long-term use, edema, GI intolerance, and impotence in men.[11, 13, 14, 20] Given the low risk of adverse effects, MA should be considered a treatment option for patients with a predicted life of weeks to months.[11, 13]

Successful corticosteroid use for treatment of anorexia and other supportive care symptoms in patients with a very short life expectancy has been reported.[6, 11, 13, 14, 21] Those steroidal agents that have been most frequently investigated for this indication are dexamethasone, methylprednisolone, and prednisolone.[13, 21] Prednisolone and dexamethasone have been studied in randomized trials that demonstrated improved appetite compared to placebo.[6, 13, 21] Dexamethasone has been investigated more frequently in cancer patients.[13] Patients who received dexamethasone 0.75 mg orally 4 times daily had similar effects on weight gain and appetite compared to those who received MA.[17] However, a larger number of patients who received dexamethasone withdrew from the study because of adverse effects from the medication. In general, the risk of adverse effects, such as myopathy, hyperglycemia, edema, insomnia, GI upset, and immunosuppression, outweighs any nutritional advantage with long-term use of corticosteroids.

Terminal patients with poor performance status may be considered potential candidates for corticosteroid intervention because the positive pharmacologic effects on other symptoms associated with end-stage cancer may outweigh the risks associated with the negative adverse effects. A corticosteroid agent such as dexamethasone should be considered for treatment of CC in patients with a predicted remaining life of days to weeks or in those patients with a history of thrombolic disease.[9–11, 17]

Other agents investigated as potential appetite stimulants have been studied less often and have demonstrated less successful results. Dronabinol is a synthetic oral form of tetrahydrocannabinol (THC), which is the active agent in marijuana thought to be responsible for its antiemetic and appetite stimulant properties.[22, 23] Dronabinol is approved by the FDA for treatment of anorexia associated with weight loss in patients with AIDS and for nausea and vomiting associated with cancer chemotherapy in patients who have failed to respond adequately to conventional antiemetic treatments.[24] Until recently, variable effects on appetite with little to no effect had been reported in investigations of this agent in small numbers of cancer patients.[13, 22] More recent investigations that include larger numbers of patients appear to confirm dronabinol's lack of efficacy as an appetite stimulant or weight enhancement agent.[17, 23] In a placebo-controlled trial, cancer patients who received 800 mg/day MA liquid reported improved appetite and weight compared to patients who received 2.5 mg dronabinol twice daily or both MA and dronabinol.[17] Another placebo-controlled trial comparing the effects of whole-plant cannabis extract and THC in cancer patients reported no differences in appetite, quality of life, or weight between groups.[23] The recommended dose for initiating dronabinol is 2.5 mg orally twice daily. This dose is associated with less adverse effects such as sedation, confusion, drowsiness, and altered mood compared to higher doses of up to 20 mg daily.[17, 23, 24] However, routine dronabinol use for first-line therapy as appetite stimulate in cancer patients is not recommended.[13, 19]

The omega-3 (Ω-3) fatty acids EPA and docosahexanoic acid (DHA) provided by fish oils have been investigated in cancer patients with CC for their anti-inflammatory activity and effects on weight loss, quality of life, and survival.[25, 26] Uncontrolled trials of fish oil provided alone or as a part of a liquid nutritional supplement in patients with pancreatic cancer and CC reported positive effects on weight gain and performance status. Unfortunately, controlled trials have demonstrated less promising results.[14, 25–28] A placebo-controlled trial of an EPA-containing liquid supplement in cancer patients with CC demonstrated no difference in appetite, weight changes, or survival between groups.[27] Similar results were reported in a placebo-controlled comparison trial of an EPA-containing supplement and MA.[28] In this study, patients were randomized to receive an EPA-containing liquid supplement with MA placebo; 600 mg/day MA and an isonitrogenous, isocaloric placebo liquid; or 600 mg/day MA and the EPA-containing liquid supplement. Patients in the single-agent MA group demonstrated better weight gain compared to the other groups. The effect on appetite was dependent on the assessment tool used and either was not different between groups or favored the single-agent MA group. No differences in survival, quality of life, or toxicity between groups were observed. Finally, a recent meta-analysis of 5 randomized, controlled trials (3 trials that compared oral EPA and placebo, and 2 trials that compared EPA-containing supplements) concluded that there were insufficient data to establish whether oral EPA was better than placebo for CC treatment.[24]

The role of Ω-3 fatty acids in the treatment of CC remains unclear.[13, 19] Some sources have recommended continued use of EPA and DHA in doses of at least 1.5 g/day to minimize the cachexia process and improve quality of life.[26] An important consideration with the use of Ω-3 fatty acid supplements is that, unlike many prescription medications, nutrient supplements are not considered a reimbursable expense by many third-party payers. As a consequence, use of these supplements may result in an increased financial burden for the patient.

Other agents that have been investigated should not be considered as first-line treatments for CC. For example, cyproheptadine is an antihistamine with serotonin-antagonist properties; it has been approved by the FDA for treatment of cold and allergy symptoms. This drug's serotonin-antagonist properties are thought to enhance appetite. Although it has been used clinically as an appetite stimulant for anorexia, cyproheptadine has not been subjected to extensive investigation in cancer patients.[13, 14] In one study, patients with advanced cancer who received cyproheptadine 8 mg orally 3 times daily demonstrated no difference in weight gain compared to a control group who received placebo.[29] Sedation is an undesirable side effect of this drug that may limit its usefulness. Routine use of cyproheptadine as an appetite stimulant in CC patients is not recommended.[13, 19]

Use of the antidepressant mirtazapine in patients with CC has also been proposed. This drug may be useful for treating multiple problems in patients with end-stage cancer including depression, anxiety, and insomnia. Mirtazapine may also demonstrate antiemetic effects because it also has $5HT_3$-antagonist properties.[30] However, its use in cancer patients has not been well studied. Additionally, sedation is a common adverse effect that may limit this drug's usefulness in some patients. The role of mirtazapine as an appetite stimulant requires further study before its routine use can be recommended in cancer patients.[14, 31]

Other anticytokine agents such as pentoxyphylline, melatonin, and thalidomide should be considered for investigational use only based on currently available data. Anabolic steroids should not be prescribed as appetite stimulants, and they require further study before their routine use as a CC treatment can be considered.[13, 19]

Chemotherapy-Induced Nausea and Vomiting

Nausea and vomiting are two of the most stressful and feared side effects of chemotherapy for both patients and their caregivers.[32–35] Advances in preventive treatments for chemotherapy-induced nausea and vomiting (CINV) over the past 25 years have improved symptom management for many patients. Indeed, development of the 5-hydroxytryptamine type 3 receptor (5HT$_3$) antagonists was a pivotal contribution to antiemetic options, and these drugs are now considered the gold standard antiemetic for CINV prevention.[32, 34, 36]

However, despite the development of newer antiemetics, CINV remains one of the most difficult side effects for practitioners to manage. Poorly controlled CINV frequently has negative effects on patients' quality of life, nutrition and hydration status, and therapy compliance or ability to continue therapy.[34, 37] Fortunately, CINV can be prevented in approximately 70–80% of patients receiving chemotherapy, especially if clinical guidelines for prophylactic antiemetic use are followed.[32]

Nausea is a subjective symptom characterized by flushing, tachycardia, and the urge to vomit.[35, 38] In general, nausea occurs more frequently than vomiting; however, the incidence of nausea correlates with the incidence of vomiting.[39] Vomiting, or emesis, is a physical phenomenon involving the contraction of abdominal muscles, descent of the diaphragm, and expulsion of stomach contents.[35, 38] Vomiting tends to be associated with worse potential metabolic and physiologic adverse effects such as acid–base imbalances, fluid and electrolyte abnormalities, and mucosal damage within the GIT.

The most commonly proposed mechanism for CINV is thought to be a complex interaction between the vomiting center and signals from a variety of other sources including the chemoreceptor trigger zone (CTZ), central responses to senses such as smell and taste, vestibular responses, and peripheral signals from the vasculature and visceral organs such as the GIT. These signals are modulated by neurophysiologic interactions that include neurotransmitters such as dopamine, histamine, endorphins, acetylcholine, cannabinoids, gamma aminobutyric acid (GABA), substance P, and serotonin or 5HT$_3$. These neurotransmitters are released in response to circulating chemotherapy or end-organ cellular damage and stimulate afferent impulses from the CTZ, pharynx, GIT, and cerebral cortex, which are in turn sent to the vomiting center. Vomiting occurs when the efferent impulses are sent from the vomiting center to the salivation center, abdominal muscles, respiratory center, cranial nerves, and salivary centers, as well as to the abdominal muscles, diaphragm, and esophagus.[35, 37, 38]

Risk factors for developing CINV include age younger than 50 years, female gender, negative alcohol and tobacco history, and prior history of nausea and vomiting, especially with pregnancy or previous chemotherapy.[32, 38] Female patients have higher risk for developing CINV because they are less likely to have a history of high alcohol intake, they tend to receive more highly emetogenic chemotherapy regimens, and they may have a history of pregnancy.[35] The emetogenic potential of the chemotherapy agents used is also a primary risk factor for developing CINV.[32] Previous categories of emetogenicity ranked chemotherapeutic agents according to 5 levels.[40] Recent changes outlined in the most recent National Comprehensive Cancer Network (NCCN) and American Society of Clinical Oncology (ASCO) guidelines have established 4 categories of emetogenicity, based on a regimen's percentage of emetic risk if antiemetics were not given; these categories are outlined in Table 15.3.[37, 39] Other factors that may affect risk of CINV include the chemotherapy administration schedule (consecutive days or single day), intravenous infusion rate (continuous or intermittent infusion), and the number of chemotherapy agents used in the regimen (combination or single-agent chemotherapy). Poorly controlled anxiety and low socioeconomic status are also risk factors for developing CINV in cancer patients.[35, 38]

CINV may be characterized by the timing of onset (acute or delayed onset) and response to treatment. Acute CINV occurs within the first 24 hours after initiation of chemotherapy but typically manifests within the first 8 hours.

Table 15.3 *Emetogenic Risk Categories for Chemotherapy*

High	Emesis risk > 90% without antimetics	Carmustine, cisplatin, cyclophosphamide (> 1500 mg/m^2), dacarbazine, dactinomycin, lomustine (> 60 mg/m^2), mechlorethamine, pentostatin, streptozocin
Moderate	Emesis risk 30–90% without antiemetics	Altretamine, cyclophosphamide (< 1500 mg/m^2), cytarabine (> 1 g/m^2), daunorubicin, doxorubicin, epirubicin, idarubicin, ifosfamide, irinotecan, lomustine (< 60 mg/m^2), melphalan, mitoxantrone (12 mg/m^2), oxaliplatin, procarbazine, temozolamide
Low	Emesis risk 10–30% without antiemetics	Aldesleukin, asparaginase, bortezomib, cetuximab, cytarabine (< 1 g/m^2), docetaxel, etoposide, 5-fluorouracil, gemcitabine, methotrexate, mitomycin, mitoxantrone (< 12 mg/m^2), paclitaxel, pegasparaginase, pemetrexed, teniposide, thiotepa, topotecan, traztuzumab
Minimal	Emesis risk < 10% without antiemetics	Bleomycin, bevacizumab, busulfan, capecitabine, cladribine, cytarabine (< 100 mg/m^2), erlotinib, fludarabine, hydroxyurea, imatinib mesylate, geftinib, interferon, melphalan, mercaptopurine, methotrexate (< 100 mg/m^2), rituximab, thioguanine, vinblastine, vincristine, vinorelbine

Source: Jordan K, Kasper C, Schmoll H. Chemotherapy-induced nausea and vomiting: Current and new standards in the antiemetic prophylaxis and treatment. *Eur J Cancer.* 2005;41:199–205.

The most emetogenic chemotherapeutic agents induce vomiting within 1–2 hours after their administration. Acute nausea is primarily mediated by serotonin release from the enterochromaffin cells in the GIT.[32, 38] Receptors for serotonin or $5HT_3$ are located on vagal nerve terminals in the periphery and centrally in the CTZ in the area postrema. Chemotherapeutic agents produce nausea and vomiting by stimulating serotonin release from the enterochromaffin cells of the small intestine, which in turn activate $5HT_3$ receptors located on the vagal afferents to initiate the vomiting reflex.[38]

Delayed CINV occurs 24 hours after chemotherapy administration and can persist for as long as 5 days or more.[32, 38] Delayed CINV is commonly associated with high doses of cisplatin and cyclophosphamide, but may also occur with anthracycline and carboplatin therapy.[38] The mechanism for delayed CINV has not been definitively established, although it is likely not the same as that proposed for acute CINV. For example, there is no evidence of increased serotonin release more than 8 hours following cisplatin-based chemotherapy, so activity through $5HT_3$ pathways is unlikely.[38, 41] Delayed CINV may be primarily mediated by substance P and neurokinin 1 (NK-1) receptors; however, other mechanisms have been investigated including blood–brain barrier disruption, GI motility abnormalities, and altered adrenal hormonal activity.[32]

Successful treatment of acute CINV lowers the risk of developing both severe, delayed CINV and anticipatory nausea.[38] Failure to control acute CINV is associated with an increased risk of developing delayed CINV. The control of delayed nausea is frequently overestimated, and the symptoms are often undertreated.[34, 42, 43] Agents that have demonstrated effectiveness in preventing acute nausea, such as the $5HT_3$ antagonists, are less effective for preventing delayed CINV. Indeed, the $5HT_3$ antagonists are no longer recommended for prevention of delayed nausea in the most recent NCCN and ASCO guidelines for treating CINV.[38, 39] Delayed CINV is more likely to respond to treatment with a dexamethasone-containing antiemetic regimen that may include a substance P/NK-1 receptor antagonist such as aprepitant.[37] Patients receiving high-emetic-risk chemotherapy or a regimen including an anthracycline and cyclophosphamide should receive combination therapy with a $5HT_3$ antagonist, dexamethasone, and aprepitant on day 1 of chemotherapy for prevention of acute CINV. Combination therapy with dexamethasone and aprepitant on days 2–3 of chemotherapy is recommended for treatment of delayed CINV associated with high-emetic-risk chemotherapy.[39]

Anticipatory CINV occurs before a new cycle of chemotherapy is administered when at least 1 previous cycle of chemotherapy has been associated with nausea and vomiting. Approximately 30% of patients will experience anticipatory CINV by the fourth cycle of chemotherapy after experiencing emetic episodes with previous cycles.[32] Anticipatory CINV is a conditioned reflex that may be triggered by taste, odor, sight, sounds, or thoughts. Increased patient anxiety due to a history of poor response to antiemetics may worsen the risk of anticipatory CINV,[32] and the incidence of this problem increases with the duration of chemotherapy.[44] Optimizing antiemetics with initial courses of chemotherapy is the cornerstone to prevention of anticipatory CINV. Lorazepam is the drug of choice for prevention and treatment of anticipatory CINV.[37–39]

Breakthrough or refractory CINV are symptoms that occur despite appropriate preventive antiemetic therapy. Previously used antiemetics are unlikely to be effective in treating such cases; instead, use of agents from a different pharmacologic class is often necessary.[35, 38] Currently available classes of antiemetics are described in Table 15.4.

$5HT_3$-receptor antagonists are the most effective agents for prevention of acute CINV.[37, 39] Members of this class are equally efficacious and safe at equivalent doses, so the agents are interchangeable for clinical use. The most commonly experienced adverse effects are usually mild and include

Table 15.4 *Classes of Antiemetics*

Class	*Drug*
$5HT_3$-receptor antagonists	Ondansetron Granisetron Dolasetron Palonosetron
Corticosteroids	Dexamethasone Methylprednisolone
Neurokinin-1 (NK1)-receptor antagonists	Aprepitant
Dopamine-receptor antagonists	Prochlorperazine Promethazine Metoclopramide Haloperidol
Benzodiazepines	Lorazepam
Cannabinoids	Dronabinol Nabilone
Antihistamines	Diphenhydramine

Sources: Wiser W, Berger A. Practical management of chemotherapy-induced nausea and vomiting. *Oncology.* 2005;19:1–14; Ettinger DS, Kloth DD, Noonan K, et al. *NCCN Clinical Practice Guidelines in Oncology: Antiemesis.* Version 2.2006.

headache and constipation. The lowest effective dose should be used because higher doses result in receptor saturation and do not enhance efficacy. Single-daily-dose regimens are as effective as multiple-dose regimens. In addition, oral and intravenous formulations have comparable efficacy.[32, 38]

Corticosteroids are often used in combination with $5HT_3$ antagonists and NK-1 antagonists to potentiate the antiemetic efficacy of each agent.[32, 38] The mechanism of action for the antiemetic activity of corticosteroids is unknown, although prostaglandin antagonism, tryptophan depletion, or changes in the permeability of the cerebrospinal fluid (CSF) to serum proteins may be involved. There is no difference in efficacy between members of the corticosteroid class, although dexamethasone is the agent most frequently investigated and allows for easy dosing. Adverse effects of corticosteroids depend on dose and the duration of therapy. The most commonly experienced adverse effects are insomnia, hyperglycemia, and psychosis.[32]

NK-1-receptor antagonists act centrally to inhibit CINV by crossing the blood–brain barrier and occupying NK-1 receptors, and selectively block the binding of substance P in the central nervous system.[37, 38] These agents enhance the response of both the $5HT_3$ antagonists and dexamethasone and are effective in combating both acute and delayed CINV.[32] The most commonly reported adverse effects are diarrhea, dizziness, nausea, and mild anorexia.[38] However, aprepitant is eliminated by CYP3A4 and is a substrate and moderate inhibitor of CYP3A4, which increases the risk for potential drug interactions. Dosing adjustments or use with caution may be necessary, as many common medications are metabolized through this pathway.[32]

Other pharmacologic agents that have been recommended for use to treat refractory or anticipatory CINV include the dopamine-receptor antagonists. These agents act centrally by blocking dopamine receptors in the CTZ and vomiting center.[38] They are not recommended for use as first-line therapy, but they may be useful for treating patients who are intolerant or refractory to standard therapy.[39] The most commonly experienced adverse effects associated with dopamine-receptor antagonists are extrapyramidal symptoms (particularly at higher doses), sedation, and orthostatic hypotension.[2]

Cannabinoids have been used for their antiemetic properties, but are not recommended as first-line agents in patients undergoing chemotherapy. They exert their effects at the cannabinoid receptors located in the brain stem.[32, 45] Their utility is limited by the high incidence of adverse effects associated with their use, including dizziness, dysphoria, and hallucinations. Cannabinoids are most effectively used for treatment of breakthrough or refractory CINV.[32]

The benzodiazepines are a useful adjuvant class of antiemetics, particularly for anticipatory CINV. However, they are not recommended for use as single agent therapy because of limited effectiveness as antiemetics when used alone in cancer patients.[32]

The antihistamines are usually reserved for use as adjunctive medications to prevent dystonic reactions when using higher doses of the dopamine-receptor antagonists. They are also useful for treating nausea that is mediated by the vestibular system and for managing motion sickness. The agents primarily used for these indications are the histamine receptor 1 (H_1) antagonists, such as diphenhydramine and hydroxyzine. Their use is also limited by adverse effects such as drowsiness, dry mouth, and blurry vision.[32, 39]

Other complementary and alternative nonpharmacologic therapies have been explored for their role in preventing or managing CINV (see Table 15.5). Currently, clinical evidence supporting the efficacy of these interventions for CINV is limited. In general, they may offer some benefit when used in conjunction with standard pharmacologic antiemetic therapy, although further studies are needed to define their role as adjuncts to conventional antiemetic therapy.[46]

Table 15.5   *Selected Complementary Therapies for Chemotherapy-Induced Nausea and Vomiting*

Acupuncture
Acupressure
Guided imagery
Music therapy
Progressive muscle relaxation
Hypnosis
Massage and aromatherapy
Acustimulation with wristband device
Ginger

Source: Tipton JM, McDaniel RW, Barbour L, et al. Putting evidence into practice: Evidence-based interventions to prevent, manage, and treat chemotherapy-induced nausea and vomiting. *Clin J Oncol Nurs.* 2007;11:69–78.

Stomatitis/Mucositis

Oropharyngeal mucositis is a common side effect of chemotherapy or radiation therapy that is potentially treatment-limiting, and is associated with other negative outcomes such as increased risk of infection, decreased quality of life, and increased cost of care. Oropharyngeal mucositis is defined as erythematous or ulcerative lesions in the oral mucosa.[47] The terms *stomatitis* and *mucositis* are frequently used interchangeably. However, mucositis is a more general term that refers to inflammatory processes involving mucous membranes of the mouth and the entire GIT, while stomatitis refers to inflammatory diseases of the mouth including the mucosa, dentition, periapices, and periodontium.[48]

The incidence of mucositis ranges from 10% to 75% in patients receiving chemotherapy and is as high as 75% in patients receiving hematopoietic stem cell transplantation (HSCT). Oropharyngeal mucositis is considered an inevitable consequence in virtually all head and neck cancer patients who receive combined chemoradiation treatment, and the mucositis is often more severe and longer in duration. Increased intensity and duration of mucositis occurs more commonly in patients receiving hyperfractionated radiotherapy.[49] The potential clinical consequences of oropharyngeal mucositis include detrimental effects on oral nutritional intake, mouth care, treatment of the disease, and ultimately the patient's performance status. Patients who are unable to maintain adequate oral feedings may require intestinal feeding tubes or parenteral nutrition.

Ulcerated mucositis in immunocompromised patients is thought to facilitate systemic entry by bacteria, resulting in potentially life-threatening infections.[50] Patients who have mucositis with chemotherapy have been reported to have twice the infection rate than those who did not develop this complication.[47] Severe mucositis and other related complications may result in delayed treatments and reduced treatment doses, which may have negative effects on tumor treatment.[48]

Several risk factors for developing mucositis have been identified, which are directly related to the drug class, dose, and method of administration of the chemotherapy agent, and intensity and dose of radiation a patient receives.[47] Complete turnover of the epithelial lining of the GIT occurs every 7 to 14 days. This cycle parallels the usual chemotherapy nadir, which begins approximately 5 to 7 days after a course of chemotherapy. Mucositis is more common with continuous infusion regimens as compared to shorter chemotherapy infusions. All chemotherapy agents can cause mucositis; however, the worst offenders are methotrexate, 5-fluorouracil (5-FU), etoposide (more common with oral administration than with IV infusion), and the anthracyclines. Dose, scheduling, and sequencing of chemotherapy affect the risk of developing mucositis.

Radiation-induced mucositis usually becomes evident 5 to 7 days after radiation therapy is initiated. A history of heavy alcohol and tobacco use increases the risk for experiencing worse radiation-induced mucositis. Other risk factors associated with development of mucositis after chemoradiation include preexisting oropharyngeal infection, poor dental hygiene or ill-fitting dentures, hyposalivation, lower baseline neutrophil counts, elevated serum urea nitrogen and serum creatinine concentrations, and extremes of age (e.g., children and the elderly).[49, 51] Chemoradiation-induced myelosuppression may also predispose patients to mucositis caused by fungal or viral infections such as oropharyngeal candidiasis or herpes simplex virus (HSV).[49]

The pathogenesis of mucositis is characterized by four phases.

Phase 1: Initiation of tissue injury

Phase 2: Signal amplification as a primary response to tissue injury, which is manifested as upregulation of pro-inflammatory cytokines such as tumor necrosis factor-alpha

Phase 3: Mucosal ulceration with barrier loss and significant inflammation

Phase 4: Healing and repair process, characterized by renewal of epithelial proliferation and tissue differentiation[47, 49]

Clinically, mucositis manifests as an erythematous oral mucosa that may progress to erosion and ulceration. These changes often occur bilaterally and may be accompanied by a foul odor and necrotic debris. The healing process usually occurs two to four weeks after administration of the last dose of therapy. Symptomatically, patients most commonly complain of pain.[47, 49] Oral mucositis is typically classified into five grades according to the World Health Organization (WHO) grading system; Table 15.6 outlines these categories.

Mucositis is generally treated with supportive care interventions such as pain control and mouth care. Pain control often requires opioids, provided in alternative forms such as liquid or intravenous solutions. Topical mouth rinses containing anesthetics are also used for pain relief.

However, prevention of mucositis is the most important component of mucositis management. Good oral hygiene is the primary preventive measure, as it reduces the oral microbial load, which in turn minimizes the likelihood of gingivitis and oral mucositis in high-risk patients. Basic oral care includes brushing teeth with a soft toothbrush, regular flossing, use of bland rinses, application of lip moisturizers, and regular assessment of the oral cavity. Pretreatment dental assessment is important to identify and treat any preexisting conditions before initiating cancer treatment in patients. Lastly,

Table 15.6 *World Health Organization Grading System for Oral Mucositis*

Oral Mucositis Grade	Description
Grade 0	Absence of mucositis
Grade I	Presence of painless ulcer, erythema, or mild sensitivity
Grade II	Presence of painful erythema or ulcers that do not interfere with the patient's ability to take food
Grade III	Confluent ulceration that interferes with the patient's ability to take solid food
Grade IV	Severe symptoms requiring enteral or parenteral nutrition support

Source: Volpato LER, Silva TS, Oliveira TM, Sakai VT, Machado M. Radiation therapy and chemotherapy-induced oral mucositis. *Rev Bras Otorhinolaringol.* 2007;73:562–568.

use of alcohol, tobacco, and irritating foods that may be spicy, hot, rough, or acidic should be discouraged.[47–49, 52]

A variety of other therapies have been suggested as potential treatments for prevention of mucositis, although no one intervention has shown to be any more efficacious than good basic mouth care. Guidelines regarding recommendations for prophylactic treatment of mucositis are available from the Multinational Association of Supportive Care in Cancer/International Society for Oral Oncology (MASCC/ISOO).[53]

Cryotherapy, or administration of ice chips to the oral cavity during chemotherapy administration, has been used to produce local vasoconstriction and reduce blood flow. This intervention is recommended for patients receiving chemotherapy agents with short half-lives, such as intravenous bolus administration of 5-FU and melphalan. Ice chips may be taken and held in the mouth 5 minutes before chemotherapy administration and replenished as needed for as long as 30 minutes.

Rinsing the mouth with a 0.9% saline or bicarbonate solution is often suggested, even though there are no studies to date demonstrating its effectiveness. Patients should be cautioned against using mouthwashes containing alcohol and phenol, because these rinses may cause mucosal irritation and dehydrate the mouth. Although supportive evidence from clinical trials is lacking, coating agents such as milk of magnesia, kaopectate, aluminum hydroxide, and sucralfate may be used alone or in combination with diphenhydramine or other anesthetics such as lidocaine for local oral comfort. Inconclusive results have been reported with use of a combination agent containing polyvinylpyrrolidone, hyaluronic acid, and glycyrrhetinic acid

(Gelclair®) as a treatment option in patients with chemoradiation-induced mucositis.[54, 55]

Growth factors are a newer method used for management of oral mucositis. Palifermin (Kepivance®) is an intravenous recombinant human keratinocyte growth factor-1 (KGF), approved by the FDA for use in patients with hemato-logic malignancies who receive myelotoxic therapy and subsequent HSCT.[56] Palifermin binds to KGF receptors, resulting in epithelial cell proliferation, differentiation, and migration in multiple tissues throughout the GIT.[47, 49, 57] Fibroblast growth factor 10 (velafermin) is currently in development for use in patients who undergo HSCT.

Glutamine is an amino acid that is important for intestinal epithelial metab-olism. It has been investigated for its potential to affect GI toxicity related to chemotherapy and radiation positively. Glutamine is available in a variety of oral forms; however, intravenous glutamine is not commercially available in the United States. The role of glutamine in prevention or treatment of chemotherapy- or radiation-induced mucositis is not clear. Currently, routine use of systemic glutamine is not recommended for prevention of mucositis.[47]

Amifostine, a free-radical scavenger, is FDA approved for use in reducing the incidence and severity of xerostomia in patients undergoing postopera-tive radiation therapy for head and neck cancer.[58] Reducing xerostomia may be helpful in reducing dental caries, oral infections, and osteonecrosis, and in improving patients' eating and speaking abilities.[42]

The MASCC/ISOO guidelines also provide recommendations *against* sev-eral other interventions for prevention or treatment of mucositis.[53] Routine use of topical antimicrobials or sucralfate is not recommended for prevention of radiation-induced oral mucositis. Acyclovir and its analogues should not be used routinely for mucositis prevention in patients receiving standard-dose chemotherapy regimens. Chlorhexidine should not be used to treat established oral mucositis in patients receiving standard-dose chemotherapy regimens. However, topical antimicrobials may be useful to reduce second-ary infections when tissue damage has occurred. Antiviral prophylaxis with acyclovir or an acyclovir analogue should be used in patients who have expe-rienced a prior HSV episode, or are receiving chemotherapy treatment for leukemia or HSCT because of the high rate of viral reactivation in patients receiving those treatments.[49]

Treatment-Related Diarrhea

Treatment-related diarrhea (TRD) is a common toxicity of cancer treatment that is poorly recognized in clinical practice. TRD often leads to significant morbidity and mortality as well as dose reductions in chemotherapy or radiation, treatment delays, or discontinuation of therapy. The reported incidence of all grades of diarrhea is as high as 82%. The severity of diarrhea has been characterized by the National Cancer Institute (NCI), as shown in Table 15.7. Severe diarrhea (grades 3–4) is reported in approximately one-third of those who experience TRD, and its impact on patient's quality of life can be significant.[59] For example, patients with severe diarrhea may require hospitalization because of significant fluid and electrolyte imbalances, dehydration, nutritional deficiencies, renal insufficiency, and infectious complications that can lead to sepsis and even death. Financial costs associated with TRD frequently exceed the cost of other treatment-related toxicities that require hospitalization, such as febrile neutropenia and cardiotoxicity.[59, 60]

Several risk factors for TRD have been identified, such as presence of a primary tumor, past history of chemotherapy-induced diarrhea (CID), chemotherapy administered during the summer months, older age, and female gender. Other significant risk factors include resection of a primary bowel tumor, irinotecan-based chemotherapy, and treatment in the adjuvant setting. In addition, deficiency of dihydropyrimidine dehydrogenase (DPD), an enzyme important in 5-FU metabolism, or presence of polymorphisms of uridine diphosphate glucuronyl transferase (UGT), an enzyme that affects glucuronidation of the irinotecan metabolite SN-38, may be risk factors for TRD. The incidence of grades 3 and 4 diarrhea has been reported to be as high as 70% in patients with the UGT1A1 isoenzyme compared to 15% in patients with normal alleles.[59] Routine clinical use of testing for DPD deficiency is limited; however, testing for the UGT1A1 isoenzyme is potentially clinically beneficial for tailoring patient-specific treatment plans. For example, irinotecan therapy may be initiated at a lower dose in patients known to be homozygous for UGT1A1 polymorphisms.[59]

Several types of diarrhea may result from chemoradiation, including osmotic, secretory, malabsorption, exudative, infectious and dysmotile diarrhea, as well as steatorrhea.[61, 62] Despite multiple investigations, the mechanism of CID is not clear. In general, CID occurs because of lower GIT irritation. It is unknown whether the resultant increased stooling occurs because of a relative decrease in intestinal absorptive capacity secondary to treatment-induced epithelial destruction, or because of altered osmotic gradients caused by cytotoxicity and associated enzymatic changes that result in decreased absorption and increased fluid and electrolyte secretion. The effect of different chemotherapy agents or combination regimens is also not well understood.[60] The chemotherapy agents that most commonly cause diarrhea are irinotecan, 5-FU, methotrexate, capecitabine, gemcitabine, topotecan, cytarabine, cisplatin, cisplatin with docetaxel, oxaliplatin, high-dose interleukin-2, gefitinib, and erlotinib. In addition, the risk of severe diarrhea

Table 15.7 *National Cancer Institute's Toxicity Criteria for Diarrhea*

Grade	0	1	2	3	4	5
Patients with colostomy	None	Increase of < 4 stools/day over pretreatment	Increase of 4–6 stools/day or nocturnal stools	Increase of ≥ 7 stools/day or incontinence; or need for parenteral support for dehydration	Physiologic consequences requiring intensive care; or hemodynamic collapse	Death
Patients without colostomy	None	Mild increase in loose water colostomy output compared with pretreatment	Moderate increase in loose watery colostomy output compared with pretreatment, but not interfering with normal activity	Severe increase in loose watery colostomy output compared with pretreatment, interfering with normal activity	Physiologic consequences requiring intensive care; or hemodynamic collapse	Death
HSCT Patients	None	> 500 mL to ≤ 1000 mL of diarrhea/day	> 1000 mL to ≤ 1500 mL of diarrhea/day	> 1500 mL of diarrhea/day	Severe abdominal pain with or without ileus	Death

HSCT = Hematopoietic stem cell transplant.

Source: Kornblau S, Benson AB, Catalano R, et al. Management of cancer treatment-related diarrhea: Issues and therapeutic strategies. *J Pain Symptom Manage.* 2000;19(2):118–129.

is greater with continuous 5-FU infusions compared to bolus administration of this medication.

Diarrhea occurs in 60–80% of patients who receive irinotecan. Irinotecan-induced diarrhea may be acute or delayed. Acute diarrhea occurs within the first 24 hours after irinotecan administration. It is usually a secretory diarrhea mediated by cholinergic receptors. The drug of choice for treatment of acute diarrhea is atropine, an anticholinergic drug. Delayed diarrhea usually occurs 24 or more hours after chemotherapy administration and is usually a secretory diarrhea as well.[61] Loperamide, the drug of choice for treatment of delayed diarrhea, is a non-analgesic opioid that decreases intestinal motility by directly affecting smooth muscle of the intestine. The usual dose is 4 mg, followed by 2 mg every 4 hours until the patient is diarrhea-free for 12 hours, to a maximum of 16 mg/day (to minimize adverse effects). The dose may be increased to 2 mg every 2 hours for patients with severe irinotecan-induced diarrhea.[60] Other options for treatment of delayed diarrhea include atropine-diphenoxalate, octreotide, and tincture of opium.[26, 39] Octreotide acts on epithelial cells, and inhibits gut hormones such as serotonin, vasoactive intestinal peptide, and gastrin; it also increases intestinal transit time and promotes electrolyte absorption, thereby decreasing mesenteric blood flow.[44, 61]

The incidence and severity of radiation-induced diarrhea is specific to the site being irradiated and the dose being administered.[63] Pelvic or abdominal radiation causes enteritis, which is manifested as abdominal cramping and diarrhea in approximately 50% of patients.[60] Life-threatening diarrhea occurs in as many as 3% of patients, and chronic post-treatment diarrhea is seen in 26% to 49% of patients who undergo radiotherapy.[63] Symptoms usually occur during the third week of fractionated radiotherapy, and the incidence is increased when the radiation is given with concomitant chemotherapy. Unfortunately, there is no clearly effective preventive therapy for radiation-induced diarrhea.[60]

A variety of pharmacological, physical, and environmental factors should be considered when assessing a patient who presents with diarrhea after antitumor treatment. Patients should be evaluated for other possible causes of diarrhea, such as medications (laxatives, antibiotics), diet, partial intestinal obstruction, fecal impaction, surgery, and comorbid infection, in addition to consideration of a chemotherapy- or radiotherapy-induced source.[59] Management of TRD requires prompt assessment and expeditious intervention. Patients should be counseled about bowel rest, appropriate hydration, and diet modifications. They should be discouraged from eating foods that may contribute to diarrhea, such as milk, high-fat foods, spicy foods, insoluble-fiber-rich foods, high-sorbitol juices, caffeinated beverages, and alcohol.[59, 64] They should be encouraged to eat small, frequent meals; drink a daily amount equal to at least 30–35 mL/kg of iso-osmotic calorie-containing beverages that are cool or warm (not hot or cold); ingest adequate soluble fiber; and eat protein-rich foods. Herbal supplements that can cause diarrhea—such as aloe, buckthorn, cascara, flaxseed, manna, milk thistle, panax ginseng, psyllium seed, rhubarb root, and senna—should be avoided.[64] Healthcare providers should warn their patients about other side effects that may accompany severe diarrhea, such as nausea, vomiting, anorexia, abdominal cramping, dehydration, neutropenia, fever, and electrolyte imbalances. Patients should be instructed to keep a detailed history of their diarrhea, including frequency, consistency, color, volume, presence or absence of blood, and any other symptoms accompanying the diarrhea.[60, 61] In addition, weekly assessment for GI toxicity during at least the first cycle of chemotherapy has been recommended, particularly for elderly patients.[60]

Mild to moderate diarrhea should initially be treated with dietary modifications and loperamide. If diarrhea persists beyond 48 hours, octreotide 100–150 mcg subcutaneously (SQ) three times daily is recommended or tincture of opium may also be initated. Complicated diarrhea (grade 3 or 4) oftentimes requires hospitalization for intravenous hydration and antibiotic support, and further evaluation for the etiology of diarrhea, including blood and stool culture collection. Oral antibiotics are recommended for patients who have diarrhea that persists beyond 24 hours.

Specific guidelines for treating CID in patients receiving irinotecan, 5-FU, and leucovorin (IFL) are outlined in Table 15.8. Discontinuing or holding

Table 15.8 *Treatment Recommendations for Chemotherapy-Induced Diarrhea in Patients Receiving Irinotecan, 5-Fluorouracil, and Leucovorin (IFL)*

Clinical Presentation	Intervention
Diarrhea, any grade	Oral loperamide (2 mg every 2 hours) and continue until diarrhea free for ≥ 12 hours
Diarrhea persists on loperamide > 24 hours	Oral fluoroquinolone × 7 days
Diarrhea persists on loperamide > 48 hours	Stop loperamide; hospitalize patient; administer IV fluids
ANC < 500 cells/μL, regardless of fever or diarrhea	Oral fluoroquinolone and continue until resolution of neutropenia
Fever with persistent diarrhea, even in the absence of neutropenia	Oral fluoroquinolone and continue until resolution of fever and diarrhea

ANC = Absolute neutrophil count; IV = intravenous.

Source: Benson AB, Ajani JA, Catalano RB, et al. Recommended guidelines for the treatment of cancer treatment-induced diarrhea. *J Clin Oncol.* 2004;22(14):2918–2926.

chemotherapy until complete resolution of symptoms for at least 24 hours without antidiarrheal therapy has been recommended for patients receiving IFL who experience significant diarrhea.[60]

The pathophysiology of diarrhea induced by graft-versus-host disease (GVHD) differs from TRD resulting from chemoradiation. High-dose chemotherapy and donor-derived alloreactive cytotoxic T lymphocytes cause intestinal mucosal damage, which is primarily limited to the distal ileum and proximal colon, in GVHD. The pharmacologic approach to treating GVHD-induced diarrhea is continuing immunosuppressants such as cyclosporine or tacrolimus, adding corticosteroids or increasing the current corticosteroid dose, and initiating octreotide. Response to octreotide intervention should occur within 3 to 4 days. Second-line immunosuppressants should be considered if there is no response within 3 to 4 days after starting corticosteroids.[65]

Treatment-Related Constipation

Constipation may occur in cancer patients for a variety of reasons, including physiologic abnormalities caused by the tumor such as obstruction or dysmotility. However, constipation may also occur as a result of chemotherapy treatments or other supportive care medications such as opioid pain medications, antiemetics with anticholinergic side effects, or over-aggressive antidiarrheal therapy. Treatment-induced metabolic abnormalities, such as dehydration from decreased oral intake, or electrolyte abnormalities, such as hypercalcemia, may also contribute to development of constipation. Environmental conditions or performance status may increase risk of developing constipation as a result of decreased exercise.

Chemotherapy-induced constipation is characterized by reduced frequency of bowel motility and increased stool consistency. Unfortunately, the mechanisms underlying its emergence are poorly defined; however, a variety of GI metabolic abnormalities have been described that contribute to development of constipation. For example, chemotherapy can alter normal gut function and cause constipation by decreasing motility, and increasing water reabsorption, contributing to development of autonomic neuropathy, and, in severe cases, contributing to development of ileus.[61] The severity of constipation has been characterized by the NCI, as outlined in Table 15.9.

The vinca alkaloids (vincristine, vinblastine, and vinorelbine) and thalidomide are the chemotherapeutic agents most frequently associated with chemotherapy-induced constipation, which can progress to an ileus if not treated appropriately. Cancer patients often receive concomitant opioids or $5HT_3$ antagonists as a part of their treatment, which can also worsen or cause constipation.

Treatment of chemotherapy-induced constipation often includes supportive care measures. Patients are recommended to ensure adequate hydration, increase fiber intake, and increase physical activity if possible. Frequently, these measures alone are not adequate so laxatives are an important addition to therapy[44] (see Table 15.10).

The NCCN has suggested guidelines for treating cancer patients with constipation.[66] In general, prophylactic measures include routine use of a stimulant laxative and stool softener. Symptomatic patients should be evaluated for the cause and severity of constipation. Fecal impaction and obstruction should be ruled out, and any underlying metabolic abnormalities that may contribute to constipation, such as electrolyte abnormalities or hypothyroidism, should be treated. Medications should be reviewed for any agents that might potentially contribute to the development of constipation.

Initial treatment for constipation includes addition of bisacodyl to the therapeutic regimen. If constipation persists after maximizing bisacodyl therapy, additional laxatives such as bisacodyl suppositories, polyethylene glycol, lactulose, sorbitol, or magnesium citrate should be considered. Other options

Table 15.10 *Laxatives for Treatment-Induced Constipation in Cancer Patients*[69]

Category	Example
Surfactant/stool softener	Docusate
Lubricant	Mineral oil
Saline	Magnesium citrate, sodium phosphates
Stimulant	Bisacodyl, castor oil, senna
Hyperosmotic	Glycerin, sorbitol, lactulose, polyethylene glycol
Prokinetic	Metoclopramide
Opioid-receptor antagonists	Naloxone, methylnaltrexone

Sources: McNicol ED, Boyce D, Schumann R, Carr DB. Mu-opioid antagonists for opioid-induced bowel dysfunction. *Cochrane Database of Systematic Reviews.* 2008;2:CD006332; Laxatives: Classification and properties. Lexi-Drugs Online. Hudson, OH: Lexi-Comp. Accessed September 10, 2008.

include phosphasoda or tap water enema and addition of a prokinetic agent to the drug regimen. Patients with impactions should be treated with a glycerin suppository with an optional mineral oil retention enema.[66] Some patients may require manual disimpaction. Saline laxatives such as magnesium citrate, magnesium hydroxide, and sodium phosphates should be used with caution in elderly patients or patients with renal insufficiency, because these agents may potentially cause electrolyte imbalances such as hyperphosphatemia or hypermagnesemia.[67, 68]

Other pharmacologic alternatives have been investigated in cancer patients with opioid-induced constipation, such as the opioid antagonist naloxone; to date, these drugs have produced inconsistent results in studies.[69, 70] Methylnaltrexone (Relistor®), a selective peripheral mu-opioid receptor antagonist, has been approved by the FDA for the treatment of opioid-induced constipation in patients with advanced illness who are receiving palliative care, when response to laxative therapy has not been sufficient.[71] Further study is needed to clarify the role of selective mu-opioid receptor antagonists as options for alleviating treatment-related constipation in cancer patients.[69]

SUMMARY

GI toxicities are an unfortunate consequence of many cancer treatments. Frequently, management of these toxicities requires supportive care with pharmacologic agents.[72] Multiple medications are available to ameliorate patient discomfort and prevent potentially serious metabolic complications. In addition, practice guidelines are available to help direct clinicians tailor use of these medications based on patient-specific criteria.[32, 37, 39, 53, 59, 60] Future research for GI toxicities associated with cancer treatments is focused on preventing or minimizing these therapies' adverse effects on GI function through use of less toxic antitumor therapies such as targeted cancer treatments and use of predictive markers for severe toxicities.[2, 72, 73] Continued research for preventing or treating unintentional weight loss is directed toward a variety of approaches to modulating metabolic abnormalities thought to be associated with inflammation, such as abnormalities in appetite regulation and cytokine-induced catabolism.[5-10] These supportive care interventions for minimizing GI toxicities and unintentional weight loss associated with cancer should complement future antitumor therapies.

REFERENCES

1. Espey DK, Wu XC, Swan J, et al. Annual report to the nation on the status of cancer, 1975–2004, featuring cancer in American Indians and Alaska Natives. *Cancer.* 2007;110:2119–2152.

2. Bentzen SM, Trotti A. Evaluation of early and late toxicities in chemoradiation trials. *J Clin Oncol.* 2007;25:4096–4103.

3. Yabroff KR, Lawrence WF, Clauser S, Davis WW, Brown ML. Burden of illness in cancer survivors: Findings from a population-based national sample. *J Natl Cancer Inst.* 2004;96:1322–1330

4. Schattner M, Shike M. Nutrition support of the patient with cancer. In: Shils ME, Shike M, Ross AC, Caballero B, Cousins RJ, eds. *Modern Nutrition in Health and Disease.* 10th ed. Baltimore, MD: Lippincott Williams & Wilkins; 2006:1290–1313.

5. Komurcu S, Nelson KA, Walsh D, Bradley R, Ford B, Rybicki LA. Gastrointestinal symptoms among inpatients with advanced cancer. *Am J Hosp Palliat Care.* 2002; 19:351–355.

6. Palesty JA, Dudrick SJ. What we have learned about cachexia in gastrointestinal cancer. *Dig Dis.* 2003;21:198–213.

7. Dewys WD, Begg C, Lavin PT, et al. Prognostic effect of weight loss prior to chemotherapy in cancer patients. *Am J Med.* 1980;68:491–497.

8. Dahele M, Fearon KCH. Research methodology: cancer cachexia syndrome. *Palliat Med.* 2004;18:409–417.

9. Laviano A, Meguid MM, Rossi-Fanelli F. Cancer anorexia: Clinical implications, pathogenesis, and therapeutic strategies. *Lancet Oncol.* 2003;4:686–694.

10. Seligman PA, Fink R, Massey-Seligman EJ. Approach to the seriously ill or terminal cancer patient who has poor appetite. *Semin Oncol.* 1998;25:33–34.

11. Jatoi A. Pharmacologic therapy for the cancer anorexia/weight loss syndrome: A data-driven, practical approach. *J Support Oncol.* 2006;4:499–502.

12. Berenstein EG, Ortiz A. Megestrol acetate for treatment of anorexia–cachexia syndrome. *Cochrane Database of Systemic Reviews.* 2005;2:CD004310.

13. Yavuzsen T, Davis MP, Walsh D, et al. Systematic review of the treatment of cancer-associated anorexia and weight loss. *J Clin Oncol.* 2005;23:8500–8511.

14. Mattox TW. Treatment of unintentional weight loss in patients with cancer. *Nutr Clin Pract.* 2005;20:400–410.

15. Chvetzoff G, Tannock IF. Placebo effects in oncology. *J Natl Cancer Inst.* 2003;95: 19–29.

16. Megace [package insert]. Princeton, New Jersey: Bristol-Myers Squibb; 2007.

17. Jatoi A, Windschitl HE, Loprinzi CL, et al. Dronabinol versus megestrol acetate versus combination therapy for cancer-associated wasting: A North Central Cancer Treatment Group study. *J Clin Oncol.* 2002;20:567–573.

18. Jatoi A, Rowland K, Loprinzi CL, et al. An eicosapentaenoic acid supplement versus megestrol acetate versus both for patients with cancer-associated wasting: A North Central Cancer Treatment Group and National Cancer Institute of Canada collaborative effort. *J Clin Oncol.* 2004;22:2469–2476.

19. Desport JC, Gory-Delabaere G, Blanc-Vincent MP, et al. Standards, options and recommendations for the use of appetite stimulants in oncology. *Br J Cancer.* 2003; 89(suppl 1):S98–S100.

20. Lopez AP, Roque I, Figuls M, Cuchi GU, et al. Systematic review of megestrol acetate in the treatment of anorexia–cachexia syndrome. *J Pain Symptom Manage.* 2004;27:360–369.

21. Woolridge JE, Anderson CM, Perry MC. Corticosteroids in advanced cancer. *Oncology.* 2001;15:225–236.

22. Martin BR, Wiley JL. Mechanism of action of cannabinoids: How it may lead to treatment of cachexia, emesis and pain. *J Support Oncol.* 2004;2:305–316.

23. Strasser F, Luftner D, Possinger K, et al. Comparison of orally administered cannabis extract and delta-9 tetrahydrocannabinol in treating patients with cancer-related anorexia–cachexia syndrome: A multicenter, phase III, randomized, double-blind, placebo-controlled clinical trial from the Cannabin-in-Cachexia Study Group. *J Clin Oncol.* 2006;21:3394–3400.

24. Dronabinol capsules [package insert]. High Point, NC: Banner Pharmacaps; 2007.

25. Dewey A, Baughan C, Dean T, Higgins B, Johnson I. Eicosapentanoic acid (EPA, an omega-3 fatty acid from fish oils) for the treatment of cancer cachexia. *Cochrane Database of Systemic Reviews.* 2007;1:CD004597.

26. Colomer R, Moreno-Nogueira JM, Garcia-Luna PP, et al. *n*-3 fatty acids, cancer and cachexia: A systematic review of the literature. *Br J Nutr.* 2007;97:823–831.

27. Fearon KCH, von Meyenfeldt MF, Moses AGW, et al. Effect of a protein and energy dense *n*-3 fatty acid enriched oral supplement on loss of weight and lean tissue in cancer cachexia: A randomized double blind trial. *Gut.* 2003;52:1474–1486.

28. Jatoi A, Windschitl HE, Loprinzi CL, et al. An eicosapentaenoic acid supplement versus megestrol acetate versus both for patients with cancer-associated wasting: A North Central Cancer Treatment Group and National Cancer Institute of Canada collaborative effort. *J Clin Oncol.* 2004;2469–2476.

29. Kardinal CG, Loprinzi CL, Schaid DJ, et al. A controlled trial of cyproheptadine in cancer patients with anorexia and/or cachexia. *Cancer.* 1990;65:2657–2662.

30. Theobald DE, Kirsh KL, Holtsclaw E, Donaghy K, Passik SD. An open label, cross-over trial of mirtazapine (15 and 30 mg) in cancer patients with pain and other distressing symptoms. *J Pain Symptom Manage.* 2002;10:110–116.

31. Kast RE. Mirtazapine may be useful in treating nausea and insomnia of cancer chemotherapy. *Support Care Cancer.* 2001;9:469–470.

32. Jordan K, Kasper C, Schmoll H. Chemotherapy-induced nausea and vomiting: Current and new standards in the antiemetic prophylaxis and treatment. *Eur J Cancer.* 2005;41:199–205.

33. Coates A, Abraham S, Kaye SB, et al. On the receiving end: Patient perception of the side-effects of chemotherapy. *Eur J Cancer Clin Oncol.* 1983;19:203–208.

34. Thein HO, Hesketh PJ. Drug insight: New antiemetics in the management of chemotherapy-induced nausea and vomiting. *Oncology.* 2005;2(4):196–201.

35. Wiser W, Berger A. Practical management of chemotherapy-induced nausea and vomiting. *Oncology.* 2005;19:1–14.

36. de Boer-Dennert M, de Wit R, Schmitz PL, et al. Patient perceptions of the side-effects of chemotherapy: The influence of $5HT_3$ antagonists. *Br J Cancer.* 1997;76:1055–1061.

37. Ettinger DS, Kloth DD, Noonan K, et al. NCCN clinical practice guidelines in oncology: Antiemesis. Version 2.2006. Available at www.NCCN.org. Accessed November 15, 2007.

38. Grunberg SM. Chemotherapy-induced nausea and vomiting: Prevention, detection, and treatment—how are we doing? *J Supp Oncol.* 2004;2(suppl 1):1–12.

39. Kris MG, Hesketh PJ, Somerfield MR, et al. American Society of Clinical Oncology guideline for antiemetics in oncology: Update 2006. *J Clin Oncol.* 2006;24:2932–2947.

40. Schwartzberg LS. Chemotherapy-induced nausea and vomiting: Which antiemetics for which therapy? *Oncology.* 2007;21:1–12.

41. Schmoll HJ, Aapro MS, Poli-Bigelli S., et al. Comparison of an aprepitant regimen with a multiple-day ondansetron regimen, both with dexamethasone, for antiemetic efficacy in high-dose cisplatin treatment. *Ann Oncol.* 2006;17:1000–1006.

42. Schwartzberg L. Chemotherapy-induced nausea and vomiting: State of the art in 2006. *J Supp Oncol.* 2006;4(2)(suppl 1):3–8.
43. Grunberg SM, et al. Incidence of chemotherapy-induced nausea and emesis after modern antiemetics. *Cancer.* 2004;100:2261–2268.
44. Ludwig H, Zojer N. Supportive care. *Ann Oncol.* 2007;18(suppl 1):i37–i44.
45. Sharma R, Tobin P, Clarke SJ. Management of chemotherapy-induced nausea, vomiting, oral mucositis, and diarrhea. *Lancet Oncol.* 2005;6:93–102.
46. Tipton JM, McDaniel RW, Barbour L, et al. Putting evidence into practice: Evidence-based interventions to prevent, manage, and treat chemotherapy-induced nausea and vomiting. *Clin J Oncol Nurs.* 2007;11:69–78.
47. Lalla RV, Peterson DE. Treatment of mucositis, including new medications. *Cancer J.* 2006;12:348–354.
48. Eilers J, Million R. Prevention and management of oral mucositis in patients with cancer. *Semin Oncol Nurs.* 2007;23(3):201–212.
49. Epstein JB. Mucositis in the cancer patient and immunosuppressed host. *Infect Dis Clin N Am.* 2007;21:503–522.
50. Volpato LER, Silva TS, Oliveira TM, Sakai VT, Machado M. Radiation therapy and chemotherapy-induced oral mucositis. *Rev Bras Otorhinolaringol.* 2007;73:562–568.
51. Keefe DM. Intestinal mucositis: Mechanisms and management. *Curr Opin Oncol.* 2007;19:323–327.
52. Quinn B, Potting C, Stone R, et al. Guidelines for the assessment of oral mucositis in adult chemotherapy, radiotherapy and haematopoietic stem cell transplant patients. *Eur J Cancer.* 2007;44:61–72.
53. Keefe DM, Schubert MM, Elting LS, et al. Updated clinical practice guidelines for the prevention and treatment of mucositis. *Cancer.* 2007;109:820–831.
54. Gelclair indications. http://www.gelclair.com/hpc-indications.htm. Accessed September 16, 2008.
55. Barber C, Powell R, Ellis A, Hewett J. Comparing pain control and ability to eat and drink with standard therapy vs Gelclair: A preliminary, double centre, randomised controlled trial on patients with radiotherapy-induced oral mucositis. *Support Care Cancer.* 2007;15(4):427–440.
56. Kepviance [package insert]. Thousand Oaks, CA: Amgen Manufacturing; 2004–2005.
57. Fliedner M, Baguet B, Blankart J, et al. Palifermin for patients with haematological malignancies: Shifting nursing practice from symptom relief to prevention of oral mucositis. *Eur J Oncol Nurs.* 2007;11:S19–S26.
58. Kouvaris JR, Kouloulias VE, Vlahos LJ. Amifostine: The first selective-target and broad-spectrum radioprotector. *Oncologist.* 2007;12:738–747.
59. Maroun JA, Anthony LB, Blais N, et al. Prevention and management of chemotherapy-induced diarrhea in patients with colorectal cancer: A consensus statement by the Canadian Working Group on Chemotherapy-Induced Diarrhea. *Curr Oncol.* 2007;14:13–20.
60. Benson AB, Ajani JA, Catalano RB, et al. Recommended guidelines for the treatment of cancer treatment-induced diarrhea. *J Clin Oncol.* 2004;22(14):2918–2926.
61. Gibson RJ, Keefe DMK. Cancer chemotherapy-induced diarrhea and constipation: Mechanisms of damage and prevention strategies. *Support Care Cancer.* 2006;14:890–900.
62. Viele CS. Overview of chemotherapy-induced diarrhea. *Semin Oncol Nurs.* 2003;19(4)(suppl 3):2–5.

63. Gwede CK. Overview of radiation and chemoradiation-induced diarrhea. *Semin Oncol Nurs.* 2003;19(4)(suppl 3):6–10.

64. Stern J, Ippoliti C. Management of acute cancer treatment-induced diarrhea. *Semin Oncol Nurs.* 2003;19(4)(suppl 3):11–16.

65. Kornblau S, Benson AB, Catalano R, et al. Management of cancer treatment-related diarrhea: Issues and therapeutic strategies. *J Pain Symptom Manage.* 2000;19(2):118–129.

66. Levy MH, Block S, Weinstein SM, et al. NCCN clinical practice guidelines in oncology: Palliative care—constipation. Version 1.2008. Available at www.NCCN.org. Accessed September 10, 2008.

67. Beloosesky Y, Grinblat J, Weiss A, et al. Electrolyte disorders following oral sodium phosphate administration for bowel cleansing in elderly patients. *Arch Int Med.* 2003;163:803–808.

68. Zaman F, Abreo K. Severe hypermagnesemia as a result of laxative use in renal insufficiency. *South Med J.* 2003;96:102–103.

69. McNicol ED, Boyce D, Schumann R, Carr DB. Mu-opioid antagonists for opioid-induced bowel dysfunction. *Cochrane Database of Systematic Reviews.* 2008; 2:CD006332.

70. Thomas J, Karver S, Cooney GA. Methylnatrexone for opioid-induced constipation in advanced illness. *N Engl J Med.* 2008;358:2332–2343.

71. www.relistor.com [package insert]. Philadelphia, PA: Wyeth Pharmaceuticals; 2008.

72. Keefe MK. Supportive care silos: Time to forge cross-links, using mucositis as an example. *Curr Opin Supp Palliat Care.* 2007;1:40–42.

73. Lenz HJ. Molecular markers in gastrointestinal cancer: Targeted therapy and tailored chemotherapy. *Onkologie.* 2004;27:12–14.

Chapter 16

Integrative Oncology

Mary Marian, MS, RD, CSO

INTRODUCTION

Integrative oncology is an evolving area of oncologic care that seeks to address the use of evidence-based complementary and alternative therapies in conjunction with traditional antineoplastic therapies. Many patients with cancer are pursuing complementary and alternative medicine (CAM) to address perceived deficits in their care. Fortunately, most people do so in concert with obtaining traditional medicine. Currently, between $36 million and $47 million is spent annually on a variety of CAM modalities,[1] which generally are not covered by insurance.

Patients employ these therapies for a number of reasons, but in general seek them out for the following reasons:

- To enhance wellness
- To relieve symptoms of the disease and the side effects of conventional treatments, or to cure disease
- To take control over treatment
- To improve quality of life
- Because of the perception that "natural" is better
- Because of a preference for "natural" remedies
- Greater rapport between CAM practitioner and patient
- Conventional medicine is too expensive
- A conventional medicine practitioner recommended CAM therapy

Many people with cancer experience pain, anxiety, and mood disturbance. For some, conventional treatments do not always relieve these symptoms to their satisfaction and the side effects of the conventional treatments might be more than they can tolerate.

The most comprehensive data regarding CAM use by Americans come from the 2002 National Health Survey conducted by the National Center for Health Statistics (an agency of the Centers for Disease Control and Prevention).[2] The survey, which tallied responses from more than 31,000 adults, revealed that 75% used some form of CAM. When prayer for health reasons was excluded, 50% of respondents still used some type of CAM therapies.

CAM users also tend to have certain traits in common: being female, being married, being older, having a higher level of education, and having a higher socioeconomic status.[2] Barnes and colleagues found in a nation-wide survey that almost 50% of adults older the age of 18 reported using some form of CAM (excluding prayer) during their lifetime; 36% of adults reported CAM use in the past year, with people aged 50 to 59 being the most likely to report use of CAM modalities.[2] Furthermore, 61–72% of these individuals did not discuss their CAM use with their physician. The primary reason cited was "The physician never asked," but additional reasons included "There wasn't enough time to discuss" and respondents often did not know that they should discuss this topic with their healthcare providers. Moreover, CAM users generally report a belief that their physicians will disapprove of, do not care about, or are knowledge deficit about such therapies.[3] Satisfaction levels with CAM therapies are typically high; likewise, most users of these modalities believe CAM is cost-effective.[4]

The most commonly used CAM modalities are prayer (43%), natural products (18.9%), deep breathing (11.9%), meditation (7.6%), chiropractic therapies (7.5%), yoga (5.1%), massage (5.0%), and diets (3.5%).[2] Although many of these therapies appear "harmless," the concern about the trend toward greater use of CAM therapies is that many patients fail to inform their physicians about these measures. Vapiwala and colleagues recently surveyed oncology patients regarding their use of CAM therapies following cancer diagnosis, during treatment, or after completing treatment.[4] Eighty-one percent of breast cancer survivors reported using vitamins or antioxidants, while 29% used herbal or botanical supplements. In comparison, the usage levels for patients with prostate cancer were vitamins/antioxidants, 73%, and herbals/botanicals, 37%; for patients with colorectal cancer, they were vitamins/antioxidants, 81%, and herbals/botanicals, 59%. Within the CAM-user group, a significant number of patients reported that using multiple therapies, with one-third of users using 3 or more CAM modalities simultaneously. Throughout the 1990s, visits to CAM practitioners reportedly exceeded the total number of annual visits to all primary care providers during this same time period.[5]

Although the usage of CAM therapies is common, not all patients have access to the full range of CAM, as these therapies are rarely covered by insurance. This lack of coverage is unfortunate because patients with intractable symptoms are among the heaviest users of healthcare services, and beneficial complementary therapies can relieve symptoms, promote self-care, and decrease healthcare costs. However, not all complementary therapies are appropriate or useful, and even helpful complementary modalities may not be optimal under some circumstances.

This chapter reviews the evidence for common CAM therapies pursued by patients with cancer to provide guidance to clinicians considering integrating such therapies into oncological practice.

Complementary versus Alternative Medicine

It is important to distinguish the difference between complementary and alternative medicine. Over time, many of the current therapies coined "CAM" have evolved from previous references such as "snake oil" or "quackery." To address this issue, Congress established the Office of Alternative Medicine in 1991; in 1998, this office was reestablished as the National Center for Complementary and Alternative Medicine (NCCAM). The primary responsibility of NCCAM is to conduct and support basic and clinical research; funding is available for clinical trials to examine the efficacy of various CAM therapies.[6]

Current practice favors the terminology *complementary* versus *alternative*. To delineate this distinction, NCCAM developed the following definitions:

- **Complementary medicine** is used **together with** conventional medicine. An example of a complementary therapy is using aromatherapy to help lessen a patient's discomfort following surgery.
- **Alternative medicine** is used **in place of** conventional medicine. An example of an alternative therapy is using a special diet to treat cancer instead of undergoing surgery, radiation, or chemotherapy that has been recommended by a conventional doctor.

In the oncology realm, the use of complementary therapies versus alternative therapies may be a pivotal decision if individuals with cancer are planning to undergo treatments with no scientific basis and if they delay beginning evidence-based treatments for their cancer.

As complementary therapies are proven safe and effective, they are typically "integrated" into care—hence the practice of integrative medicine. In the oncology field, the integration of CAM therapies into treatment for cancer is commonly referred to as *integrative oncology*. In general, complementary therapies are not used to "treat" cancer but rather to address the symptoms associated with cancer or cancer treatment(s). The types of therapies considered complementary or alternative are in a perpetual state of flux. Integrative oncology, however, combines treatments from conventional medicine and CAM therapies for which there is some high-quality evidence of safety and effectiveness.

The NCCAM classifies CAM therapies into five domains plus the practice of *whole medicine*, which includes all five domains (see Table 16.1). Evidence is accumulating that some of the therapies can help; in contrast, some have been proven not to help, and for others there is little or no evidence to support their use. Because similar symptoms affect patients across the cancer spectrum, most CAM therapies can be used by a variety of patients—not just by individuals with one particular type of cancer.

Biologically Based Therapies

Nutrition, and specifically medical nutrition therapy, was previously thought of as one of the many CAM modalities available to patients with cancer. However, the importance of nutrition in both primary and secondary disease

Table 16.1 *National Center for Complementary and Alternative Medicine's Domains for CAM Therapies*

Biologically Based Therapies
Nutritional supplements, orthomolecular medicine (high-dose vitamin/mineral therapies), herbal medicine, shark cartilage, therapeutic diets

Mind–Body Practices
Meditation, imagery, hypnosis, prayer, yoga, art therapies

Manipulative and Body-Based Methods
Osteopathic manipulation, physical therapy, chiropractic, massage, rolfing, Feldenkrais

Energy Therapies
Bio-field therapies (e.g., Reiki, qi gong, therapeutic touch), bio-electromagnetic-based therapies (e.g., magnet therapy, pulsed fields)

Whole Medical Systems (based on systems of theory and practice)
Homeopathic medicine
Naturopathic medicine
Traditional Chinese medicine
Ayurveda

Source: National Center for Complementary and Alternative Medicine. Available at http://nccam.nih.gov. Accessed February 12, 2008.

prevention is now widely accepted, making nutrition intervention an integral part of therapy.

A variety of diet-centered therapies advertising to "cure" cancer have been aimed at cancer patients. Examples include Gerson nutrition therapy, the Johanna Brandt grape cure diet, the Dr. Johanna Budwig diet, and macrobiotic diets, to name a few. Additionally, several national cancer organizations have issued their own nutrition recommendations, as summarized in Table 16.2. Survivors should be encouraged to follow these evidence-based dietary recommendations instead of engaging in diets promoted to "cure" cancer. This strategy will enable them to avoid following diets that can have adverse effects.

Table 16.2   *Nutrition Recommendations for Cancer Patients and Survivors*

American Cancer Society[1]
Maintain a healthy weight throughout life.
- Balance caloric intake with physical activity.
- Avoid excessive weight gain throughout the life cycle.
- Achieve and maintain a healthy weight if currently overweight or obese.

Adopt a physically active lifestyle.
- Adults: Engage in 30 minutes of moderate-to-vigorous physical activity on 5 or more days per week.
- Children and adolescents: Engage in at least 60 minutes of moderate-to-vigorous activity on 5 or more days per week.

Consume primarily a plant-based diet.
- Choose foods and beverages that help maintain a healthy weight.
- Consume 5 servings of fruits and vegetables daily.
- Consume whole grains over processed carbohydrates.
- Limit consumption of red and processed meats.

Limit consumption of alcoholic beverages.
- Women: Limit intake to 1 alcoholic drink/day.
- Men: Limit intake to 2 drinks/day.

American Institute of Cancer Research[2]
Choose mostly plant foods, limit red meat, and avoid processed meat.
Be physically active every day in any way for 30 minutes or more.
Aim to be a healthy weight throughout life.

National Cancer Institute[3]
Reduce fat intake to 30% of calories or less.
Increase fiber to 20–30 g/day with an upper limit of 35 g.
Include a variety of fruits and vegetables in the daily diet.
Avoid obesity.
Consume alcoholic beverages in moderation, if at all.
Minimize consumption of salt-cured, salt-pickled, and smoked foods.

[1]American Cancer Society. Available at www.cancer.org. Accessed February 14, 2008.

[2]American Institute for Cancer Research. Available a: www.aicr.org. Assessed February 14, 2008.

[3]National Cancer Institute. *Eating hints for cancer patients: Before, during, and after treatment.* Washington, DC: U.S. Department of Health and Human Services; 2006.

Dietary Supplements

Many patients with cancer and long-term survivors of cancer become interested in taking dietary supplements after being diagnosed. More cancer patients and survivors take multiple vitamin and mineral (MVM) supplements as compared to the general population, with estimates of use in the former populations ranging from 64% to 81%.[4, 7]

Whether dietary supplementation in general can reduce treatment-related symptoms or improve survival is unclear. Additionally, the guidelines from national cancer organizations regarding MVM use are also conflicting. The American Cancer Society (ACS) states that while MVM use during treatment is controversial and potentially harmful, taking a daily MVM in amounts equal to the Recommended Daily Value (RDV) would probably be a benefit during those times when it is difficult to consume a healthy diet.[8] The use of high doses of vitamins, minerals, or other dietary supplements is not recommended, however, because excess amounts of some supplements can increase cancer risk. In fact, the National Cancer Institute (NCI) encourages patients to avoid MVM supplements while undergoing treatment or to take supplements only when recommended by a physician.[9, 10]

Given that many cancer patients and survivors take a variety of dietary supplements, it is important to encourage patients to open up a dialog on this topic with the healthcare team so that providers can discern whether such supplements are beneficial or harmful. Recently, an increased risk for prostate cancer in conjunction with MVM use was found in 2 consecutive reports from the Cancer Prevention Study II, which suggested that multivitamin use was associated with a higher risk of fatal prostate cancer.[11, 12] In the first report,[11] supplement users (men consuming multivitamins for 5 or more years) compared with nonusers were at increased risk of fatal prostate cancer (RR = 1.31, 95% CI = 1.04–1.66). An updated analysis[12] reported that multivitamin use of 15 or more times per month was associated with a marginally increased risk of fatal prostate cancer (RR = 1.07, 95% CI = 0.99–1.15) compared with nonusers.

Similarly, the results of the National Institutes of Health (NIH)–AARP Diet and Health Study, a large prospective study including 295,344 men, showed that while multivitamin use was unrelated to overall risk of total and organ-confined prostate cancer,[13] risk of advanced and fatal prostate cancer increased among those who took multivitamins more than seven times per week compared with never-users. Additionally, the risk of advanced prostate cancer and prostate cancer mortality associated with heavy multivitamin use was highest in men who reported concomitant use of selenium, beta-carotene, or zinc supplements, or who had a positive family history of prostate cancer. Although multivitamin use was not significantly correlated with the incidence of localized prostate cancer, an increased risk of localized prostate cancer was found among subjects taking multivitamins more than 7 times per week versus never taking them, in men also taking vitamin E, selenium, or folate supplements.

Conversely, in their observational study, Dong et al.[14] found that use of 1 or more multivitamin supplements daily was associated with a significantly decreased risk of esophageal adenocarcinoma in patients previously diagnosed with Barrett's esophagus. Significant inverse associations were also noted between risk and supplemental vitamin C ($\geq$ 250 mg/day versus none: hazard ratio [HR] = 0.25; 95% CI = 0.11–0.58), and between risk and supplemental vitamin E ($\geq$ 180 mg/day versus none: HR = 0.25; 95% CI = 0.10–0.60).

Similar to the concerns surrounding the use of multivitamin/mineral supplements, the ingestion of some botanical supplements has been shown to result in harmful interactions. For example, St. John's wort has been found to reduce plasma levels of the chemotherapeutic agents irinotecan and imatinib.[15, 16] Mathijssen and colleagues[15] found that plasma levels of irinotecan were reduced by 42% in patients taking St. John's wort. In addition, healthy subjects taking imatinib combined with this herb experienced a 43% greater clearance of imatinib.[16] St. John's wort is known to induce the cytochrome P450 hepatic enzyme system.[15] More than half of the chemotherapeutic agents now used are broken down by the cytochrome system, including the vinca alkaloids and the antineoplastic agents etoposide, teniposide, anthracycline, paclitaxel, docetaxel, and tamoxifen. Given that St. John's wort is often used by consumers as a "natural" remedy for the treatment of depression, patients should be screened for use of this herb as well as other botanicals prior to beginning chemotherapy. Other top-selling herbal supplements, such as garlic, ginkgo, ginseng, and kava, are also known to interact with commonly prescribed medications such as anticoagulants, diuretics, and tranquilizers.

Supplement Use During Cancer Treatment

The use of high doses of antioxidants in the form of dietary supplements during antineoplastic therapy (e.g., radiation, chemotherapy) is very controversial. Patients with cancer have been found to have lower circulating plasma antioxidant levels before therapy than do controls. Whether this phenomenon is due to the cancer or results from reduced oral intake by these patients has not been determined.[17] Conversely, other studies have reported opposite findings.[18, 19] Observational studies have reported that antioxidant status is depleted during chemotherapy[20–22] due to the significant degree of oxidative stress induced by the administration of antineoplastic drugs.

Theoretically, antioxidants could serve as beneficial agents that might enhance the cytotoxicity of antineoplastic therapy by potentially blocking the generation of reactive oxidant species (ROS), thereby protecting the DNA of healthy cells from oxidative damage induced by treatment. Lipid ROS are an essential component of life: They participate in cell signaling, which is part of the cascade of events that spurs phagocytes to begin their bactericidal activity. At the same time, ROS result in oxidative stress, which has been implicated in the etiology and progression of many disease processes. ROS are usually controlled by an extensive antioxidant defense system, but under some conditions this system can be depleted. Antioxidants (primarily beta-carotene and vitamins A, C, and E) generally work in tandem with one another through a series of oxidation–reduction reactions to quench ROS. When each of these nutrients is present in adequate amounts, it can be restored to its active antioxidant form following a reaction with the active oxidant species.

For patients undergoing antineoplastic therapy, this restoration is an important issue because in some cases chemotherapy induces a greater level of stress than the cancer itself. During chemotherapy, levels of lipid peroxidation products increase, thereby reducing the free-radical-trapping capacity of blood plasma and resulting in diminished plasma levels of antioxidants such as vitamins C and E, and beta-carotene. Elevated levels of oxidative stress during chemotherapy are thought to overcome the oxidative defenses of cancer cells and their specialized systems that normally decrease lipid peroxidation. As a consequence, increasing lipid peroxidation reduces or stops cancer cell proliferation and interferes with the activity of chemotherapy.[17] This may have an important effect on the response to chemotherapy—specifically, individuals with depleted antioxidant levels may not respond to treatment.[17] Indeed, it has been hypothesized that supportive nutritional therapy with antioxidants during chemotherapy, which diminishes the generation of lipid peroxides, can overcome the growth-inhibiting effects of oxidative stress and help maintain patients' responsiveness to chemotherapeutic agents.

Of note, in vitro and preclinical studies in animal models have suggested that maintaining micronutrient levels can improve the antitumor activity of chemotherapeutics modalities.[23, 24] Several studies have shown that high doses of individual antioxidant micronutrients, such as vitamins A, C, and E, and carotenoids, including beta-carotene, both inhibit the growth of and promote apoptosis in cancer cells in vitro.[25] These antioxidants also reduce the growth of tumors in animal models and certain human tumors (cervical and oral cancers) without affecting the growth of healthy cells.[25] Finally, it is believed that antioxidants may reduce the toxicity associated with chemotherapy.[17]

Radiation therapy causes damage to both normal and cancer cells, primarily through the production of free radicals and, to a lesser extent, through direct ionization. Some researchers suggest that if radiation-modifying agents could either selectively protect normal cells (but not tumor cells) against radiation damage or selectively enhance the effect of irradiation on tumor cells (but not healthy cells), the efficacy of radiation therapy could be improved. Thus far, however, such agents have been found to be ineffective.[25] It has also been hypothesized that antioxidants might be the most useful of the nontoxic, selective radiation-modifying agents. Researchers and clinicians are divided on this issue: Some believe that antioxidants may protect both cancerous and healthy cells, whereas others suggest antioxidants might improve the efficacy of radiation therapy by increasing tumor response and reducing some of the toxic effects on normal cells.[25]

A few case reports and small studies have reported that high doses of micronutrients, including antioxidants, have been well tolerated by patients with cancer who were receiving radiation therapy and chemotherapy. Moreover, several clinical studies have noted small decreases in treatment-related symptoms with the concurrent administration of antioxidant supplements during neoplastic treatments.[26–28] An in-depth discussion of these studies is beyond the scope of this chapter. Nevertheless, note that Simone and colleagues,[29] in their review of the literature addressing the use of antioxidant supplements during oncological therapies, summarize the results of these studies and reach two conclusions: (1) antioxidants and other nutrients do not interfere with chemotherapy or radiation, and (2) these supplements are associated with improved survival.

When providing recommendations for clinical practice, the results of prospective, randomized, controlled clinical trials (PRCT) are generally considered the gold standard for supporting evidence. Many of the studies cited by Simone and colleagues in making their recommendations are small observational studies that did not follow the same rigorous study design or include sufficient numbers of subjects to obtain an adequate sample size.

In the most recent review of antioxidant supplement use during neoplastic treatment, Lawenda et al.[30] evaluated data only from published PRCT and came to a conclusion that was the exact opposite to that reached by Simone and colleagues. Specifically, these authors stated that antioxidant supplements should not be used during radiation or chemotherapy because of the potential for tumor protection and reduced survival.

Bairati and colleagues[31] randomized 540 patients receiving radiation for head and neck cancer to receive either alpha-tocopherol (400 IU/day of dl-alpha-tocopherol), alpha-tocopherol and beta-carotene, or alpha-tocopherol and placebo supplements. The beta-carotene supplement arm was discontinued after 156 patients were enrolled due to ethical concerns regarding beta-carotene supplementation. Although a statistically significant decrease (38%) in acute, severe treatment-related impact symptoms was observed, the rate of local recurrence was greater in the supplement arm (HR = 1.37, 95% CI = 0.93–2.02). Additionally, in those patients who continued to smoke throughout treatment and follow-up, supplementation was associated with an increase in both disease recurrence (HR = 2.41, 95% CI = 1.25–4.46) and cancer-related mortality.[32] No increase in adverse outcomes for nonsmokers in any of the groups was observed.

In another study, overall survival was dramatically affected for patients with head and neck cancers who used vitamin E rinses during radiation as therapies for mucositis. During the 2 years of post-treatment follow-up, Ferreira et al.[33] noted that survival was reduced in the treatment group versus the placebo group (32% with vitamin E versus 63% with placebo; $P = .13$). Lesperance and colleagues recently reported that patients with unilateral, nonmetastatic breast cancer who took megadoses of beta-carotene, vitamin C, niacin, selenium, coenzyme Q10, and zinc experienced shorter survival and disease-free survival times when compared to matched controls.[34] Other non-controlled clinical trials have found no changes in antioxidant levels with supplementation during therapy, and no reduction in toxicity-related symptoms (i.e., mucositis, alopecia, stomatitis). Studies have also demonstrated that cancer cells readily absorb vitamins and contain higher vitamin C concentrations than the surrounding healthy tissue.[35, 36]

Guidelines for Practice

Standardized guidelines for the use of dietary supplements are lacking, although certain patient populations are known to have a higher risk for developing nutritional deficiencies (see Table 16.3). Dietary supplements, as classified under the Dietary Supplement Health and Education Act of 1994,[37] are not required to undergo the same stringent approval process required for prescription and over-the-counter medications. Put simply, makers of dietary supplements are not required to prove the safety and efficacy of these products before marketing them. To help providers determine the risk–benefit ratio for dietary supplementation, patients should be encouraged

Table 16.3 *Patients at Higher Risk of Nutritional Deficiencies*

The elderly: These patients' risk may be increased by poor dietary intake and inability to digest some vitamins and minerals.

Vegans: Vegan diets exclude animal products. Unless fortified vegan foods are consumed, such diets usually contain inadequate amounts of vitamin B_{12}, calcium, and vitamin D.

Alcoholics: Individuals who consume large amounts of alcohol are at risk of nutritional deficiencies because of poor dietary intake and compromised absorption of some vitamins.

Individuals with autoimmune conditions and malabsorption problems: Patients with conditions such as Crohn's disease, ulcerative colitis, and irritable bowel syndrome are at increased risk because the need for antioxidants may be increased with inflammation. Patients with GI pathologies may also develop malabsorption problems, which may increase their risk of nutritional deficiencies.

Lactose-intolerant individuals: Unless non-dairy foods fortified with calcium and vitamin D are consumed, supplements providing these micronutrients may be necessary to prevent deficiencies.

Individuals on low-calorie diets: Consuming a low-calorie diet (1,200 calories/day or less) may make it difficult to obtain the micronutrients in adequate levels.

Members of the following groups also have unique nutritional requirements, requiring specific tailoring of dietary supplement recommendations:
- **Pregnant and lactating women:** Requirements increased.
- **Adolescents:** Due to poor dietary intake.
- **Women of childbearing age:** Vitamin supplements can provide the folic acid (400 mcg/day) needed for the prevention of neural tube defects.

to communicate openly with all members of their healthcare team regarding their use of any dietary supplements—whether vitamins, minerals, botanicals, or anything else.[38]

For some populations, the use of dietary supplements, such as vitamins and/or minerals, can be useful in meeting their daily adequate intake recommendations and reducing their risk for disease. Table 16.4 provides an overview of commonly used biological and pharmacologic therapies by cancer patients, based on data from a variety of sources.[39–65] Considering the currently available science on this topic, individuals with cancer should refrain from using high doses of antioxidants during treatment, and relying on dietary sources of these nutrients, until the results from prospective randomized trials are available.

Table 16.4 *Overview of Commonly Used Biological and Pharmacologic Therapies by Cancer Patients*

Biologic/ Pharmacologic Therapies	Also Known as	Health Claims	Administration	Adverse Effects/ Possible Risks	Claims Scientifically Proven?
Antineoplastons	Burzynski therapies developed by Stanislaw Burzynski	Group of synthetic compounds isolated from the blood and urine believed to have immune properties to fight against tumors.	Administered as an injection; only available at the Burzynski Institute in Houston.	Rashes, gas, chills, fever, and blood pressure changes have been reported. Potential adverse effects currently being studied by NCI.	NCI clinical trials initiated in 1993, but halted in 1995 due to procedural issues. The Burzynski Research Institute continues to conduct NCI registered trials; see the NCI Web site for more information.[39]
Coenzyme Q10	Ubiquinone, ubiquinol CoQ	Cancer prevention, immunostimulation, and cardioprotection from some chemotherapies, including adriamycin/doxyrubicin.[40]	Oral supplements such as tablets, capsules, or gelcaps.	No significant side effects reported, although nausea, diarrhea, insomnia, and decreased appetite have been reported.	Case reports of breast cancer remission with intake of 90–390 mg/day.[40, 41]
Hydrazine sulfate	Hydrazine, hydrazine monosulfate	Promoted for treatment of cancer cachexia.	Oral and IV forms available.	Potential side effects: nausea, dizziness, neuropathies, and hypoglycemia.	Several large clinical trials have failed to show any clinical benefits.[40]
Omega-3 fatty acids	Fish oils, eicosapentaenoic acid (EPA)/ docosahexaenoic acid (DHA), α-linolenic acid	Epidemiologic studies report that omega-3 fatty acids may reduce the risk of breast, colon, or prostate cancers.	Consumption of fatty fish such as salmon, tuna, sardines, mackerel, or fish oil supplements; walnuts, soy foods, and flaxseeds.	Intake ≥ 3 g/day may increase risk of bleeding; GI upset and decreased blood pressure have also been reported.	Increased efficacy of doxorubicin, epirubicin, 5-FU, mitomycin C, tamoxifen, and arabinosylcytosine; rodents/cell lines; weight gain and improved quality of life with supplementation in pancreatic cancer.[42, 43]

Selenium	Selenomethionine, selenocysteine	Research suggests that selenium may decrease the risk for prostate, colon, GI, and lung cancers.	Brazil nuts, seafood, cereals, grains and supplements.	Adverse effects: GI upset and toxicity (muscle weakness, fatigue, peripheral neuropathy) in doses > 1,000 mcg/day.	Clinical trial is under way to examine selenium's role in cancer prevention. It is reportedly effective for reducing therapy-related lymphedema.[44] May decrease hair loss, abdominal pain, and anorexia in ovarian cancer patients undergoing chemotherapy.[26, 40]
Herbal/Plant-Based Therapies				
Amygdalin	Laetrile, vitamin B17, apricot pits. Amygdalin is a naturally occurring substance found in nuts, plants, and the pits of certain fruits, primarily apricots.	It was previously thought that cancer cells would metabolize amygdalin into cyanide, causing cell death. Deficiency of vitamin B17 was also thought to cause cancer.	Injectable and oral forms available. Not approved for use in the United States. Popular in Mexico.	Amygdalin is metabolized to cyanide, prunasin, and benzaldehyde. Its oral administration has resulted in cyanide toxicity, coma, and death. Additional adverse effects reported include nausea, vomiting, headache, and mental obtundation.	Found to be ineffective in clinical trial.[40, 45]

(continues)

Table 16.4 *Overview of Commonly Used Biological and Pharmacologic Therapies by Cancer Patients, Continued*

Herbal/Plant-Based Therapies	Also Known as	Health Claims	Administration	Adverse Effects/Possible Risks	Claims Scientifically Proven?
Astragalus	*Astragalus membranaceus*, Huang Chi, milk vetch	Useful as a chemoprotective and hepatoprotective agent, and as an immunostimulant[40]	Oral and IV forms available.	No adverse effects reported. May decrease immunosuppression following treatment with cyclophosphamide. May antagonize the effect of immuno-suppressants such as cyclosporine and tacrolimus.	Clinical trial in patients with end-stage renal disease found increased interleukin 2 (IL-2) levels with use of IV astragalus compared to placebo.[47] A Chinese herbal product that contained astragalus increased the effectiveness of platinum-based chemotherapy for advanced non-small-cell lung cancer in a meta-analysis, although many studies were of low quality.[47]
ECGC (green tea)	*Camellia sinensis*, green tea extract, green tea polyphenols	The primary active ingredient is epigallo-catechin-3-gallate (EGCG), which accounts for 40% of total polyphenol content. EGCG may reduce risk for prostate, breast, esophageal, lung pancreatic, bladder, and skin cancers, as EGCG has been shown to modulate vascular endothelial growth *(continues)*	Primarily consumed as a dietary beverage.	Considered safe. Tannins may decrease absorption and the bioavailability of iron, codeine, and atropine. Insomnia, irritability, and anxiety can result from the beverage's caffeine content.	Green tea consumption is associated with decreased risk for a variety of cancers. Studies are currently under way to assess the effectiveness of green tea extracts in the treatment of cancers.

		factor, induce apoptosis, and stimulate tumor antiangiogenesis.[40]			
Essiac	Tea consisting of four botanicals: burdock root, powdered sheep sorrel root, powdered slippery elm bark, and powdered rhubarb root	Promoters purport the tea boosts the immune system, treats cancer, and acts as a general tonic.	Consumed as a tea.	Patients with renal or hepatic insufficiency should avoid this product. Adverse effects include nausea/vomiting, diarrhea, contact dermatitis, and anaphylaxis.	No scientific data to support claims.
Flaxseed and flaxseed Oil	*Linum usitatissimum*	Lignan properties possess possible estrogen-receptor (ER) agonist/antagonist properties, thereby reducing risk for breast cancer.	Flaxseeds or flaxseed oil.	Early evidence suggests that the α-linolenic acid component of flaxseed may be associated with increased risk for prostate cancer. Women with history of ER-positive breast cancer/other hormonal conditions should use these products with caution due to their potential phytoestrogenic effects. Side effects may include mild GI distress, and anaphylaxis has been reported. May increase bleeding time.	Pilot data suggest consumption reduces PSA levels and suggest reduced cellular proliferation.[40,48]

(continues)

Table 16.4 *Overview of Commonly Used Biological and Pharmacologic Therapies by Cancer Patients, Continued*

Herbal/Plant-Based Therapies	Also Known as	Health Claims	Administration	Adverse Effects/Possible Risks	Claims Scientifically Proven?
Ginger	*Zingiber officinale,* Ginger root	Used for treatment of nausea/vomiting and other GI symptoms. Thought to stimulate the flow of saliva, gastric secretions, and bile; to inhibit gastric contractions; and to improve intestinal peristalsis.	Available as a dietary supplement, tea, ginger candies, and ginger ale.	Adverse effects include heartburn, dermatitits, CNS depression, and arrhythmias with overdoses. May also increase the risk of bleeding.	NCCAM is currently recruiting patients for a randomized phase II/III trial to determine the effectiveness of antiemetic drugs with or without ginger in treating nausea in patients receiving chemotherapy.
Indole-3-carbinol	I3C, indole-3-methanol	I3C is a specific compound found in cruciferous vegetables (broccoli, kale, cabbage, Brussels sprouts) that is known to stimulate detoxifying enzymes in the gut and liver. It may decrease the risk for breast and prostate cancers by arresting the cell cycle for, and promoting apoptosis of, cancer cells.	Available in food sources and as an oral dietary supplement. Supplementation is needed to consume the amounts shown to be beneficial in clinical studies (300 mg/day).[49]	Evidence suggests that I3C may promote tumor growth in animals exposed to carcinogens. Generally well tolerated.	NCCAM has completed a phase I trial evaluating I3C and breast cancer; the results have not yet been published. I3C may decrease the risk for ER-sensitive breast cancer,[49] and it may prevent progression of precancerous cervical lesions.[50] I3C has been shown to act synergistically with tamoxifen.[51] Data from animal studies are conflicting regarding the benefits; for this reason, use of I3C supplements is not recommended.

Maitake mushrooms	*Grifola frondosa;* active component thought to be beta-glucan polysaccharide; king of mushrooms, dancing mushrooms, cloud mushrooms	Sold as immune stimulant.	Available in capsules, tables, or liquid extract, or as raw mushrooms.	Have not been thoroughly studied in humans and side effects are not well known. May lower blood sugar and blood pressure levels.	Have been shown to enhance bone marrow colony formation and to reduce doxorubicin toxicity in vitro. A small, noncontrolled study found tumor regression or significant improvement in symptoms in 50% of patients using Maitake extract.[5,52]
Melatonin	N-acetyl-methoxytryptamine, pineal hormone	May be beneficial for cancer patients through antioxidant, anti-inflammatory, immune-enhancing, hormonal, antiangiogenic, apoptotic, or direct cytotoxic properties.	Available in oral, IV, or injectable (into muscle) doses.	Generally regarded as safe for short-term use. Reported side effects include irritability, fatigue, dizziness, and decreased prothrombin time.	Human trials found IV or injectable melatonin decreased incidence of neuropathies, stomatitis, cachexia, and thrombocytopenia with various chemotherapy agents.[54,55] Melatonin suppresses ER gene, modulates several estrogen-dependent regulatory proteins and pro-oncogenes, inhibits cell proliferation, and impairs the metastatic capacity of MCF-7 human breast cancer cells.[56] Further studies are needed to better elucidate its efficacy.

(continues)

Table 16.4 *Overview of Commonly Used Biological and Pharmacologic Therapies by Cancer Patients, Continued*

Herbal/Plant-Based Therapies	Also Known as	Health Claims	Administration	Adverse Effects/ Possible Risks	Claims Scientifically Proven?
Milk thistle (MT)	*Silybum marianum*, holy thistle, lady's thistle	Advertised to reduce drug-induced hepatotoxicity and to prevent cancer. Potential mechanism of action: provides hepatocellular protection by stabilizing hepatic cell membranes, thereby preventing liver toxins from penetrating the outer cellular membrane. Other studies report that flavonoids in milk thistle produce anticancer effects by inducing G1 and S phase arrest in cells.[57]	Available as a dietary supplement.	Inhibits cytochrome p450 3A4; as a consequence, increased levels of medications metabolized via this route may occur.[17] Adverse effects include GI upset, laxative effects, and allergic reactions.	In vitro studies show silibinin, a component of milk thistle, is protective against the nephrotoxicity associated with cisplatin and vincristine; dose-dependent inhibition of ovarian and breast cancer cell growth occurred in conjunction with use of silybin (primarily as a flavonoid in methotrexate MT should be milk thistle instead of methotrexate) and doxorubicin.[40,58]
Shark cartilage (SC)	Carticin, Cartilade, BeneFin, Neovastat (highly purified form not available to the general public)	Three principal mechanisms of action have been proposed to explain how SC prevents/treats cancer: (1) SC kills cancer cells directly; (2) it possesses immunostimulatory *(continues)*	Oral forms as extracts of shark cartilage are available.	SC may be contraindicated in patients with liver disease. Adverse effects include nausea, vomiting, diarrhea, anorexia, dyspepsia, and constipation. *(continues)*	Results from clinical trials are inconclusive. Small, randomized phase I/II trials report longer survival in patients with refractory renal cancer and non-small-cell lung cancer.[60,61] Patients with advanced cancers *(continues)*

	properties; or (3) it prevents formation of new blood vessels that allow tumors to grow in an unrestricted manner.[59]		Commercially available SC supplements may contain variable amounts of SC. Many contain a high percentage of fillers.		experienced no benefits with SC supplements.[62] NCCAM trials have been completed, but the results have not been published. Neovastat has shown efficacy against psoriasis through its antiangiogenic effect.[63]
Soy	*Glycine max,* soya, tofu, miso, tempeh	Decreased risk for breast, colon, prostate, and endometrial cancers due to the presence of phytoestrogens and other anticarcinogenic phytochemicals (isoflavones, saponins, phytates, phytosterols, and protease inhibitors).	Soybeans, soy flour, soy milk, tofu, soy protein isolate, soy oil.	Allergic response, flatulence.	Not clear from laboratory studies if the isoflavones in soy stimulate or block the effects of estrogen. Genistein inhibits the growth of androgen-dependent and -independent human prostate cancer cell lines.[64]
St. John's wort	*Hypericum perforatum,* goat weed, Klamath weed	Used for depression and sleep disorders.	Flowering tops used in teas; OTC supplements available.	Headache, nausea, abdominal discomfort, constipation.	May alter chemotherapy levels due to alterations in metabolism, resulting in increased toxicity and reduced efficacy, particularly with irinotecan[15] and possibly cyclophosphamide, paclitaxel, and etoposide.

(continues)

Table 16.4 *Overview of Commonly Used Biological and Pharmacologic Therapies by Cancer Patients, Continued*

Herbal/Plant-Based Therapies	Also Known as	Health Claims	Administration	Adverse Effects/Possible Risks	Claims Scientifically Proven?
Turmeric/curcumin	*Curcuma longa,* Indian saffron, curcumin	Purported to prevent cancer, infections, and inflammation. Its mechanism of action has not been clearly elucidated; its anti-inflammatory action may be due to inhibition of leukotrienes. Also acts as an antioxidant and free-radical scavenger.	Used as a spice for seasoning foods or available as an oral dietary supplement. Bioavailability is 60–65%.	Potentially inhibits antitumor effects of some chemotherapies such as cyclo-phosphamide (in treatment of breast cancer).[65] Contraindicated for patients with GI disorders, bile duct obstruction. and gallstones. Adverse effects include allergic response, convulsions, cyanosis, GI distress, nausea/vomiting, and death. Use with anticoagulants may increase risk of bleeding.	In vitro and animal studies suggest turmeric possesses antiproliferative and preventive anticarcinogenic properties. Human studies are lacking.

Table 16.5 provides a summary of the NIH 2006 State-of-the-Science Conference Statement on Multivitamins[38]; Table 16.6 (page 430) describes the potential risks associated with the use of multivitamin/mineral supplements. Table 16.7 (page 431) provides suggestions for the evaluation of supplements before purchasing.

Mind–Body Practices

Once diagnosed, many individuals with cancer experience anxiety, depression, and other mood disturbances due to fear of death, disfigurement from oncologic interventions, disruption of relationships, fatigue, and overall deterioration in quality of life. Depression is common in patients with cancer, though this condition often goes undiagnosed. Mind–body therapies include a variety of techniques designed to enhance the mind's capacity to affect bodily function and symptoms. Some techniques used to reduce anxiety and depression were considered complementary or alternative therapies in the past, but have since become integrated into conventional cancer care (e.g., patient support groups and cognitive-behavioral therapy). Clinical services in a number of oncology programs around the country have evolved to offer techniques such as acupuncture, massage, Reiki, therapeutic touch,

Table 16.5 *National Institutes of Health 2006 State-of-the-Science Conference Statement on Multivitamins*

1. Multivitamins may not be as "safe" as the public thinks they are.
2. Given that the vitamin levels in multivitamins often exceed the daily recommended intake and that levels of vitamins are increased in fortified foods, there is higher likelihood for adverse effects.
3. The Dietary Supplement Health and Education Act (DSHEA 1994) may contribute to points 1 and 2, and should be revised.
4. Randomized controlled trials on multivitamin use for the prevention of chronic disease have many deficits and are few in number.
5. Many of the studies do not provide strong evidence for beneficial health-related effects of supplements taken as single agents, in pairs, or in combinations of three or more.
6. Overall conclusion: "There is insufficient evidence to recommend for or against the use of multivitamins by the American public to prevent chronic disease."

Source: Huang HY, Caballero B, Chang S, et al. The efficacy and safety of multivitamin and mineral supplement use to prevent cancer and chronic disease in adults: A systematic review for a National Institutes of Health State-of-the-Science Conference. *Ann Intern Med.* 2006;145:364–371.

Table 16.6   *Risks Associated with Multivitamin and Mineral Supplements*

• Supplementation with beta-carotene with or without vitamin A increases the incidence of lung cancer in persons with asbestos exposure or in smokers.
• Vitamin A supplementation moderately increases serum triglyceride levels.
• Calcium supplementation may increase the risk of kidney stones.
• Vitamin E supplementation may increase the risk for all-cause mortality.
• Recent trials have found an increased risk of advanced and fatal prostate cancer among men taking multivitamins compared with never users. Additionally, the risk of advanced prostate cancer and prostate cancer mortality associated with heavy multivitamin use was highest in men who reported concomitant use of selenium, beta-carotene, or zinc supplements—particularly among men with a family history.

Sources: Watkins ML, Erickson JD, Thun MJ, et al. Multivitamin use and mortality in a large prospective study. *Am J Epidemiol.* 2000;152:149–162; Stevens VL, McCullough ML, Diver WR, et al. Use of multivitamins and prostate cancer mortality in a large cohort of US men. *Cancer Causes Control.* 2005;16:643–650; Lawson KA, Wright ME, Subar A, et al. Multivitamin use and risk of prostate cancer in the National Institutes of Health-AARP Diet and Health Study. *J Natl Cancer Inst.* 2007;99:754–764; Alpha-Tocopherol BCCPSG. The effect of vitamin E and beta carotene on the incidence of lung cancer and other cancers in male smokers. *N Engl J Med.* 1994;330(15):1029–1035; Evidence Report/Technology Assessment. Number 139. Multivitamin/mineral supplements and prevention of chronic disease. Available at http://www.ahrq.gov/downloads/pub/evidence/pdf/multivit/multivitpdf. Accessed August 11, 2008; Jackson RD, LaCroix AZ, Gass M, et al. Calcium plus vitamin D supplementation and the risk of fractures. *N Engl J Med.* 2006;354:669–683.

meditation, and guided imagery; yoga, tai chi, and qi gong are also being offered onsite. These therapies and a number of others—including music therapy, art therapy, and prayer—are some of the most common mind–body practices pursued by cancer patients and survivors.

Mind–body interventions such as acupuncture, massage therapy, and music therapy have been studied as treatments for mood disturbance. Relaxation techniques, guided imagery, and meditation have also been investigated in several randomized, controlled trials that showed they improved anxiety, depression, and other symptoms of distress.[66–69] In a meta-analysis of 116 studies, Devine and Westlake[70] reported that mind–body modalities could reduce anxiety, depression, and mood disturbances in cancer patients. Additionally, Speca and colleagues found that a seven-week mindfulness-based stress reduction program significantly improved symptoms of stress and mood disturbances in 109 patients with cancer.[67]

Other mind–body therapies may reduce stress and pain. Hypnosis was associated with a reduction in postsurgical pain and stress in studies involving women undergoing excisional breast biopsies or children undergoing

Table 16.7   *Assessing Multivitamin/Mineral Supplements*

Claims of "High Potency"

Claims of high potency do not necessarily result in a superior product. The FDA allows multivitamin/mineral supplement (MVM) manufacturers to use this claim if at least two-thirds of their additives have 100% of the Daily Value (DV). Thus some products will increase their provision of vitamin C or the B vitamins while containing only small amounts of other nutrients, such as magnesium, zinc, and chromium. Many people think that a "high-potency" supplement contains significantly greater amounts of nutrients than are found in a general MVM. Carefully reading the label may show that 100% of the DV for vitamins is provided, but the supplement may not contain any minerals or such small amounts that the supplement is really worthless. Choosing a supplement that contains 100% of the RDA for both vitamins and minerals is generally a good choice. High-potency supplements generally cost more without providing significant additional benefits.

Serving Size

It is important to evaluate the serving size necessary to obtain 100% of the DV. Does 1 tablet meet these needs, or are more tablets needed? Many consumers take only 1 tablet when the serving size may require 3 or 4 tablets.

Evaluating Specific Nutrients

Vitamin A

Avoid supplements with 100% of the vitamin A provision from synthetic vitamin A (vitamin A palmitate, vitamin A acetate, or retinol palmalate) to avoid increased risks for hip fractures. (Choose supplements that provide some percentage of the vitamin A as beta-carotene). Many MVM supplements contain vitamin A as beta-carotene. While beta-carotene is not toxic and does not cause birth defects, doses greater than 33,000 IU/day may increase the risk for cancer in people who smoke. Consumption of foods with rich beta-carotene content is recommended over taking high doses of beta-carotene from a supplement. Supplements containing a mixture of carotenoids (beta-carotene *plus* zeaxnthin, astaxantin, lutein, lycopene, alpha-, or gamma-carotenes) may provide additional benefits while avoiding overloading on just one type of nutrient.

Vitamin C

The RDA for vitamin C is 75 mg/day for women, 90 mg/day for men, and an additional 35 mg/day for people who smoke. However, 250–500 mg/day is often needed to obtain saturation of tissue levels. Because most of the population does not consume at least 5 to 9 servings of fruits and vegetables per day (the recommended intake), selecting a vitamin supplement with at least 100% of the RDA and increasing fruit and vegetable intake should enable individuals to achieve optimal tissue levels. A level of 1,000–3,000 mg/day, from a separate vitamin C supplement, may facilitate recovering from a cold faster, but only when started with the first signs of a cold. Supplements claiming superiority because they contain certain types of vitamin C, such as EsterC, do not provide any greater benefits.

(continues)

Table 16.7 *Assessing Multivitamin/Mineral Supplements, Continued*

Vitamin D

Vitamin D is available as cholecalciferol (D_3) and ergocalciferol (D_2). D_3 is the preferred form of vitamin D, as it can be easily used by the body and does not require additional hydroxylation. Ergocalciferol (D_2) is the form added to most foods, such as cereals and milk, but it requires the additional hydroxylation step by the kidneys and is not the most bioavailable form of vitamin D. Also, D_3 may increase blood levels of usable vitamin D for a longer period of time than does D_2; D_2 is 33% less potent than D_3. One instance in which dietitians may recommend D_2 instead of D_3 is for a strict vegetarian or vegan patient. D_2 is made from yeast, whereas D_3 is made from lanolin or fish oil.

Vitamin E

Vitamin E supplements that contain a mixture of the four tocopherols and four tocotrienols may be the best options. Although eight forms of vitamin E exists, alpha-tocopherol (the natural form is designated by D-alpha-tocopherol on the label) is the most common form found in the body as well as dietary supplements. In general, synthetic vitamin E, which is less biologically active and less expensive that the natural version, is designated by DL-alpha-tocopherol on the label. Most multivitamin supplements contain this type.

Vitamin B$_{12}$

Approximately 10–30% of people older than age 50 may malabsorb the vitamin B_{12} when it is bound in food. Taking a daily MVM supplement containing at least 25 mcg of vitamin B_{12} is recommended for the prevention of megaloblastic anemia in this population. For individuals younger than age 50, obtaining the RDA (6 mcg/day) is recommended.

Thiamin (Vitamin B1), Riboflavin (Vitamin B2), Niacin, and Vitamin B$_6$

Choosing a MVM supplement based on the amount of thiamin, riboflavin, niacin, and vitamin B_6 is not necessary. While consuming the higher amounts of these nutrients found in many supplements is generally safe, extremely high doses of niacin (500 mg) and vitamin B_6 (250 mg) may be harmful. Doses greater than the RDA for niacin should be taken only under a physician's care. Doses of vitamin B_6 greater than 250 mg/day may result in toxicity.

Calcium

A number of calcium supplements are available (e.g., chewables, tablets, liquids, powders). When recommending supplements, consideration should be given to the calcium source—that is, whether calcium carbonate or citrate is preferred. Also, the serving size should be taken into account. Additionally, it must be determined whether concurrent supplementation with vitamin D and magnesium be desirable. Calcium citrate does not require the presence of food in the GI tract to be absorbed; calcium carbonate does. Calcium carbonate also tends to induce constipation to a greater degree.

Zinc

Excess intake of zinc can cause copper depletion. A zinc-copper ratio of 10:1 is recommended. The RDA for zinc is 15 mg/day, and healthy individuals should avoid taking supplements containing greater amounts.

(continues)

Table 16.7   *Assessing Multivitamin/Mineral Supplements, Continued*

Selenium

Toxicity may potentially occur with selenium supplementation, as this nutrient has a narrow therapeutic range. The usual daily dose is 200 mcg. The Institute of Medicine has set the upper intake level at 400 mcg/day. Supplementation may be beneficial in some individuals, especially those with the following medical conditions: HIV, cancer (especially prostate, lung, colorectal, and liver), heart disease, and rheumatoid arthritis.

Fish Oil Supplements

The American Heart Association advises individuals with cardiovascular disease (CVD) to consume 1 g/day of eicosapentaenoic acid (EPA) plus docosahexaenoic acid (DHA), either from consumption of oily fish or as a dietary supplement under a physician's supervision. Patients who need to lower serum triglycerides may take 2 to 4 g/day of EPA + DHA supplements under a physician's care. To obtain the levels outlined above, the amount of both EPA and DHA per serving on the label should be calculated; the goal is to consume 1,000 mg/day of EPA + DHA.

Flaxseeds

Prospective studies have evaluated the relationship between alpha-linolenic acid intake and CVD; each 1 g/day increase in dietary ALA intake has been associated with a 16% reduction in the risk of CVD. Flaxseed may also decrease C-reactive protein (CRP) levels. However, the conversion of alpha-linolenic acid, which is obtained from plant sources such as freshly ground flaxseeds, canola oil, and walnuts, is thought to be predicated on the levels of the omega-6 fatty acid linoleic acid (ALA) because ALA and the omega-6 fatty acids compete for rate-limiting enzymatic processes. Therefore, this process is not considered an efficient process; estimates of the rate of conversion range from 2% to 15%. To obtain the optimal benefits associated with omega-3 fatty acid consumption, eating cold-water fish at least 2 times per week or using fish oil supplements daily is recommended.

Flaxseed Oil: One meta-analysis found an association between either flaxseed oil intake or high blood levels of alpha-linolenic acid and increased risk of prostate cancer. Whether this relationship reflects the removal of the lignans in flaxseed, which are thought to be a major component of its anticancer effects, is unclear. Most brands of flaxseed oil do not contain lignans. Until we know more about the association between flaxseed oil and risk of prostate cancer, men should refrain from consuming flax oil supplements or consume only oils fortified with lignans.

bone marrow aspiration or lumbar puncture procedures.[71–73] Hypnosis has also reportedly decreased oral pain due to mucositis in patients who underwent bone marrow transplant.[74] Moreover, the NIH Technology Assessment Panel found good evidence that hypnosis helps in alleviating cancer-related pain. Hypnosis is efficacious for treating anticipatory nausea for both children and adults[75]; reductions in postoperative nausea and vomiting have also been reported with use of this technique.[76]

Given the current level of evidence and the risk–benefit factor, mind–body practices should be explored with appropriate patients. Patients with mood disturbances will require an initial evaluation to uncover any problems that may necessitate an immediate psychiatric referral, such as panic attack or suicidal ideation, before complementary therapies are considered. Mind–body techniques can help these patients cope with distressful situations, such as learning the news of cancer diagnosis or recurrence. In addition, complementary therapies avoid the stigma that patients sometimes associate with psychotherapy and psychotropic mediations, and because of their noninvasive approach they (with the exception of certain dietary supplements) are quite safe. For patients with longstanding symptoms and established diagnoses of general anxiety or major depression, pharmacologic interventions remain the most effective measures. Even with these patients, however, discussions involving the use of mind–body practices can identify individuals who may be interested in and could benefit from these modalities. Mind–body techniques and massage therapies are appropriate modalities assuming they are provided by licensed, competent practitioners such as those employed in many cancer programs throughout North America. Using these therapies as complementary techniques or integrating them into conventional cancer care can also facilitate reduction of the amount of medications required.

Manipulative and Body-Based Practices

The NIH domain of manipulative and body-based practices includes massage, physical therapy, and chiropractic and/or osteopathic manipulation.[6] Manipulative and body-based practices involve manipulation of bones, joints, soft tissues, and the circulatory and lymphatic systems. Many of these practices arose from ancient traditional systems such as Oriental medicine; other practices, such as chiropractic and osteopathic manipulation, are more recent developments.

The diagnosis of cancer can prove overwhelming for the patient, as can the multitude of anticancer treatments' potential impact-symptoms, and the alterations in body image that can result from surgery and other forms of treatment. Isolation, fear of recurrence, and threat of death can also weigh heavily on the patient's psyche. Available evidence indicates that massage provides benefits such as reduction of anxiety and stress, fatigue, pain, nausea, and improvements in sleep and immune parameters, although many of these studies were small and further research is needed.[77] A variety of massage types—Swedish, Thai, and shiatsu, to name a few—are available in cancer centers, in health spas, and through privately licensed therapists. Other body-work therapies, such as yoga, tai chi, Reiki, and Pilates, are also widely available, often in the same types of facilities.

While many providers of manipulative and body-based therapies have formal training and may be certified or licensed, considerable variation in the training exists. Given this fact, both patients and practitioners should be familiar with the competency of practitioners they use personally or as referrals. It is always prudent to look for a practitioner who is licensed on the state level (if such licensing is available) or for a practitioner who is affiliated with a reliable organization or facility. For individuals with cancer, it is also preferable to find someone familiar with cancer and cancer therapy.

Energy Therapies

The NIH domain of energy therapies includes two types of energy fields: veritable and putative.[6] Veritable energy utilizes mechanical vibrations and electromagnetic forces (such as visible light, monochromatic radiation such as laser beams, magnetism, and rays from other areas of the electromagnetic spectrum).[6] Putative energy fields are based on the theory that humans have a vital life force known as *qi* (in Chinese medicine), *ki* (in Japanese medicine), or *doshas* (in Ayurvedic medicine). Practitioners of energy medicine believe that imbalances in these life forces—where the mind, body, and emotions combine to form the energy fields—result in illness. Reiki, qi gong, acupuncture, homeopathy, healing or therapeutic touch, and intercessory prayer are examples of techniques that seek to access putative energy fields. Many energy practitioners believe that these modalities can harness an individual's energy bio-fields, thereby promoting balance and restoration of health. While the use of energy therapies is considered the most nebulous of the NCCAM domains due to the lack of critical evidence supporting it, the use of energy therapies continues to increase steadily.[6]

Therapeutic touch, healing touch, and Reiki are hand-mediated CAM modalities often used interchangeably; in all of these techniques, the hands are used to direct energy fields in and around the body to facilitate healing.[6] Reiki, an ancient energetic healing practice, is a Japanese term meaning "universal life force."[78] Energy therapies are being used more often by healthcare practitioners and consumers as noninvasive interventions to obtain a number of positive outcomes, including relaxation, anxiety and stress reduction, alleviation of pain, wound healing, and improvements in sense of well-being in addition to healing.[76]

Several small studies have found favorable outcomes with therapeutic touch. A meta-analysis, which assessed 11 controlled trials investigating the use of this modality, found positive outcomes in 7 studies; 3 showed no effect; and 1 study found that members of the control group healed more quickly than members of the therapeutic touch group.[79]

Whole Medical Systems

Whole medical systems have evolved based on a variety of theories and practices from around the world. Although these systems embody different components, they share a common belief—namely, that the individual's body has the capacity to heal itself. In addition to systems such as traditional Chinese and Ayurvedic medicine, practices such as homeopathic and naturopathic medicine are considered whole medical systems. Traditional Chinese medicine (TCM) has also evolved, as other Asian countries such as Korea and Japan have developed their own systems. Practitioners utilizing these approaches to healing focus on promoting the "internal natural forces to promote integration of state and mind."[6]

According to practitioners of TCM, which dates back to 200 BCE, the body consists of a balance between two opposing forces, *yin* and *yang*. Yin comprises cold, slow, or passive principles, whereas yang exhibits hot, excited, or active principles.[6] TCM practitioners believe that good health can be achieved when yin and yang are in harmony; in contrast, disease arises when an imbalance occurs between the two. Additionally, it is thought that disease arises when an obstruction occurs in the flow of *qi* (also known as vital energy) and/or the circulatory pathways (known as meridians).[6] Acupuncture, herbal remedies, and massage are therapeutic modalities used to release obstructions and promote the flow of qi to regain yin and yang balance and health.

Ayurvedic medicine, which dates back more than 5,000 years, is a natural medicine system developed in India that suggests the mind, body, and spirit play equal roles in promoting health and wellness.[6] Nutrition, physical activity, meditation, relaxation therapies, massage, and herbal products are a few of the modalities utilized in achieving harmony and health in Ayurvedic practice. Five elements found in nature—earth, water, fire, air, and ether—represent the core qualities found in the body. Ayurveda categorizes qualities from these elements, also known as life forces, into three biologic humors called *doshas*. The three doshas have the following characteristics:[80]

- *Vata dosha* is a combination of air and space. It controls movement and basic bodily functions such as cellular division, breathing, and circulation. Individuals where vata doshas are dominant are considered thin, fast, and quick-thinking, and are susceptible to anxiety, fatigue, impatience, and other ailments.

- *Pitta dosha* is a combination of fire and water. It controls hormones and the digestive system. Individuals with pitta dosha dominance are thought to have fiery personalities and oily skin, and suffer from acne, ulcers, heart disease, and heartburn.

- *Kapha dosha* is a combination of water and earth. It controls growth, immunity, and strength. Individuals with kapha-dominant doshas are thought to be calm and stubborn, and are susceptible to weight gain, diabetes, and elevated cholesterol levels.

According to Ayurvedic medicine, all three doshas are found in a unique combination in each individual. The goals of Ayurvedic medicine are to achieve a balance between the doshas, given that manifestations of disease are though to result from imbalances; various foods and emotions are also thought to disrupt the doshas' balance. Completion of the Ayurvedic mind–body questionnaire determines one's personal dosha. In general, Ayurvedic practitioners attempt to reduce the dosha qualities that are in excess and to increase those qualities that are present in insufficient amounts. Eating guidelines are available not only to adjust dosha activities but also to aid in optimizing digestion and elimination.[80]

Herbal products are often used to achieve dosha balance. Several tested Ayurvedic herbal products manufactured in Asia have been found to contain potentially harmful levels of lead, mercury, and/or arsenic.[81, 82] Additionally, some Ayurvedic practices—such as colonic cleansings and enemas—are considered controversial and potentially unsafe.

Because of the holistic nature and application of these diverse modalities, it has proven difficult to evaluate the efficacy of any of the whole medical systems, such as TCM and Ayurvedic medicine, for individuals with cancer; the challenge arises because trials have tended to focus on individual components of the various systems, rather than on the whole system of care. Until evidence from clinical trials is available, patients should discuss use of these systems (in part or as a whole) with knowledgeable practitioners to determine the risk–benefit ratio for their health promotion.

Safety and Efficacy

The scientific jury is still out on the risk and benefits for some complementary and alternative therapies. Recently, the Society for Integrative Oncology published a set of integrative oncology practice guidelines.[83] Cassileth and Deng also recently published evidence-based clinical practice guidelines for complementary therapies and integrative oncology in lung cancer.[84]

Many cancer centers have established integrative medicine programs offering the best-studied, most-efficacious therapies. These programs serve as reliable resources and help provide guidance on CAM modalities. In addition, many centers are engaged in research to determine the safety and efficacy of less-studied modalities or therapies where the risk–benefit ratio is still in question. Table 16.8 provides reliable sources for CAM information.

Becoming a CAM Practitioner

According to the National Cancer Institute, 88% of all U.S. cancer centers had a CAM practitioner and 54% offered CAM programs in 1999.[39] Given the frequency of CAM use by individuals with cancer, and their reported hesitancy to discuss this use with their healthcare team, it is essential to

Table 16.8 *Internet Resources for Complementary and Alternative Medicine*

American Cancer Society	http://www.cancer.org
Memorial Sloan Kettering Cancer Center	http://www.mskcc.org/mskcc/html/11570.cfm
University of Texas M. D. Anderson Cancer Center	http://www.mdanderson.org/CIMER
National Cancer Institute	http://www.cancer.gov
National Center of Complementary and Alternative Medicine	http://nccam.nih.gov
Natural Medicines Comprehensive Database (subscription website)	http://www.naturaldatabase.com

incorporate questions on CAM use when discussing medical issues, health habits, and lifestyle history. Because advice on diet, dietary supplement use, and other CAM therapies can come from many different places, such as friends, family and Web sites, healthcare practitioners taking care of individuals with cancer need to open up a dialog with patients on this issue and be prepared to offer solid, evidence-based advice. Of course, this will happen only if oncology practitioners take the time and energy to learn about CAM and integrated therapies, and if they develop some appreciation for their risks and benefits in the oncology setting.

Healthcare practitioners who wish to integrate CAM therapies into their practice must think of the patient as a "whole person" if the CAM techniques are to have the optimal impact. Integration of CAM therapies into practice not only includes making recommendations for foods or dietary supplements such as vitamins or botanicals use, but also involves evaluating the individual's physical activity, sleep cycle, level of stress, emotional state, and functional abilities, in addition to the traditional practice of soliciting information about past and current medical status. Table 16.9 outlines tips for success in recognizing and using CAM in patients with cancer.

Practice must be based on the best evidence available. As described in this chapter, the strength of evidence supporting the use of CAM modalities to alleviate symptoms related to oncologic therapies such as nausea, pain, anxiety, insomnia, quality of life, and other impact-symptoms is increasing; therefore, CAM modalities should be integrated into oncological care when and where appropriate. Utilization of other, unsubstantiated modalities should be weighed based on the risk–benefit ratio before pursuing this line of treatment. Documenting outcomes associated with any technique's use is needed to determine its efficacy and safety.

Table 16.9　*CAM Practitioner Tips for Success*

• Elicit information regarding CAM use
• Serve as a reliable resource for CAM information
• Practice evidence-based medicine
• Practice patient-centered nutrition counseling using a nonjudgmental approach
• Obtain advanced-level skills
• Establish a network; engage in a dialog with other clinicians about CAM
• Monitor outcomes; help each patient achieve his or her goals

SUMMARY

Integrative oncology is a growing field that promotes the use of complementary and alternative therapies for which high-quality evidence supports their inclusion as adjunct modalities to traditional oncologic care. The use of CAM therapies is extremely common in both the U.S. population as a whole and the cancer survivor population. Many patients seek out CAM therapies to address the physical and emotional symptoms associated with cancer. Healthcare practitioners must elicit information regarding the use of such modalities if they are to provide appropriate guidance for using such therapies—not only in terms of how to obtain the optimal benefits, but also regarding how to avoid any potential adverse effects. As the realm of integrative oncology expands, clinicians should be well versed in the risks and benefits of CAM therapies.

Strong evidence exists for recommending acupuncture as a complementary therapy when both pain and nausea and vomiting are poorly controlled.[83] Quality-of-life measures can be improved with mind–body practices and with energy therapies. While not considered formal CAM therapies, the adoption of a healthy lifestyle including a healthy diet, appropriate levels of physical activity, and avoidance of tobacco use and alcohol abuse must be addressed in cancer prevention. The evidence supporting the integration of such therapies into clinical practice is evolving, and much research is still needed. Nevertheless, a significant body of evidence is accruing that supports the use of many CAM therapies, including their integration into oncological supportive care services on a routine basis.

REFERENCES

1. Tindle HA, David RB, Phillips RS, Eisenberg DM. Trends in the use of complementary and alternative medicine by U.S. adults. *Altern Ther Health Med.* 2005; 11:42–49.
2. Barnes PM, Powell-Griner E, McFann K, Nahin RL. Complementary and alternative medicine use among adults: United States, 2002. *CDC Advance Data Report* #343. 2004.
3. Adams M, Jewel AP. The use of complementary and alternative medicine by cancer patients. *Intl Semin Surg Oncol.* 2007;4(10):4–10.
4. Vapiwala N, Mick R, Hampshire MK, et al. Patient initiation of complementary and alternative medical therapies (CAM) following cancer diagnosis. *Cancer J.* 2006;12(6):467–474.
5. Eisenberg DM, Davis RB, Ettner SL, et al. Trends in alternative medicine use in the United States, 1990–1997: Results of a follow-up national survey. *JAMA.* 1998; 280(18):1569–1575.
6. National Center for Complementary and Alternative Medicine. http://nccam.nih.gov. Accessed February 12, 2008.

7. Velicer CM, Ulrich CRM. Vitamin and mineral supplement use among US adults after cancer diagnosis: A systematic review. *J Clin Oncol.* 2008;26:665–673.

8. American Cancer Society. http://www.cancer.org. Accessed February 14, 2008.

9. American Institute for Cancer Research. http://www.aicr.org. Assessed February 14, 2008.

10. National Cancer Institute. *Eating hints for cancer patients: Before, during, and after treatment.* Washington, DC: US Department of Health and Human Services; 2006.

11. Watkins ML, Erickson JD, Thun MJ, et al. Multivitamin use and mortality in a large prospective study. *Am J Epidemiol.* 2000;152:149–162.

12. Stevens VL, McCullough ML, Diver WR, et al. Use of multivitamins and prostate cancer mortality in a large cohort of US men. *Cancer Causes Control.* 2005;16:643–650.

13. Lawson KA, Wright ME, Subar A, et al. Multivitamin use and risk of prostate cancer in the National Institutes of Health–AARP diet and health study. *J Natl Cancer Inst.* 2007;99:754–764.

14. Dong LM, Kristal AR, Peters U, et al. Dietary supplement use and risk of neoplastic progression in esophageal adenocarcinoma: A prospective study. *Nutr Cancer.* 2008;60(1):39–48.

15. Mathijssen RH, Verweij J, de Bruijn P, et al. Effects of St. John's wort on irinotecan metabolism. *J Natl Cancer Inst.* 2002;94:1247–1249.

16. Meijerman I, Beijnen JH, Schellens JHM. Herb–drug interactions in oncology: Focus on mechanisms of induction. *Oncologist.* 2006;11(7):742–752.

17. Drisko JA, Chapman J, Hunter VJ. The use of antioxidant therapies during chemotherapy. *Gynecol Oncol.* 2003;88(3):434–439.

18. Thangaraju M, Vijavalakshmi T, Sachdanandam P. Effect of tamoxifen on lipid peroxide and antioxidative system in postmenopausal women with breast cancer. *Cancer.* 1994;74(1):78–82.

19. Vernie LN, De Vries M, Benckhuijsen C, De Goeii JJ, Zegers C. Selenium levels in blood and plasma, and glutathione peroxidase activity in blood of breast cancer patients during adjuvant treatment with cyclophosphamide, methotrexate and 5-fluorouracil. *Cancer Lett.* 1983;18(3):283–289.

20. Dürken M, Herrnring C, Finckh B, et al. Impaired plasma antioxidative defense and increased nontransferrin-bound iron during high-dose chemotherapy and radiochemotherapy preceding bone marrow transplantation. *Free Radic Biol Med.* 2000;28(6):887–894.

21. Dürken M, Agbenu J, Finckh B, et al. Deteriorating free radical-trapping capacity and antioxidant status in plasma during bone marrow transplantation. *Bone Marrow Transplant.* 1995;15:757–762.

22. Erhola M, Nieminen MM, Kellokumpu-Lehtinen P, et al. Plasma peroxyl radical trapping capacity in lung cancer patients: A case-control study. *Free Radic Res.* 1997;26(5):439–447.

23. Spronck JC, Kirkland. Niacin deficiency increases spontaneous and etoposide-induced chromosomal instability in rat bone marrow cells in vivo. *Mutat Res.* 2002; 508(1–2):83–97.

24. Caffrey PB, Frenkel GD. Selenium compounds prevent the induction of drug resistance by cisplatin in human ovarian tumor xenografts in vivo. *Cancer Chemother Pharmacol.* 2000;46(1):74–78.

25. Prasad KN, Cole WC, Kumar B, Che Prasad K. Pros and cons of antioxidant use during radiation therapy. *Cancer Treat Rev.* 2002;28(2):79–91.

26. Sieja K, Talerczyk M. Selenium as an element in the treatment of ovarian cancer in women receiving chemotherapy. *Gynecol Oncol.* 2004;93:320–327.

27. Conklin KA. Coenzyme Q10 for prevention of anthracycline-induced cardiotoxicity. *Integr Cancer Ther.* 2005;4(2):110–130.

28. Pace A, Savarese A, Picardo M, et al. Neuroprotective effect of vitamin E supplementation in patients treated with cisplatin chemotherapy. *J Clin Oncol.* 2003;21 (5):927–931.

29. Simone CB 2nd, Simone NL, Simone V, Simone CB. Antioxidants and other nutrients do not interfere with chemotherapy or radiation therapy and can increase kill and increase survival, part 2. *Altern Ther Health Med.* 2007;13(2):40–46.

30. Lawenda BD, Kelly KM, Ladas EJ, et al. Should supplemental antioxidant administration be avoided during chemotherapy and radiation therapy? *J Natl Cancer Inst.* 2008;100:773–783.

31. Bairati I, Meyer F, Gélinas M, et al. A randomized trial of antioxidant vitamins to prevent secondary primary cancers in head and neck cancer patients. *J Natl Cancer Inst.* 2005;97(7):481–488.

32. Meyer F, Bairati I, Fortin A, et al. Interaction between antioxidant vitamin supplementation and cigarette smoking during radiation therapy in relation to long-term effects on recurrence and mortality: A randomized trial among head and neck cancer patients. *Intl J Cancer.* 2008;122:1679–1683.

33. Ferreira PR, Fleck JF, Diehl A, et al. Protective effect of alpha-tocopherol in head and neck cancer radiation-induced mucositis: A double-blind randomized trial. *Head Neck.* 2004;26(4):313–321.

34. Lesperance ML, Olivotto IA, Forde N, et al. Mega-dose vitamins and minerals in the treatment of non-metastatic breast cancer: An historical cohort study. *Breast Cancer Res Treat.* 2002;76(2):137–143.

35. Agus DB, Vera JC, Golde DW. Stromal cell oxidation: A mechanism by which tumors obtain vitamin C. *Cancer Res.* 1999;59(18):4555–4558.

36. Langemann H, Torhorst J, Kabiersch A, et al. Quantitative determination of water- and lipid-soluble antioxidants in neoplastic and non-neoplastic human breast tissue. *Intl J Cancer.* 1989;43(6):1169–1173.

37. Dietary Supplement Health and Education Act of 1994; Public Law 103-417. U.S. Food and Drug Administration Web site. Available at http://www.fda.gov/opacom/laws/dshea.html. Accessed May 7, 2008.

38. Huang HY, Caballero B, Chang S, et al. The efficacy and safety of multivitamin and mineral supplement use to prevent cancer and chronic disease in adults: A systematic review for a National Institutes of Health State-of-the-Science Conference. *Ann Intern Med.* 2006;145:364–371.

39. National Institute of Cancer. U.S. National Institutes of Health. http://www.cancer.gov. Accessed December 4, 2007.

40. Review of therapies: Biologic/organic/pharmacologic therapies. http://www.md anderson.org. Accessed January 19, 2004.

41. Lockwood K, Moesgaard S, Folers K. Partial and complete regression of breast cancer in patients in relation to dosage of coenzyme Q10. *Biochem Biophys Res Comm.* 1994;199:1504–1508.

42. Hardman WE. (n-3) Fatty acids and cancer therapy. *J Nutr.* 2004;134:3427S–3430S.

43. Fearon KC, Barber MD, Moses AG, et al. Double-blind, placebo-controlled, randomized study of eicosapentaenoic acid diester in patients with cancer cachexia. *J Clin Oncol.* 2006;24(21):3401–3407.

44. Micke O, Bruns F, Mucke R, et al. Selenium in the treatment of radiation-associated secondary lymphedema. *Intl J Radiat Oncol Biol Phys.* 2003;56:40–49.

45. Moertel CG, Ames MM, Kovach JS, Moyer TP, Rubin JR, Tinker JH. A pharmacologic and toxicological study of amygdalin. *JAMA.* 1981;245:561–564.

46. Qun K. Effects of astragalus on IL-2/IL-2R system in patients with maintained hemodialysis. *Clin Neph.* 1999;52:333–334.

47. McCulloch M, See C, Shu XJ, et al. Astragalus-based Chinese herbs and platinum-based chemotherapy for advanced non-small-cell lung cancer: Meta-analysis of randomized trials. *J Clin Oncol.* 2006;24(3):419–430.

48. Demark-Wahnefried W, Robertson CN, Walther PJ, et al. Pilot study to explore effects of low-fat, flaxseed-supplemented diet on proliferation of benign prostatic epithelium and prostate-specific antigen. Urology. 2004;63:900–904.

49. Wong GY, Bradlow L, Sepkovic D, et al. Dose-ranging study of indole-3-carbinol for breast cancer prevention. *J Cell Biochem Suppl.* 1997;29:111–116.

50. Bell MC, Crowley-Nowick P, Bradlow HL, et al. Placebo-controlled trial of indole-3-carbinol in the treatment of CIN. *Gynecol Oncol.* 2000;78(2):123–129.

51. Cover CM, Hsieh SJ, Cram EJ, et al. Indole-3-carbinol and tamoxifen cooperate to arrest the cell cycle of MCF-7 human breast cancer cells. *Cancer Res.* 1999;59: 1244–1251.

52. Kodama N, Komuta K, Nanba H. Can Maitake MD-fraction aid cancer patients? *Altern Med Rev.* 2002;7:236–239.

53. Lin II, She YII, Cassileth BR, et al. Maitake beta-glucan MD-fraction enhances bone marrow colony formation and reduces doxorubicin toxicity in vitro. *Intl Immunopharmacol.* 2004;4:91–99.

54. Lissoni P, Barni S, Mandala M, et al. Decreased toxicity and increased efficacy of cancer chemotherapy using the pineal hormone melatonin in metastatic solid tumour patients with poor clinical status. *Eur J Cancer.* 1999;35:1688–1692.

55. Lissoni P, Tancini G, Barni S, et al. Treatment of cancer chemotherapy-induced toxicity. *Support Care Cancer.* 1997;5:126–129.

56. Srinivasan V, Spence DW, Pandi-Perumal SR, et al. Melatonin, environmental light, and breast cancer. *Breast Cancer Res Treat.* 2008;108(3):339–350.

57. Tyagi AK, Agarwal C, Chan DC, Agarwal R. Synergistic anti-cancer effects of silibinin with conventional cytotoxic agents doxorubicin, cisplatin and carboplatin against human breast carcinoma MCF-7 and MDA-MB468 cells. *Oncol Rep.* 2004; 11:493–499.

58. Venkataramanan R, Ranachandran V, Komoroski BJ, et al. Milk thistle, a herbal supplement, decreases the activity of CYP3A4 and uridine diphosphoglucoronosyl transferase in human hepatocyte cultures. *Drug Metab Dispos.* 2000;28: 1270–1273.

59. Oikawa T, Ashino-Fuse H, Shimnamura M et al. A novel angiogenic inhibitor derived from Japanese shark cartilage (I): Extraction and estimation of inhibitory activities toward tumor and embryonic angiogenesis. *Cancer Lett.* 1990;51: 181–186.

60. Latreille J, Batist G, Laberge F, et al. Phase I/II trial of the safety and efficacy of AE-941 (Neovastat) in the treatment of non-small-cell lung cancer. *Clin Lung Cancer.* 2003;4(4):231–236.

61. Batist G, Patenaude F, Champagne P, et al. Neovastat (AE-941) in refractory renal cell carcinoma patients: Report of a phase II trial with two dose levels. *Ann Oncol.* 2002;13(8):1259–1263.

62. Loprinzi CL, Levitt R, Barton DL, et al. Evaluation of shark cartilage in patients with advanced cancer: A North Central Cancer Treatment Group trial. *Cancer.* 2005;104(1):176–182.

63. Sauder DN, Dekoven J, Champagne P, et al. Neovastat (AE-941), an inhibitor of angiogenesis: Randomized phase I/II clinical trial results in patients with plaque psoriasis. *J Am Acad Dermatol.* 2002;47:535–541.

64. Holzbeierlein JM, McIntosh J, Trasher JB. The role of soy phytoestrogens in prostate cancer. *Curr Opin Urol.* 2005;15:17–22.

65. Somasundaram S, Edmund NA, Moore DT, et al. Dietary curcumin inhibits chemotherapy-induced apoptosis in models of human breast cancer. *Cancer Res.* 2002;62:3868–3875.

66. Petersen RW, Quinlivan JA. Preventing anxiety and depression in gynaecological cancer: A randomised controlled trial. *Br J Obstet Gynaecol.* 2002;109:386–394.

67. Speca M, Carlson LE, Goodey E, Angen M. A randomized, wait-list controlled clinical trial: The effect of a mindfulness meditation-based stress reduction program on mood and symptoms of stress in cancer outpatients. *Psychosom Med.* 2000;62: 613–622.

68. Targ EF, Levine EG. The efficacy of a mind–body–spirit group for women with breast cancer: A randomized controlled trial. *Gen Hosp Psychiatry.* 2002;24:238–248.

69. Carlson LE, Ursuliak Z, Goodey E, et al. The effects of a mindfulness meditation-based stress reduction program on mood and symptoms of stress in cancer outpatients: 6-month follow-up. *Support Care Cancer.* 2001;9:112–123.

70. Devine EC, Westlake SK. The effects of psychoeducational care provided to adults with cancer: Meta-analysis of 116 studies. *Oncol Nurs Forum.* 1995;22:1369–1381.

71. Montgomery GH, Weltz CR, Seltz M, et al. Brief presurgery hypnosis reduces distress and pain in excisional breast biopsy patients. *Intl J Clin Exp Hypn.* 2002;50:17–32.

72. Liossi C, Hatira P. Clinical hypnosis versus cognitive behavioral training for pain management with pediatric cancer patients undergoing bone marrow aspirations. *Intl J Clin Exp Hypn.* 1999;47:104–116.

73. Richardson J, Smith JE, McCall G, Pilkington K. Hypnosis for procedure-related pain and distress in pediatric cancer patients: A systematic review of effectiveness and methodology related to hypnosis interventions. *J Pain Symptom Manage.* 2006;31(1):70–84.

74. Syrjala KL, Cummings C, Donaldson GW. Hypnosis or cognitive behavioral training for the reduction of pain and nausea during cancer treatment: A controlled clinical trial. *Pain.* 1992;48:137–147.

75. Integration of behavioral and relaxation approaches into the treatment of chronic pain and insomnia: NIH Technology Assessment Panel on Integration of Behavioral and Relaxation Approaches into the Treatment of Chronic Pain and Insomnia. *JAMA.* 1996;276:313–318.

76. Faymonville ME, Mambourg PH, Joris J, et al. Psychological approaches during conscious sedation: Hypnosis versus stress reducing strategies: A prospective randomized study. *Pain.* 1997;73:361–367.

77. Russell NC, Sumier SS, Beinhorm CM, Frenkel MA. Role of massage therapy in cancer care. *J Altern Complement Med.* 2008;14(2):209–214.

78. Vitale A. An integrative review of Reiki touch therapy research. *Holist Nurs Pract.* 2007;21(4):167–179.

79. Winstead-Fry P, Kijek J. An integrative review and meta-analysis of therapeutic touch research. *Altern Ther Health Med.* 1999;5(6):58–67.

80. Clements M. Ayureveda: The mother of traditional medicine. In: Marian MJ, Williams-Mullen P, Bowers JM, eds. *Integrating Therapeutic and Complementary Nutrition.* Boca Raton, FL: CRC Press, Taylor & Francis; 2007:15–28.

81. Centers for Disease Control and Prevention. Lead poisoning associated with Ayurvedic medications—five states, 2000–2003. *Morbid Mortal Weekly Rep.* 2004; 53:582–584.

82. Saper RB, Kales SN, Paquin J, et al. Heavy metal content of Ayurvedic herbal medicine products. *JAMA.* 2004;292:2868–2873.

83. Deng GE, Cassileth BR, Cohen L, et al. Integrative oncology practice guidelines. *J Soc Integr Oncol.* 2007;5(2):65–84.

84. Cassileth BR, Deng G. Complementary and alternative therapies for cancer. *Oncologist.* 2004;9:80–89.

Index